DATE DUE

Adolescent Sleep Patterns

Recent years have witnessed a growing concern for insufficient sleep, particularly in the United States. In the early 1990s a congressionally mandated commission noted that insufficient sleep is a major contributor to catastrophic events, such as the nuclear disaster at Chernobyl and the grounding of the *Exxon Valdez*, as well as personal tragedies, such as automobile accidents. Adolescents appear to be among the most sleep-deprived populations in our society, although they are rarely included in sleep assessments. This book explores the genesis and development of sleep patterns at this stage of the life-span. It examines biological and cultural factors that influence sleep patterns, presents risks associated with lack of sleep, and reveals the effects of environmental factors such as work and school schedules on sleep. *Adolescent Sleep Patterns* will appeal to psychologists and sociologists of adolescence who have not yet considered the important role of sleep in the lives of our youth and to educators who work regularly with young people.

Mary A. Carskadon is Professor of Psychiatry and Human Behavior at Brown Medical School and Director of Sleep and Chronobiology Research at the E. P. Bradley Hospital. A former president of the Sleep Research Society, Dr. Carskadon is a Fellow of the American Academy of Sleep Medicine, recipient of the Nathaniel Kleitman Award for Distinguished Service, a member of the Sleep Disorders Research Advisory Board of the National Heart, Lung, and Blood Institute and the National Space Biomedical Research Institute Advisory Board, and associate editor of the journals *Sleep* and *Behavioral Sleep Medicine*.

Adolescent Sleep Patterns

Biological, Social, and Psychological Influences

Edited by

MARY A. CARSKADON

Brown Medical School

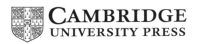

CAMBRIDGE UNIVERSITY PRESS

PUBLISHED BY THE PRESS SYNDICATE OF THE UNIVERSITY OF CAMBRIDGE
The Pitt Building, Trumpington Street, Cambridge, United Kingdom

CAMBRIDGE UNIVERSITY PRESS
The Edinburgh Building, Cambridge CB2 2RU, UK
40 West 20th Street, New York, NY 10011-4211, USA
477 Williamstown Road, Port Melbourne, VIC 3207, Australia
Ruiz de Alarcón 13, 28014 Madrid, Spain
Dock House, The Waterfront, Cape Town 8001, South Africa

http://www.cambridge.org

First published 2002

Printed in the United Kingdom at the University Press, Cambridge

Typeface Palatino 10/13 pt.   *System* LATEX 2$_\varepsilon$ [TB]

A catalog record for this book is available from the British Library.

Library of Congress Cataloging in Publication data
Adolescent sleep patterns : biological, social, and psychological influences / edited by
Mary A. Carskadon.

    p. cm.
    Includes bibliographical references and index.
    ISBN 0-521-64291-4
    1. Sleep disorders in children.   2. Health behavior in adolescence.   3. Sleep.
I. Carskadon, Mary A.
    RJ506.5.S55 A364   2002
    616.8'498 – dc21   2001037541

ISBN 0 521 64291 4 hardback

Contents

Contributors

Christine Acebo, Brown Medical School

Miriam Andrade, University of São Paulo

Mary A. Carskadon, Brown Medical School

Flavia Cortesi, University "La Sapienza," Rome

Ronald E. Dahl, University of Pittsburgh

William C. Dement, Stanford University

Sanford M. Dornbusch, Stanford University

Flavia Giannotti, University "La Sapienza," Rome

Mari S. Golub, University of California, Davis

Reut Gruber, Tel-Aviv University

Tana M. Hoban-Higgins, University of California, Davis

James T. McCracken, UCLA Neuropsychiatric Hospital, Los Angeles

Melissa K. Melby, Emory University

L. Menna-Barreto, University of São Paulo

Gary S. Richardson, Henry Ford Hospital, Detroit

Roger H. Rosa, U.S. Department of Health and Human Services,
  Cincinnati

Avi Sadeh, Tel-Aviv University

Peter T. Takeuchi, University of California, Davis

Barbara A. Tate, Children's Hospital of Boston

Kyla L. Wahlstrom, University of Minnesota

Amy R. Wolfson, College of the Holy Cross

Carol M. Worthman, Emory University

Foreword

WILLIAM C. DEMENT

Adolescence is the great and terrifying transition from childhood to adulthood. It is in the interest of a civilized society that a mature, responsible, and well-educated young adult emerges from this transition. Along with mental and physical maturation, a triumvirate of preventive health should be inculcated during adolescence as a permanent philosophy of living. The practice of nutritional health will ensure the best possible outcome during the process of growing older. Exercise and physical fitness, likewise, will also foster health and quality of life. Healthy adequate sleep will foster longevity and particularly the optimal use of our waking hours. We are not healthy unless our sleep is healthy. Sadly (perhaps the raison d'être of this volume), the inculcation of this third member of the triumvirate of preventive health is absent. Furthermore, its absence can have many known and as yet unknown deleterious effects on human life.

A recent report of an exhaustive study on adolescence, *Great Transitions: Preparing Adolescents for a New Century* prepared by the Carnegie Corporation of New York (1995), exemplifies the puzzling and frustrating blind spot regarding sleep issues by even the best of the best. While excellent, thorough, and future-oriented in every other area, the report did *not* mention adolescent sleep or biological rhythms.

It has been my great privilege to be associated for many years with the editor and progenitor of this book. I knew her first as a family member (a cousin of my wife), and then I was very lucky that a unique concatenation of events brought her to Stanford University in 1970. She directed a truly pioneering program on the scientific study of daytime sleepiness in the Stanford University Summer Sleep Camp from 1975 to 1985. The studies in this remarkable facility established the scientific basis of our current understanding of the critical dimension of waking sleepiness-alertness and its nocturnal determinants. In addition, and of great importance to the topic of this book, she directed a longitudinal study of a cohort of children as they went through the great transition of adolescence.

At the beginning of this remarkable decade of research, the gold standard of assessing daytime sleepiness, the multiple sleep latency test (MSLT), was developed and applied. Using this test each summer on the longitudinal cohort, it was established that sleep need does not change or may even increase during the great transition. The MSLT also allowed an assessment of the effect of sleep restriction on daytime alertness; for the first time, it was clear that the impact of lost sleep accumulates from day to day. This accumulation is often referred to as the "sleep debt." Finally, the great disparity between MSLT measures of sleep need in adolescents versus questionnaire data on actual sleep obtained at home during the school year allows us to conclude that many, if not most, adolescents must be severely, chronically sleep deprived. The data bases are very small, but students falling asleep in class are a familiar sight to middle school and, particularly, high school teachers. This situation is further complicated by the biological tendency for phase delay of circadian rhythms and the markedly increased prevalence of students holding extracurricular jobs, usually in the evening, to earn money.

During much of 1990 and 1991, Dr. Carskadon and I served on the National Commission on Sleep Disorders Research, which carried out a congressionally mandated study of the role of sleep deprivation and sleep disorders in American society. One of the areas that we examined was whether the facts about sleep that we have known for more than two decades have actually been integrated into the educational system and the health care system. Unfortunately, crucial education about sleep need and biological rhythms and sleep disorders likely to occur in adolescence was completely absent. It is my very strong opinion that all human beings become victims of the lack of awareness about sleep during the great transition and, to some extent, for the rest of their lives. Although data on sleep disorders in latency-age children are limited, the studies conducted by Dr. Carskadon, particularly for children in middle- and upper-class environments, suggest that sleep needs are generally fulfilled at this age with a resulting optimal daytime alertness and performance.

In terms of developing a society in which healthy sleep is a priority, the optimal target may be the developing adolescent. Crucial material about sleep, sleep deprivation, biological rhythms, and sleep disorders can be readily taught at this age level. It might also be possible to introduce effective interventions to promote positive schedule strategies that allow more time for sleep. For example, a great deal can be accomplished by using the "bully pulpit" of driver training, a key issue for all adolescents.

Another area pioneered by Dr. Carskadon and to some extent revealed during the early days of the Stanford University Sleep Disorder clinic is what is now called the delayed sleep phase syndrome. In the Stanford studies and more recently in her research at Brown and in the work of others, it has become clear that there is a major biological rhythm problem in adolescence, and this problem clearly exacerbates the sleep loss problem. This knowledge has come onto the radar screen in recent years with sporadically successful efforts to change the starting time in high schools to a later hour. Accomplishing this initiative is uniquely difficult because of the complexity of forces determining the school schedule. Preliminary data where the starting time has been successfully delayed have been promising.

Finally, it is time to address the pervasive adolescent problem of school schedule–biological clock mismatch in some effective manner. There is an urgent need for researchers and clinicians in the area covered by this volume to cooperate, to arrive at a consensus, and to provide leadership both in adding to the necessary scientific data bases to foster change, and to provide leadership in advocating wise public policy in this crucial area. Leadership is needed at every level, including local school boards, county and state organizations, and even at the federal level. Dr. Carskadon is certainly the outstanding leader in this area, and she has assembled a tiny band of other leading researchers to produce a very important and long-overdue book.

Preface

MARY A. CARSKADON

The maturation of sleep patterns in teens has been a focus of my research for 25 years – long enough for the teens I first studied to have teenagers of their own. I often wonder why we don't know it all yet, and then I step into the world and am reminded of the complexity of life and the accelerating rate of change in opportunities, expectations, technology, and social mores. Developing humans are at the center of it all, with sleep's core behavioral role at the mercy of these factors and many more.

I am humbled by the task of attempting to understand the phenomena we observe, and I am inspired by the process of scientific investigation. As in other fields, progress is usually neither linear nor direct; it is affected by the evolution of methodologies and ideas, and the flow of knowledge can be entirely redirected by conceptual breakthroughs. My research in the area of adolescent sleep patterns has benefited from several such major reconstructive conceptual shifts. The first seism occurred in the longitudinal Summer Sleep Camp study at Stanford – inspired by William Dement and Thomas Anders – in which we not only failed to confirm the predicted reduction of sleep need across adolescent development but also showed a restructuring of sleep so that pubertal adolescents sleeping no less than before were actually *sleepier* in the afternoon. The conclusion: teens don't need less sleep.

A second movement of our conceptual tectonic plates fractured the assumption that the delay in the timing of sleep in adolescents, especially later bedtimes, was purely a psychosocial phenomenon. Instead, we now find that the brain's mechanisms controlling the timing of sleep appear to undergo a shift at adolescence that is permissive of and in some may drive the teen phase delay. The conclusion: teens cannot simply decide to fall asleep or wake up.

The major theoretical contribution that allows us to frame a biological context for these investigations began with A. A. Borbély's articulation of the two-process model of sleep (in *Human Neurobiology*, 1982), a model that allows us to predict and examine the principal biological components regulating sleep. Combined with new methods and measures, the theoretical advances in understanding these biological factors provide exciting opportunities. The story of adolescent sleep goes beyond biology, however, and the contributors to this book provide stepping-stones leading to the future development of this ever challenging area of study.

The birthplace of this project was an international symposium on Contemporary Perspectives on Adolescent Sleep held in Marina del Rey, California, in April 1997. The symposium was sponsored by the University of California at Los Angeles, Youth Enhancement Services (YES), under the leadership of Michael Chase, Ph.D., and supported by an unrestricted educational grant from the Anheuser-Busch Foundation. Many of the attendees at the symposium have authored chapters in this book. We are indebted to Dr. Chase and the Anheuser-Busch Foundation for assembling us to begin this project.

I can never thank Bill Dement, M.D., Ph.D., adequately for all of his enthusiastic support and encouragement over many years of mentorship. I am again indebted to him for writing the Foreword to this book and providing such a persuasive reminder of the importance of this work in his usual charismatic style.

One clear gap in understanding the place of sleep in the lives of teens has been its integration with social roles and societal forces that influence teens. I am grateful to Dr. Sanford Dornbusch for his chapter, which discloses so eloquently the blind eye that the field of adolescent sociology has turned toward sleep and acknowledges the likely importance the assessment of sleep may hold for sociologists.

I tried to provide some scaffolding for subsequent chapters in a broad overview of "Factors Influencing Sleep Patterns of Adolescents," Chapter 2. An outline of issues from home, to work, to school, to basic biological concepts precedes the description of our field-lab study in 9th and 10th grade students. This particular study clarifies most strongly for me the enormous burden an early school start time places on adolescents given no support to make appropriate adjustments.

The overview of "Endocrine Changes Associated with Puberty and Adolescence" by Gary Richardson and Barbara Tate adds to the scaffold with a clear explanation of human neuroendocrine system changes during this critical developmental phase and how these changes influence brain mechanisms that contribute to the control of sleep and wakefulness.

The idea for chapters on comparative biology of adolescent sleep patterns was inspired by an e-mail from Mari Golub in 1996 asking me to help interpret activity pattern findings from her adolescent Rhesus monkeys. I was working at the time with Barbara Tate to develop a rodent model (*Octodon degus*) to examine similar issues. The explorations of adolescent activity patterns in these species in Chapters 4 and 5 offer interesting counterpoints to the human condition and add strength to the hypothesis that biological changes at the adolescent transition assist a phase delay.

In the course of a research career, certain moments in time hold salient places in our intellectual development or scientific yearning. One such moment for me came during the challenge of grant writing while collecting data at the Stanford Sleep Camp in the summer of 1979. This striking image includes an overwhelming sense of urgency to know about sleep patterns from the viewpoint of an anthropologist: what *is* the developmental pattern of sleep in non-Westernized cultures? I remember vividly my desire to know right then and there and my wish that I could do the field work myself. Of course, this urgency dissipated in the throes of ongoing work, but the yearning for this knowledge has remained. Thus, one of my most gratifying experiences was meeting Dr. Carol Worthman at the symposium, and I am thrilled to include her scholarly presentation, "Toward a Comparative Developmental Ecology of Human Sleep," in this book. Carol's chapter is the first comprehensive assessment of human sleep from the perspective of an anthropologist, and it is stunning in its scope and analysis. Worthman and her colleague, Melissa Melby, have embraced this effort with enthusiasm, and I am both grateful for and a bit in awe of their accomplishment. I am also delighted to know that Carol has recently completed the first field study specifically to examine sleep, the first of what I hope are many to follow.

Two views of adolescent sleep patterns from disparate contemporary "Westernized" societies are provided in the chapters by Miriam Andrade and Luiz Menna-Barreto, who examine the sleep of teens in São Paolo, and by Flavia Gianotti and Flavia Cortesi, who probe sleep patterns and sleep problems of Italian teens. These chapters stand in contrast to the anthropological perspective and as introduction to the issues of sleep patterns and school schedules in North American adolescents.

Before considering these concerns, however, our journey through the world of adolescent sleep takes two brief side trips to explore related but more tangential issues. I have wanted to summarize the data from our adolescent driving risk surveys for a number of reasons. First, they hold an inherent message about drowsy driving in teens. In addition, I have wanted to honor the cherished memory of and say farewell to my dear friend, Helen Bearpark, Ph.D., who shared in this research and for whom the issue of drowsy driving was a compelling concern. Thank you, Helen. Roger Rosa takes us next to Finland for an examination of adult workers who experience early-morning shift schedules. His research points out not only difficulties associated with such work shifts but also the challenges of making life-style choices to accommodate sleep under those circumstances. Adolescents with early school start times face similar challenges.

To my knowledge, Kyla Wahlstrom is the first career educator to have embraced a research interest at the interface of school schedules and teen sleep. I marvel at the complexities of school systems that Kyla's chapter charts for us, as she examines step by step the structures that impact decisions about the school schedule. The tantalizing tales of the Edina, Minnesota, experience only whet our appetites for results from Kyla's longitudinal assessments of the Minneapolis "experiment." A preliminary summary of those findings is included as an appendix to her chapter.

Amy Wolfson's chapter takes aim at the challenges that face teenagers as this century progresses and provides useful suggestions that may help reverse societal, family, and life-style trends providing the pressure to shrink adolescent sleep. This insightful presentation gives us fair warning and prescriptive recommendations.

I find Christine Acebo's assessment of adolescent sleep patterns in "Influence of Irregular Sleep Patterns on Waking Behavior" very important in its unique examination of sleep's impact while controlling for other important factors. This chapter acknowledges that such outcomes as grades, depressed mood, injuries associated with alcohol or drugs, and absenteeism are multidetermined. The subsequent analytical models then include sleep predictors in multiple regressions that allow us to identify clearly the significant impact of sleep amount and regularity, even when accounting for age, sex, race, educational expectations, learning disabilities, and substance use. These findings highlight the crucial role of sleep and provide a strong introduction for the final chapters.

The last three chapters of this book provide more clinical perspectives of adolescent sleep patterns. Avi Sadeh and Reut Gruber write of the ways stressful events in adolescents' lives can impinge on sleep. The case vignettes concluding their chapter put real faces to the theoretical models and predictions. James McCracken is a practicing psychiatrist and researcher who has studied depression in adolescence. He summarizes for the clinical scientist the ways in which adolescents' sleep and depressed mood are intertwined and speculates on neural substrates. Ronald Dahl writes compellingly of the challenges an adolescent's brain faces to achieve a successful integration of cognitive and emotional development and how this process is impacted by and has an impact on the sleep patterns of adolescents.

I thank all these authors for their thoughtful contributions to this book and their patience with the process. I believe we have assembled a set of perspectives that will enlighten and inform. I must also especially thank Christine Acebo and Amy Wolfson for helping bring this work to fruition and Marian "Max" Elliott for her many hours of labor and solicitous forbearance of my moods.

Adolescent Sleep Patterns

1. Sleep and Adolescence: A Social Psychologist's Perspective

SANFORD M. DORNBUSCH

My immediate reaction to reading the chapters in this book is shame. Generations of researchers have studied the psychological and social lives of adolescents, and their main tools have been time-use studies. Among numerous examples, how much time each day or week does the adolescent spend watching television, hanging out with friends, or engaging in extracurricular activities? What is the relation of such time expenditures to measures of academic performance, deviance, or other indicators of adolescent functioning?

The emphasis has been completely on the waking hours, and this book impressively underscores the importance of hours spent sleeping. An undergraduate friend, with whom I had discussed some of the findings in various chapters, immediately provided a real-life illustration of the interaction between the physiological imperatives of sleep and the social perceptions by which we structure our lives. She had been accustomed to staying up very late and sleepily forcing herself to attend her morning classes. In general, she found Stanford professors boring. Now she is getting more sleep and finding her teachers more interesting.

A constant theme of life in society is determining the causes of the phenomena we perceive. Often, there is a choice to be made between internal causes and external causes. For example, I was once feeling sick in Guatemala City and, feeling dizzy, I decided that I was even sicker than I had believed. I was one of the few persons who was relieved to discover that I was experiencing a minor earthquake. A different example occurs in the study of hyperactive children, some of whose restlessness in school may be a product of boring teachers.

Let me use an example of considerable importance in the lives of American adolescents. Part-time employment while attending high school is more common in the United States than in other industrial societies. Those American adolescents who work a moderate number of hours each week tend to have higher grades in school than do adolescents who do not work at all. Yet, those adolescents who are employed for a large number of hours, say for more than 20 hours a week, tend to have lower grades than those in the other two groups.

The typical explanations of the negative relation between many hours of work and high school grades reflect the problems of explaining this simple association. Perhaps spending so much after-school time at work (external) prevents an appropriate investment of energy on schoolwork, or perhaps the adolescent chooses to work so much (internal) because he or she has done poorly in school and developed low educational expectations. Probably both explanations are partially correct, but neither considers the additional impact of being sleep-deprived.

Those adolescents who work long hours go to bed later and get less total sleep than do those who do not work that much. Getting insufficient sleep has an impact on the quality of the activities of adolescents and on their perceptions of the contexts in which they find themselves. The high-work group has trouble staying awake in class or while doing homework. Cross-cultural research reinforces the view that less total sleep time among adolescents is associated with inability to concentrate on schoolwork and poorer school performance, as well as with mood disorders and substance abuse.

Many years ago I did a study of gender differences in adolescents' satisfaction with their bodies (Dornbusch et al., 1984). As expected, American females were more likely to want to be thinner, but what was striking was the extent to which social class, as predicted by Thorstein Veblen (1889), led adolescent females to be increasingly dissatisfied with their bodies as they moved through puberty. The fat that normally accompanies female sexual development was negatively evaluated, whereas males were pleased with the musculature that was associated with their pubertal development. Perceptions in the social world were allowing societal standards to override biological processes.

Research on adolescent sleep is revealing a similar pattern. I must admit to my own surprise on learning that adolescents need more, not less, sleep as they move out of childhood. Neither adults nor adolescents are generally aware of the biological need for increased sleep during pubertal development. Instead, believing that sleep can be shortened for the sake of compliance with the social standards of those around them, adolescents reduce their sleep time in order to engage in activities that bring them immediate rewards. Whether for parties or jobs or cramming for examinations, adolescents engage in activities that deprive them of sleep. Adults, unaware of the sleep needs of adolescents, require them to start school earlier in the day than is required of younger children. The social norms of the wider society, as well as those of most peer groups, do not discourage patterns of behavior that displace sleep.

The sleep needs of adolescents appear similar across cultures, but there are, as is evident in these chapters, cultural differences in sleep patterns, reflecting differences in parental and peer control, in leisure activities, and in schooling. These chapters reflect a complex mixture of biological and developmental forces that are expressed within social and cultural settings. It seems obvious that, unaware of the sleep needs of adolescents, norms for behavior have developed that have unwittingly created additional problems for adolescents.

Researchers who study adolescent functioning should take advantage of this new knowledge and reshape part of the research agenda. For example, there are already hints that knowledge about sleep patterns may contribute to the study of deviant behavior, school failure, and psychological symptoms among adolescents beginning in the prepubertal period and extending into young adulthood. My prediction is that sleep time will have a small, but measurable, influence on various indicators of adolescent functioning even after controlling for the contributions of the usual variables that affect adolescent development.

Such studies also have practical consequences in the short run. Parents and adolescents may become more aware of the consequences of sleep deprivation; far more significant, policy makers may assess the negative impact of current practices in part-time employment and schooling. With so many adolescents working too many hours or too late in the evening, and adolescents starting school so early each weekday, there appears to be a need for thoughtful oversight of the demands of employers and schools. Adolescence is defined as a time for development, and harmful sleep patterns that increase risks for adolescents during that sensitive period cause adult society to pay a high price. Policy makers will soon be asked to take into account the impact of sleep deprivation on adolescents.

REFERENCES

Dornbusch SM, Carlsmith JM, Duncan PD, Gross RT, Martin JA, Ritter PL, Siegel-Gorelick B (1984). Sexual maturation, social class, and the desire to be thin among adolescent females. *Journal of Behavioral and Developmental Pediatrics* 5:308–314.
Veblen T (1889). *The Theory of the Leisure Class*. New York: Macmillan.

2. Factors Influencing Sleep Patterns of Adolescents

MARY A. CARSKADON

How I hated her method of waking me. My adolescent sleeps were long, dark and sullen. Never once in all those years did I wake of my own accord. It was Margaret, always, knocking on my door like some rodent trapped behind a wall. This would bring me to a rage of wakefulness and I would stomp into the bathroom, bad-tempered and clearly in the wrong, while Margaret, who had been up and gone to six o'clock Mass, would watch me with a silent and superior reproach. That would increase my fury; it is impossible to feel the equal of someone who's been awake longer than you.

Mary Gordon, *Final Payments*

Sleep patterns in humans emerge from a complex interplay of several distinct processes: maturation and development, behavioral phenomena, and intrinsic sleep and circadian regulatory mechanisms. Each factor likely plays an important role during the transition from childhood to adulthood, a time when significant changes in sleep patterns occur. Sleep also affects many facets of waking human life, although a definitive explanation of sleep's function(s) remains undiscovered. Unquestioned, however, is the obligatory nature of sleep and our commonsense intuition that sleep fulfills some vital role in our waking lives, a role that enhances our abilities to think, perform, feel, and interact.

This research program has received support from the National Institutes of Health grants MH45945 and MH52415. Many individuals have contributed to this research program, including Christine Acebo, Ronald Seifer, Amy Wolfson, Orna Tzischinsky, Pamela Thacher, Susan Labyak, Barbara A. Tate, Gary S. Richardson, Catherine Darley, Katherine Sharkey, Jenifer Wicks, Elizabeth Yoder, Christina Orringer, Katherine Minard, Liza Kelly, Clayton Bennett Jr., Jeffrey Cerone, Thomas Maloney, and many undergraduate trainees.

The patterns of sleep that unfold during adolescence differ markedly from those of preadolescents. Our sense is that many adolescents in the United States obtain insufficient and ill-timed sleep and that daytime functioning suffers as a consequence. This review will focus on a number of major factors that affect sleep patterns of adolescents, summarize a recent study that examines several factors in an operational setting, and speculate on major consequences of these changes.

Although large-scale epidemiologic studies of broadly generalizable samples are not available, our group is reasonably certain that many adolescents do not obtain adequate sleep, based upon self-reported sleep-wake patterns of children and adolescents investigated by a number of groups, primarily using cross-sectional sleep habits surveys (Strauch, Dubral, & Strucholz, 1973; Webb & Agnew, 1973, 1975; Zepelin, Hamilton, & Wanzie, 1977; Anders, Carskadon, Dement, & Harvey, 1978; Price, Coates, Thoresen, & Grinstead, 1978; Carskadon, 1979; White, Hahn, & Mitler, 1980; Klackenberg, 1982; Petta, Carskadon, & Dement, 1984; Bearpark & Michie, 1987; Billiard, Alperovitch, Perot, & Jammes, 1987; Henschel & Lack, 1987; Strauch & Meier, 1988; Carskadon, 1990a,b; Andrade, Benedito-Silva, & Menna-Barreto, 1992; Gau & Soong, 1995; Saarenpaaheikkila, Rintahaka, Laippala, & Koivikko, 1995; Wolfson & Carskadon, 1998). A few longitudinal survey studies have also been done (Klackenberg, 1982; Strauch & Meier, 1988; Andrade et al., 1992). Several major trends emerge from such data:

- Older teenagers sleep less than younger teenagers.
- The timing of sleep is delayed in older versus younger teenagers.
- With age, teenagers show an increasingly large discrepancy between school night and weekend sleep schedules.

This chapter focuses on the first two of these trends; the third is examined by Acebo and Carskadon (Chapter 13 in this volume).

Behavioral Phenomena

Physiological processes play an important role in regulating sleep and wakefulness. Yet, human sleep patterns are also determined by choices, often rooted in psychosocial phenomena. Such phenomena include, for example, delaying bedtime to socialize or to finish reading a good book, advancing bedtime in anticipation of an early rising, truncating sleep length with an alarm clock, and so forth. Behavioral contributions to sleep patterns are strong in both children and adolescents; however, a rapidly changing psychosocial milieu during adolescence contributes to marked alterations in the behavioral phenomena affecting sleep patterns.

Parents

One of our first studies of sleep patterns at the childhood-to-adolescent transition (Carskadon, 1979) showed a change in the influence of parents on children's sleep patterns, particularly on school days. Among other items, this sleep habits survey of 218 children asked students to describe the reasons they had for going to bed at night and waking up in the morning. Children aged 10 and 11 years were significantly more likely to report that parents set their school-night bedtimes (age 10 = 54.3%; age 11 = 48.3%) than were the 12- and 13-year-old children (age 12 = 38.5%; age 13 = 19.6%); conversely, the 12- and 13-year-olds reported more frequently (age 12 = 73.1%; age 13 = 70.2%) that parents or alarm clocks provided the morning stimulus to wake up on school mornings than did the younger children (age 10 = 45.7%; age 11 = 37.9%).

Our subsequent studies of high school students have shown that older adolescents report much later bedtimes and give such reasons for staying up late as watching television, finishing homework, and socializing. For example, our group recently undertook a survey of approximately 3,000 9th through 12th grade students from four Rhode Island school districts (Acebo & Carskadon, 1997; Wolfson & Carskadon, 1998; referred to here as "the high school survey") using an eight-page anonymously administered self-report form (reproduced at http://www.sleepforscience.org). Only 5.1% of these older teens had a school-night bedtime set by parents; 32.7% went to bed when homework (13.1%), TV viewing (8.7%), or socializing (10.9%) was finished for the day, and 44.1% reported that bedtime was set by the time they feel sleepy. Furthermore, an even higher percentage of high school than primary school students reported relying on an external source for a school-morning wake-up cue. Our high school survey data show that 87% of older teens use an alarm (59.9%) or parent (27.1%) for waking them up on school days. As summarized in Figure 2.1, these data indicate strong developmental trends: parents are more likely to set bedtimes for younger adolescents, more likely to assist with waking up older adolescents, and the younger adolescents are

Reason for Going to Sleep on School Nights

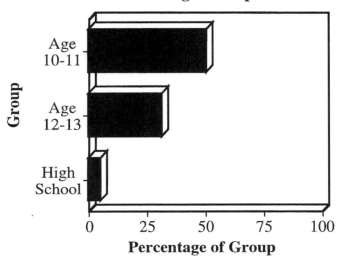

Reasons for Waking Up on School Mornings

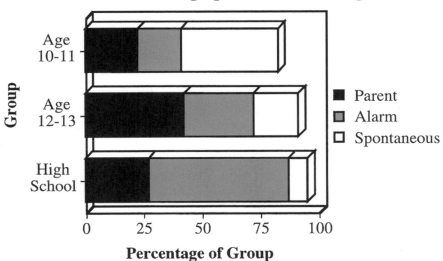

Figure 2.1. Self-report data from sleep habits surveys of younger (ages 10 and 11 years; 12 and 13 years) and older adolescents (high school students ages 14 to 18 years). The top figure shows the percentage of students who reported that their parents set their bedtimes on school nights. In the lower panel, data are similarly summarized for three of the reasons students reported for factors that determine what time they wake up on school mornings, parents (black), alarm clock (gray), or spontaneous (white, i.e., "I don't know, I just wake up") arousals.

significantly more likely than older teens to wake spontaneously on school mornings.

Peers

Although a commonly remarked feature of adolescent development is the increasing influence of peer group on behavior, we are aware of no data that directly assay this factor with regard to sleep patterns. Our recent high school survey data indicate a minor influence of school on one or two sleep variables; however, this effect may be more a result of the school schedules per se than of peer influences. The data show that evening "socializing" is a factor influencing school-night bedtimes in only 10.9%, although a case might be made that TV watching (associated with bedtimes in 8.7% of students) may have a peer-group component. These adolescents reported a significantly greater influence of social activities to account for bedtime on weekend nights, with 40.9% reporting this factor as the chief reason they choose to go to bed. One conclusion, therefore, is that the older adolescents have more social opportunities or greater access to evening social activities, and these activities have a greater influence on sleep patterns during the weekends than on school nights.

Academics

Academic obligations are often mentioned by adolescents when asked about factors affecting their sleep patterns. Our high school survey data show evidence that homework is a significant factor influencing sleep patterns for only a limited number of students. Thus, approximately 13% of the 9th through 12th grade students reported that their school-night bedtime is set according to the time they finish their homework. This relationship does not seem to reflect a developmental change, because about 15.2% of 12- and 13-year-old students in our earlier study reported staying up until homework was finished (Carskadon, 1979). Our high school survey data also indicate a rather low mean number of hours these students reported studying in the last week, on average about an hour a day (6.7 ± 5.9 hours per week). Data from students in another educational system – Taipei, Taiwan – showed that the students in more academically challenging programs reported less sleep and lower levels of alertness than those students in the less challenging program (Gau & Soong, 1995). In the United States, as well, those students on the academic fast track are likely to sleep less, although data confirming this trend are not available.

Extracurricular Club Activities and Sports

Other activities that may influence sleep patterns of adolescents include extracurricular club activities, such as chorus, band, orchestra, and scouting, as well as after school sports. Our recent high school survey examined these factors by asking students to describe the nature of these obligations. Only about one-quarter of the sample reported participating in extracurricular club activities during the preceding week, and 90% of these students took part fewer than 12 hours per week. Students in this survey reported somewhat more participation in sports, with about one-third of students involved in organized athletics in the past week, 80% of whom reported participating 12 or fewer hours per week. For the majority of the students, therefore, extracurricular club activities or after school sports were not a major factor determining sleep patterns. Future analyses will examine these issues more closely, particularly to identify students whose commitments span many activities, in which case sleep may be affected more significantly. One group most likely to experience significant sleep loss includes those students with multiple commitments who also work.

Employment

As we have indicated elsewhere (Carskadon, Mancuso, & Rosekind, 1989; Carskadon, 1990a,b), a major influence on sleep patterns of U.S. high school students is the number of hours they spend working for pay. Thus, we have previously noted that students who report working 20 or more hours per week (about 28% of our earlier high school sample) report having later bedtimes, sleeping fewer hours per night, and falling asleep in school and oversleeping more frequently than do those who either do not work or who work fewer than 20 hours per week. Our more recent high school survey, which asked students to report hours worked in the last week, shows similar findings. About half the students reported working, and the average number of hours worked was 19.5 (median = 18 hours). As further explicated in Chapter 12, the association of hours spent working with sleep parameters and other outcome variables is also similar to our previous findings. For example, number of hours worked across the week reported by the new high school sample is correlated with school-night total sleep time ($r = -.235; p < .001$) and school-night bedtime ($r = .345; p < .001$).

The developmental psychologist Laurence Steinberg and his colleagues Bradford Brown and Sanford Dornbusch (1996) make the point that the rather impressive amount of time adolescents in the United States spend working for pay is a relatively new phenomenon, appearing only in the second half of the 20th century. Furthermore, they note that the typical adolescent is neither working to save for college education or to supplement family income nor serving in a true apprenticeship position to learn valuable job skills but rather is earning money to spend on personal consumables by working as largely unskilled laborers. Hours of work are not confined to weekends but extend significantly into the school week. According to Steinberg (1996), "by the time they are seniors in high school, many students spend more time on the job than they do in the classroom" (p. 169).

School Start Time

In most U.S. school districts, the start of the school day is progressively earlier as students move from grade school to middle school to high school (Allen, 1991, 1992). Thus, adolescents are required to rise earlier in the morning than preteens in order to get to school on time. We have hypothesized that older adolescents do not adjust appropriately to these demands. As with adolescent employment, historical trends may play a role in the issue of early school start time for older teens. Preliminary data, for example, show that the starting times for U.S. high schools have moved to an earlier hour across the past 20 years (Carskadon & Acebo, 1997). Other countries are not immune to this problem, as noted in Israel, where the "zero hour" (i.e., 7:00 A.M.) for school start time has become a recent concern (Epstein, Chillag, & Lavie, 1995). Clearly for most teenagers, the school bell is a major nonnegotiable factor that mandates the termination – often premature – of nocturnal sleep.

One other important consequence of earlier school start times unrelated to sleep patterns is the amount of largely self-supervised time adolescents have when school release times are also moved earlier. Increasingly, investigators (and legislators, at least in Minnesota) are noting this phenomenon with concern. For example, Richardson, Radziszewska, Dent, and Flay (1993) note an association with after school "self-care" in adolescents and substance abuse, risk taking, depressed mood, and lower academic grades.

Intrinsic-Biological Processes

While the behavioral and psychosocial processes and exposures that adolescents undergo clearly have a marked influence on developing sleep patterns, biological processes may also contribute. The notion that physical changes associated with adolescent development may contribute to sleep patterns is relatively new. In fact, we and others had assumed for many years that the entire scope of the broad behavioral changes in sleep patterns associated with adolescence (e.g., reduced and delayed sleep) could be entirely accounted for by behavioral factors. A gradual accumulation of small pieces of evidence has led us to speculate more strongly about the influence of biological processes, which we categorize under two principal regulatory systems: the sleep mechanisms and the circadian timing system.

Intrinsic Sleep Mechanisms

Commonly referred to as sleep homeostatic mechanisms, intrinsic sleep mechanisms strongly influence the distribution and patterning of sleeping and waking. In simplest terms, the longer one goes without sleep or with minimal sleep, the greater the rebound of sleep. Data on sleep infrastructure from many groups clearly indicate that the amount of slow wave (stages 3 and 4) sleep (cf. Berger & Oswald, 1962; Williams, Hammach, Daly, Dement, & Lubin, 1964; Moses, Johnson, Naitoh, & Lubin, 1975; Webb & Agnew, 1975) and electroencephalographic (EEG) delta power during sleep (Borbély, Bauman, Brandeis, Strauch, & Lehmann, 1981; Feinberg, Fein, & Floyd, 1982) depend on the length of prior wakefulness, providing experimental evidence for and a physiological marker of the homeostatic process. We have previously shown that, like adults, children and adolescents respond to sleep restriction and sleep deprivation with increased physiological sleepiness, as well as an increase in stages 3 and 4 non–rapid eye movement (NREM) sleep during recovery (Carskadon, 1979; Carskadon, Harvey, & Dement, 1981a,b,c). Experimental support for this phenomenon was recently reemphasized in a report by Rosenthal, Roehrs, Rosen, and Roth (1993) demonstrating that graded restriction of nocturnal sleep produced graduated increases of recovery sleep during the subsequent 24 hours, as well as daytime sleepiness on the multiple sleep latency test (MSLT).[1]

---

[1] The MSLT is a test of sleep tendency or "physiological sleepiness" developed in the 1970s by the Stanford group (Carskadon & Dement, 1977b; Richardson, Carskadon,

Few data exist to indicate whether homeostatic mechanisms change at the childhood-to-adolescent transition or across adolescent development. Could adolescents find it easier to stay awake later because the sleep homeostatic mechanism undergoes developmental alterations? Known developmental changes in sleep physiology that occur in adolescence are rather subtle, largely involving the infrastructure of sleep and the pattern of sleepiness-alertness. For example, when youngsters are permitted to sleep 10 hours a night (i.e., when their sleep is not constrained to their "usual" amount), a marked linear decline in slow wave sleep occurs across adolescence, although total nocturnal sleep length is unchanged at about 9.25 hours (Carskadon, 1982). (The latter finding is often cited as evidence that the need for sleep does not decline across the teenage years.)

Studies have also shown that REM sleep latency at night is generally shorter in adolescents than in prepubertal children (Karacan, Anch, Thornby, Okawa, & Williams, 1975; Carskadon, 1982; Coble, Kupfer, Taska, & Kane, 1984). Furthermore, midpuberty is accompanied by a clear-cut augmentation of daytime sleepiness measured using the MSLT (Carskadon, Harvey, Duke, Anders, Litt, & Dement, 1980), even when sleep amount is unchanged. (This finding has been interpreted by some to indicate that teenagers may actually have an increasing need for sleep.)

One interpretation of these developmental findings is that they indicate a reduction in the intensity of sleeping (reduced slow wave sleep) and waking (increased physiological sleepiness on MSLT) processes coincident with adolescence, in other words suggesting a developmental decline in the strength of homeostatic control. The slow-wave sleep decline across adolescence, on the other hand, may simply represent an epiphenomenon of cortical maturation (dendritic pruning), with no fundamental relationship to sleep mechanisms (Feinberg, 1983).

Our previous studies of acute sleep restriction and sleep loss in adolescents and young adults showed no marked age-related differences

---

Flagg, van den Hoed, Dement, & Mitler, 1978). The measure involves assessment of the speed of falling asleep at 2-hour intervals across a day under controlled conditions. Useful in the diagnosis of narcolepsy because of the occurrence of REM sleep during the brief naps (Mitler et al., 1979), sleep latency scores on the MSLT have been categorized by the *International Classification of Sleep Disorders* (1990) as indicating severe sleepiness (< 5 minutes), moderate (5 to 10 minutes), and mild (10 to 15 minutes). Behavioral studies indicate significant performance decrements and episodes of unintended sleep in association with the severe level of sleepiness (Roth, Roehrs, Carskadon, & Dement, 1994).

either in the "sleepiness response" to these procedures or in the recovery process, although these issues were not expressly addressed in experimental design and analyses. On the other hand, using a matched comparison of prepubescent and pubertal adolescents in a carefully monitored sleep-loss study, we noted a tendency for younger children to respond with somewhat more frequent "unintentional" sleep episodes (Carskadon, Littell, & Dement, 1985). This finding also seems to indicate a reduction in the intensity of the homeostatic sleep-wake control as a function of adolescent development. Nevertheless, the question remains open whether pubertal maturation impacts on the homeostatic mechanisms controlling sleep and its consequences for waking behavior.

These intrinsic homeostatic mechanisms also provide tools to examine the neurophysiologic responses to insufficient sleep. Thus, we can use the MSLT to examine the response of the waking brain and slow-wave sleep data to assess the response of the sleeping brain. Ongoing experiments in our laboratory address these mechanisms directly. One preliminary finding (Carskadon, Acebo, & Seifer, 2001) indicates that the slow-wave sleep response to sleep deprivation in pubertal teenagers is reduced versus prepubertal youngsters. Our most current model integrates developmental changes in the organization of the circadian timing system with sleep-wake homeostasis in ways that favor evening alertness in pubertal adolescents.

Circadian Timing System

Another factor with considerable consequences for the patterning of sleeping and waking is the circadian timing system, which affects both the infrastructure of sleep as well as the timing of sleep and waking behavior. For example, studies that involve temporal isolation or multiple sleep opportunities across a day (e.g., 90-minute or 180-minute day) show that the timing of sleep onset (Weitzman et al., 1974; Carskadon & Dement, 1977a; Zulley, Wever, & Aschoff, 1981), the length of sleep (Czeisler, Weitzman, Moore-Ede, Zimmerman, & Kronauer, 1980; Strogatz, 1986), and the timing of REM sleep (Carskadon & Dement, 1980; Czeisler, Zimmerman, Ronda, Moore-Ede, & Weitzman, 1980; Zulley, 1980) vary as a function of the phase of the circadian timing system. In most human studies, the output of the circadian oscillator is marked principally by the pattern of core body temperature, which typically rises across the day to the late afternoon or early evening and then falls across the nighttime, rising again in the early morning hours. The trough of this temperature cycle marks the peak phase for REM sleep, which seems to be tightly coupled to the circadian timing system. Human studies have also identified the predictable occurrence of daily "forbidden zones" when it is difficult to fall asleep (Strogatz, 1986) and "gates" when sleep comes most easily (Lavie, 1985). Animal studies also indicate that the circadian oscillator provides a major signal for daily activity onset (Edgar, Dement, & Fuller, 1993).

Another variable that provides access to the "hands" on the circadian clock involves the measurement of the melatonin secretory cycle. The circadian timing system controls the timing of the secretion of this hormone by the pineal gland. The melatonin secretory phase occurs during the nocturnal hours in both diurnal and nocturnal animals, and it is thus sometimes referred to as the hormone of darkness. If an animal is exposed to a bright light source during the melatonin secretory phase, the hormone's secretion is temporarily terminated. Thus, measurement of melatonin must take place in dim lighting conditions. Melatonin is available from plasma samples as well as from saliva. The onset of the melatonin secretory phase measured in dim light has been called the dim-light melatonin onset (DLMO) measure and is used by Lewy and Sack (1989) and others (e.g., Van Cauter et al., 1994) to assess the circadian system. In our laboratory, we have successfully measured a component of the circadian timing system with salivary melatonin. Figure 2.2 illustrates data obtained using this method in adolescents evaluated on two occasions separated by about 4 months.

A number of investigators have noted alterations in melatonin secretion in association with pubertal development: in general, the level of serum or salivary melatonin secretion declines during puberty. Some have speculated that melatonin may be involved in inhibiting the onset of puberty. These speculations were raised in conjunction with findings that a "dilution" of circulating nocturnal melatonin levels is associated with physical growth. Furthermore, an inverse relationship between circulating melatonin and leuteinizing hormone (LH) levels occurs across pubertal development (Waldhauser & Steger, 1986). Others have failed to confirm a direct causal association between melatonin and puberty, however, even with extensive trials (e.g., Wilson, Lackey, Chikazawa, & Gordon, 1993). These concerns are not germane in the context of our experimental protocols, in which melatonin is used to mark the phase of the circadian timing system.

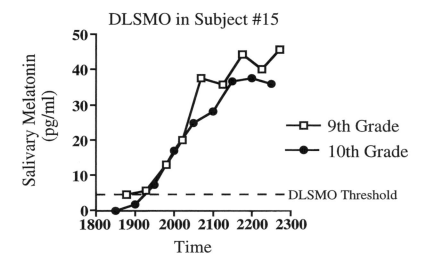

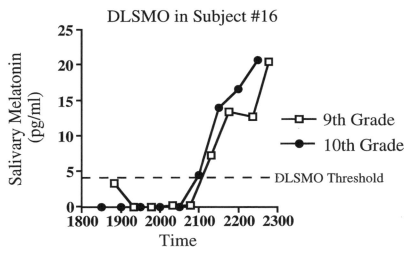

Figure 2.2. Dim-light salivary melatonin levels obtained from 30-minute evening samples obtained in dim light (< 50 lux) in two adolescent volunteers on occasions approximately 4 months apart. These adolescents were participants in the school transition project. Subject 15 is a girl who was age 14.8 years on the first (9th grade) assessment; subject 16 is a girl who was age 15.1 years on the first assessment.

Many studies have noted a clear circadian component to the timing of a variety of human behaviors. Thus, in addition to sleep and wakefulness, performance, memory function, and mood fluctuate with a circadian periodicity (cf. Monk, Fookson, Moline, & Pollack, 1985; Boivin et al., 1997). Such behaviors are also influenced by sleep deprivation (cf. Dinges & Kribbs, 1991). Thus sleep deprivation and circadian timing may both relate to vulnerability in these behavioral domains, either independently (through insufficient sleep or ill-timed behavior) or simultaneously.

Our interest was initially drawn to a possible association between the circadian timing system and adolescent development by the patterns of behavioral change revealed by surveys. As noted, sleep time shortens across the adolescent span, and this reduction of sleep time under weekday constraints is related to a delay in the phase of sleep onset and an advance in the *enforced* time of sleep offset. On weekends, sleep onset is later, as is sleep offset – if released from *enforced* arousal – in adolescents. These patterns are also associated with a change in teenagers' perceived phase preference (Andrade et al., 1992; Carskadon, Vieira, & Acebo, 1993) – that is, the degree to which youngsters recognize in themselves an increasing "evening" versus "morning" capacity for activities. An important corollary may be found in other primates, as noted Golub and her colleagues, who find a delay in the timing of activity rhythms occurring in association with puberty in female rhesus monkeys (Golub, 1996; Chapter 5 in this volume). We have also obtained data from our "long nights" studies of human adolescents indicating that a phase delay in the circadian timing system may occur in association with puberty (Carskadon, Acebo, Richardson, Tate, & Seifer, 1997). The offset phase of melatonin secretion was correlated with age ($r = .62$, $df = 12$, $p = .018$) and Tanner stage ($r = .62$, $df = 12$, $p = .02$).[2] This finding indicates that the intrinsic circadian timing system changes during adolescent development in a phase delay direction. If so, then strategies for interventions to improve adolescent sleep patterns will need to take this change into consideration.

These findings highlight the usefulness of monitoring circadian timing when assessing adolescent sleep patterns and their consequences. Certain adolescents may be profoundly affected by changes in the

---

[2] Tanner staging is a means of identifying pubertal status by physical examination of secondary sexual characteristics, in which stage 1 is prepubertal and stage 5 is mature (Tanner, 1962).

circadian timing system and others may experience a more modest effect. The project described in the next section utilized sleep and circadian measures to evaluate the response of adolescents to a behavioral event: the transition to an earlier school start time.

School Transition Study

The chief goal of this study (Carskadon, Wolfson, Acebo, Tzischinsky, & Seifer, 1998) was to examine the effects of a transition from 9th grade, where school started at 8:25 A.M., to 10th grade, where school started at 7:20 A.M. Evaluations were scheduled at three time points: spring (9th grade), summer vacation, and fall (10th grade); a subgroup was also evaluated in March of 10th grade. Participants wore small wrist monitors to measure sleeping and waking activity levels, and they also completed sleep diaries for two weeks. Saliva samples were collected on the last evening under dim light conditions, and this was followed by an overnight polysomnographic sleep study and subsequent daytime sleepiness testing using the MSLT. Forty 9th grade students were enrolled in the project. They included 15 males and 25 females, ages 14 to 16.2 (mean = 15.0 ± .47) years at the time of the first assessment. Tanner staging was performed in 34 of the students in 9th grade, and most were well advanced in pubertal development: 3 were Tanner stage 3, 12 were Tanner stage 4, and 19 were Tanner stage 5.

Sleep data were derived from the actigraphically estimated values averaged for the school nights of the week immediately preceding the laboratory study. Our measure of the circadian timing system was the phase of the dim-light salivary melatonin onset (DLSMO), derived from saliva samples obtained in dim light (approximately 20 to 30 lux) on the evening of the in-lab study and computed as the interpolated time of salivary melatonin rising above a threshold of 4 picograms per milliliter. The MSLT measures included the mean value for speed of falling asleep across the day of testing (four sleep latency tests) and the type of sleep that occurred.

Several important changes occurred across the 9th-to-10th-grade transition in these youngsters. In the 10th grade, students showed:

- Less sleep on school nights.
- Earlier rising times on school mornings.
- No change in sleep onset times on school nights.
- Later time of the DLSMO phase.

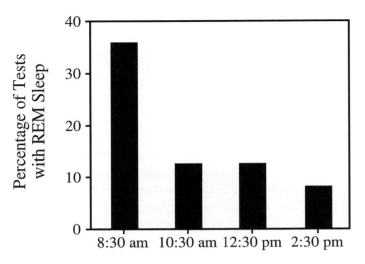

Time of Multiple Sleep Latency Test

Figure 2.3. The percentage of MSLTs with REM sleep during the 10th-grade assessment of the school transition project. The likelihood of REM sleep episodes was significantly greater in the morning than in the afternoon.

- Greater sleepiness on MSLT.
- REM sleep on MSLT in 12 of 25 students evaluated, REM occurring chiefly on morning MSLTs (see Figure 2.3) and related to a delay in the DLSMO phase (Carskadon et al., 1998).

The latter finding was striking and of particular importance: REM sleep episodes do not frequently occur on MSLTs in normal humans under normal sleep-wake conditions, but such episodes are significant for the diagnosis of narcolepsy (Richardson et al., 1978; Mitler et al., 1979; Carskadon, Dement, Mitler, Roth, Westbrook, & Keenan, 1986). In patients with narcolepsy, REM sleep occurs during daytime sleep episodes with equal likelihood at any time of day (Mitler, 1982). In our many studies of normal children, adolescents, and young adults, we have seen REM sleep rarely on MSLTs, with an incidence of less than 7% for even one REM episode in subjects studied when on schedules providing at least 8 (young adults) or 10 (children and adolescents) hours of nocturnal sleep. Rosenthal and his colleagues recently (1995) reported an REM sleep incidence of 23% on MSLTs in nonnarcoleptic adults, more commonly in males than females and with a relatively consistent distribution across the day on naps given at 10:00 A.M., 12:00 A.M., 2:00 P.M., and 4:00 P.M.

The implications of these findings are striking. If a delay in circadian phase is related to adolescent development, then requiring older adolescents to attend school and attempt to take part in intellectually meaningful endeavors in the early morning may be biologically inappropriate. Furthermore, rapid sleep onset and early transitions to REM sleep are more indicative of a brain ready to sleep than to be awake. Data from our long-nights study showed a mean melatonin secretory duration of 634 minutes in adolescents. Thus, it is not at all unlikely that teenagers are being asked to be awake when the circadian system is in its nocturnal mode. The students may be in school, but their brains are at home on their pillows.

At face value, these data indicate that many students are not adjusting adequately to the school start time change and that nearly one-half of the students are perhaps attending school at a circadian phase that favors sleep over waking. In our protocol, the first MSLT occurred at 8:30 A.M., which places it during the time of the second school class period. At this time, students were able to fall asleep in less than 5 minutes and were likely to have REM sleep onsets. In summary, our school transition project provides compelling evidence calling into question early school start times in the absence of any positive steps to assist students to make an appropriate adjustment to such schedules. In general, the adolescents with early school start times did not obtain sufficient sleep, and many were excessively sleepy and attending school at a biologically inappropriate time.

Vulnerable Systems

We have noted two principal alterations of sleep-wake patterns during adolescence: a change in the timing of sleep, which is strongly influenced by psychosocial factors that likely occur in combination with changes in the biological sleep and circadian timing systems, all of which produce a delay in the timing of sleep onset; and a widespread pattern of insufficient sleep, which is influenced greatly by the sleep delay compounded by the nonnegotiable necessity to terminate sleep prematurely in order to attend school. The association of reduced nocturnal sleep with increased daytime sleepiness is well established. Sleepiness has also been associated with a number of behavioral consequences in adults, principally in the realm of performance decrements (cf. Dinges & Kribbs, 1991). Academic performance difficulties have been reported in adolescents (Kowalksi & Allen, 1995; Link & Ancoli-Israel, 1995; Wolfson & Carskadon, 1998). Another area recently identified is the relationship between sleep loss and the immune system, with several animal and human studies providing preliminary, as yet tentative evidence that the processes are linked (Dinges, Douglas, Hamarman, Zaugg, & Kapoor, 1995; Everson, 1995). Direct evidence of increased incidence of illness in sleep-deprived populations is not available. Danner (1993) was among the first to note that physical injury may be associated with inadequate sleep in adolescents, and Pack and his colleagues (1995) clearly indicate that teenagers and young adults are at highest risk for automobile accidents. Our recent high school survey data also indicate a small but significant association between injuries and sleep patterns in high school students (Acebo & Carskadon, 1997). Other important issues, such as relationship formation and maintenance, truancy and delinquency, and especially emotion regulation, have been inadequately studied in association with sleep patterns and insufficient sleep. Animal research, however, has found that sleep loss – in particular, REM sleep loss – is associated with marked increases in aggressive behavior and violence (cf. Hicks, Moore, Hayes, Phillips, & Hawkins, 1979; Peder, Elomaa, & Johansson, 1986; Vogel, Minter, & Woolwine, 1986).

Concern over insufficient sleep in our society has been rising, yet this concern is based principally on "disasters" that occur in sleep-deprived adults resulting largely from performance deficits – the nuclear accidents at Three Mile Island and Chernobyl, highway crashes, and so forth (e.g., Mitler, Carskadon, Czeisler, Dinges, Graeber, & Dement, 1988; Dinges, Graeber, Carskadon, Czeisler, & Dement, 1989). Our previous research has highlighted particular risks for adolescents in whom sleep need competes for time in the face of increasing social and academic pressures (Carskadon, 1990a,b). Hard data are sparse and rarely include youngsters who may confront the greatest threats to safe and adequate sleep and attendant risk factors.

Research is needed to fill these gaps and help us begin to understand more completely the role sleep plays in adolescents' daily lives. For example, if as we suspect, sleep helps to regulate emotions, may there be lasting consequences? We can only speculate about emotional consequences of insufficient sleep on a societal level. If the hypotheses of our research are supported, we will have evidence that sleepiness is related to negative emotional expression and higher levels of emotional dysregulation. An important connection may exist between the growing level of violent behavior among young people (perhaps in part a reflection of failure to regulate emotions) and our society's increasing failure to attend to our bioregulatory needs. Even if the consequences are less overt, our research may expose a more subtle risk – that insufficient sleep alters cognitive perception, literally coloring life blue. Does excessive sleepiness constitute a dark cloud hanging over adolescents (e.g., Tanz & Charrow, 1993)? Our research postulates that sleep patterns are related to successful waking adaptability and that problems with sleep jeopardize behavioral development. These issues attain increasing importance as adolescents and families are confronted by life-style changes that themselves impinge upon sleep patterns.

Because of the core nature of sleep in the human behavioral repertoire, we believe that sleep difficulties in a large segment of a population can indicate dysregulation on a broader societal level. To the extent that adolescents in our society are not able to obtain sufficient sleep at the appropriate time to facilitate their chief developmental task – that is, to become educated members of society by participating effectively in the learning process – this phenomenon marks a potentially very serious problem. Laurence Steinberg's recent treatise (1996) on the plight of adolescent education speaks eloquently about factors affecting poor school performance. Steinberg bases his conclusions on a large, longitudinal study of American schoolchildren. He concludes that "No curricular overhaul, no instructional innovation, no change in school organization, no toughening of standards, no rethinking or teacher training or compensation will succeed if students do not come to school interested in, and committed to learning" (p. 194). Steinberg cites many factors affecting students' lack of interest in schooling, including that they are falling asleep in the classroom. Our attention is obviously drawn to the sleep issue, and based on our data regarding insufficient and ill-timed sleep in adolescents, we believe that these factors may have a powerful impact on student disaffection with school and may also influence their affinity for after school jobs.

REFERENCES

Acebo C, Carskadon MA (1997). Relations among self-reported sleep patterns, health, and injuries in adolescents. *Sleep Research* 26:149.
Allen RP (1991). School week sleep lag: Sleep problems with earlier starting of senior high schools. *Sleep Research* 20:198.
    (1992). Social factors associated with the amount of school week sleep lag for seniors in an early starting suburban high school. *Sleep Research* 21:114.
Anders TF, Carskadon MA, Dement WC, Harvey K (1978). Sleep habits of children and the identification of pathologically sleepy children. *Child Psychiatry and Human Development* 9:56–63.

Andrade MMM, Benedito-Silva AA, Menna-Barreto L (1992). Correlations between morningness-eveningness, character, sleep habits and temperature rhythm in adolescents. *Brazilian Journal of Medical and Biological Research* 28:835–839.

Bearpark HM, Michie PT (1987). Prevalence of sleep/wake disturbances in Sidney adolescents. *Sleep Research* 16:304.

Berger RJ, Oswald I (1962). Effects of sleep deprivation on behavior, subsequent sleep, and dreaming. *Journal of Mental Science* 108:457–465.

Billiard M, Alperovitch A, Perot C, Jammes A (1987). Excessive daytime somnolence in young men: Prevalence and contributing factors. *Sleep* 10:297–305.

Boivin DB, Czeisler CA, Dijk DJ, Duffy JF, Folkard S, Minors DS, Totterdell P, Waterhouse JM (1997). Complex interaction of the sleep-wake cycle and circadian phase modulates mood in healthy subjects. *Archives of General Psychiatry* 54(2):145–152.

Borbély AA, Bauman F, Brandeis P, Strauch I, Lehmann D (1981). Sleep-deprivation: Effect on sleep stages and EEG power density in man. *Clinical Neurophysiology* 51:483–493.

Carskadon MA (1979). Determinants of daytime sleepiness: Adolescent development, extended and restricted nocturnal sleep. Ph.D. dissertation, Stanford University.

——— (1982). The second decade. In C. Guilleminault, ed., *Sleeping and Waking Disorders: Indications and Techniques*, pp. 99–125. Menlo Park, CA: Addison Wesley.

——— (1990a). Adolescent sleepiness: Increased risk in a high-risk population. *Alcohol, Drugs and Driving* 5–6:317–328.

——— (1990b). Patterns of sleep and sleepiness in adolescents. *Pediatrician* 17(1):5–12.

Carskadon MA, Acebo C (1997). Historical view of high school start time: Preliminary results. *Sleep Research* 26:184.

Carskadon MA, Acebo C, Richardson GS, Tate BA, Seifer R (1997). An approach to studying circadian rhythms of adolescent humans. *Journal of Biological Rhythms* 12(3):278–289.

Carskadon MA, Acebo C, Seifer R (2001). Extended nights, sleep loss, and recovery sleep in adolescents. *Archives of Italian Biology* 139:301–312.

Carskadon MA, Dement WC (1977a). Sleepiness and sleep state on a 90-minute schedule. *Psychophysiology* 14:127–133.

——— (1977b). Sleep tendency: An objective measure of sleep loss. *Sleep Research* 6:200.

——— (1980). Distribution of REM sleep on a 90-minute sleep-wake schedule. *Sleep* 2:309–317.

Carskadon MA, Dement WC, Mitler MM, Roth T, Westbrook P, Keenan S (1986). Guidelines for the multiple sleep latency test (MSLT): A standard measure of sleepiness. *Sleep* 9:519–524.

Carskadon MA, Harvey K, Dement WC (1981a). Acute restriction of nocturnal sleep in children. *Perceptual Motor Skills* 53:103–112.

——— (1981b). Multiple sleep latency tests in the development of narcolepsy. *Western Journal of Medicine* 135:414–418.

(1981c). Sleep loss in young adolescents. *Sleep* 4:299–312.

Carskadon MA, Harvey K, Duke P, Anders TF, Litt IF, Dement WC (1980). Pubertal changes in daytime sleepiness. *Sleep* 2:453–460.

Carskadon MA, Littell WP, Dement WC (1985). Constant routine: Alertness, oral body temperature, and performance. *Sleep Research* 14:293.

Carskadon MA, Mancuso J, Rosekind MR (1989). Impact of part-time employment on adolescent sleep patterns. *Sleep Research* 18:114.

Carskadon MA, Vieira C, Acebo C (1993). Association between puberty and a circadian phase delay. *Sleep* 16(3):258–262.

Carskadon MA, Wolfson AR, Acebo C, Tzischinsky O, Seifer R (1998). Adolescent sleep patterns, circadian timing, and sleepiness at a transition to early school days. *Sleep* 21(8):871–881.

Coble PA, Kupfer DJ, Taska LS, Kane J (1984). EEG sleep of normal healthy children. Part 1: Findings using standard measurement methods. *Sleep* 7:289–303.

Czeisler CA, Weitzman ED, Moore-Ede MC, Zimmerman JC, Kronauer RS (1980). Human sleep: Its duration and organization depend on its circadian phase. *Science* 210:264–1267.

Czeisler CA, Zimmerman JC, Ronda JM, Moore-Ede MC, Weitzman ED (1980). Timing of REM sleep is coupled to the circadian rhythm of body temperature in man. *Sleep* 2:329–346.

Danner F (1993). Sleep patterns and health during adolescence. *Sleep Research* 22:79.

Dinges DF, Douglas SD, Hamarman S, Zaugg L, Kapoor S (1995). Sleep deprivation and human immune function. *Advances in Neuroimmunology* 5(2): 97–110.

Dinges, DF, Graeber RC, Carskadon MA, Czeisler CA, Dement WC (1989). Attending to inattention. *Science* 245:342.

Dinges DF, Kribbs NB (1991). Performing while sleepy: Effects of experimentally-induced sleepiness. In T. Monk, ed., *Sleep, Sleepiness and Performance*, pp. 97–128. New York: John Wiley & Sons.

Edgar DM, Dement WC, Fuller CA (1993). Effect of SCN lesions on sleep in squirrel monkeys: Evidence for opponent processes in sleep-wake regulation. *Journal of Neuroscience* 13(3):1065–1079.

Epstein R, Chillag N, Lavie P (1995). Sleep habits of children and adolescents in Israel: The influence of starting time of schools. *Sleep Research* 24A:432.

Everson C (1995). Functional consequences of sustained sleep deprivation in the rat. *Behavioural Brain Research* 69:43–54.

Feinberg I (1983). Schizophrenia: Caused by a fault in programmed synaptic elimination during adolescence? *Journal of Psychiatric Research* 17(4): 319–334.

Feinberg I, Fein G, Floyd TC (1982). Computer-detected patterns of electroencephalographic delta activity during and after extended sleep. *Science* 215:1131–1133.

Gau S-F, Soong WT (1995). Sleep problems of junior high school students in Taipei. *Sleep* 18(8):667–673.

Golub MS (1996). Changes in diurnal rest-activity patterns of rhesus monkeys during adolescence. Paper presented at NIH symposium on Neurobiology of Adolescent Depression, Bethesda, MD, March 28–29.

Henschel A, Lack L (1987). Do many adolescents sleep poorly or just too late? *Sleep Research* 16:354.

Hicks RA, Moore JD, Hayes C, Phillips N, Hawkins J (1979). REM sleep deprivation increases aggressiveness in male rats. *Physiology and Behavior* 22(6):1097–1100.

International Classification of Sleep Disorders: Diagnostic and Coding Manual (1990). Diagnostic classification steering committee, MJ Thorpy, Chairman, Rochester, Minnesota, American Sleep Disorders Association.

Karacan I, Anch M, Thornby JI, Okawa M, Williams RL (1975). Longitudinal sleep patterns during pubertal growth: Four-year follow-up. *Pediatric Research* 9:842–846.

Klackenberg G (1982). Sleep behaviour studied longitudinally. *Acta Paediatrica Scandinavica* 71:501–506.

Kowalski N, Allen R (1995). School sleep lag is less but persists with a very late starting high school. *Sleep Research* 24:124.

Lavie, P (1985). Ultradian rhythms: Gates of sleep and wakefulness. *Experimental Brain Research* (suppl. 12):149–164.

Lewy AJ, Sack, RL (1989). The dim light melatonin onset as a marker for circadian phase position. *Chronobiology International* 6(1):993–1002.

Link SC, Ancoli-Israel S (1995). Sleep and the teenager. *Sleep Research* 24a:184.

Mitler MM (1982). The multiple sleep latency test as an evaluation for excessive somnolence. In C. Guilleminault, ed., *Sleeping and Waking Disorders: Indications and Techniques*, pp. 145–153. Menlo Park, CA: Addison-Wesley.

Mitler MM, Carskadon MA, Czeisler CA, Dinges D, Graeber RC, Dement WC (1988). Catastrophes, sleep, and public policy: Consensus report. *Sleep* 11:100–109.

Mitler MM, van den Hoed J, Carskadon MA, Richardson GS, Park R, Guilleminault C, Dement WC (1979). REM sleep episodes during the multiple sleep latency test in narcoleptic patients. *Electroencephalography and Clinical Neurophysiology* 46:479–481.

Monk TH, Fookson JE, Moline ML, Pollack CP (1985). Diurnal variation in mood and performance in a time-isolated environment. *Chronobiology International* 2:185–193.

Moses JM, Johnson LC, Naitoh P, Lubin A (1975). Sleep stage deprivation and total sleep loss: Effects on sleep behavior. *Psychophysiology* 12(2):141–146.

Pack AI, Pack AM, Rodgman D, Cucchiara A, Dinges DF, Schwab CW (1995). Characteristics of crashes attributed to the driver having fallen asleep. *Accident Analysis and Prevention* 27:769–775.

Peder M, Elomaa E, Johansson G (1986). Increased aggression after rapid eye movement sleep deprivation in Wistar rats is not influenced by reduction of dimensions of enclosure. *Behavioral and Neural Biology* 45(3):287–291.

Petta D, Carskadon MA, Dement WC (1984). Sleep habits in children aged 7–13 years. *Sleep Research* 13:86.

Price VA, Coates TJ, Thoresen CE, Grinstead OA (1978). Prevalence and correlates of poor sleep among adolescents. *American Journal of Diseases of Children* 132:583–586.

Richardson GS, Carskadon MA, Flagg W, van den Hoed J, Dement WC, Mitler MM (1978). Excessive daytime sleepiness in man: Multiple sleep latency measurement in narcoleptic and control subjects. *Electroencephalography and Clinical Neurophysiology* 45:621–627.

Richardson JL, Radziszewska B, Dent CW, Flay BR (1993). Relationship between after-school care of adolescents and substance use, risk taking, depressed mood, and academic achievement. *Pediatrics* 92(1):32–38.

Rosenthal L, Bishop C, Helmus T, Roehrs TA, Brouillard L, Roth T (1995). The frequency of multiple sleep onset REM periods among subjects with no EDS. *Sleep Research* 24:331.

Rosenthal L, Roehrs TA, Rosen A, Roth T (1993). Level of sleepiness and total sleep time following various time in bed conditions. *Sleep* 16(3):226–232.

Roth T, Roehrs TA, Carskadon MA, Dement WC (1994). Daytime sleepiness and alertness. In M. H. Kryger, T. Roth, & W. C. Dement, eds., *Principles and Practice of Sleep Medicine* (2d ed.), pp. 40–49. Philadelphia: W. B. Saunders.

Saarenpaaheikkila OA, Rintahaka PJ, Laippala PJ, Koivikko MJ (1995). Sleep habits and disorders in Finnish school children. *Journal of Sleep Research* 4(3):173–182.

Steinberg L with Brown B, Dornbusch S (1996). *Beyond the Classroom: Why School Reform Has Failed and What Parents Need to Do*. New York: Simon & Schuster.

Strauch I, Dubral I, Struchholz C (1973). Sleep behavior in adolescents in relation to personality variables. In U. J. Jovanovic, ed., *The Nature of Sleep*, pp. 121–123. Stuttgart: Gustav Fischer.

Strauch I, Meier B (1988). Sleep need in adolescents: A longitudinal approach. *Sleep* 11:378–386.

Strogatz SH (1986). *The Mathematical Structure of the Human Sleep-Wake Cycle*. New York: Springer-Verlag.

Tanner JM (1962). *Growth at Adolescence*. Oxford: Blackwell.

Tanz RR, Charrow J (1993). Black clouds – work load, sleep and resident reputation. *American Journal of Diseases of Children* 147(5):579–584.

Van Cauter E, Sturis J, Byrne MM, Blackman JD, Leproult R, Ofek G, L'Hermite-Baleriaux M, Refetoff S, Turek FW, Van Reeth O (1994). Demonstration of rapid light-induced advances and delays of the human circadian clock using hormonal phase markers. *American Journal of Physiology* 166 (Endocrinology and Metabolism 29):E953–E963.

Vogel GW, Minter K, Woolwine B (1986). Effects of chronically administered antidepressant drugs on animal behavior. *Physiology and Behavior* 36(4): 659–666.

Waldhauser F, Steger H (1986). Changes in melatonin secretion with age and pubescence. *Journal of Neural Transmission* 21:183–197.

Webb WB, Agnew HW (1973). *Sleep and Dreams*. Dubuque, Iowa: Wm. C. Brown Company.

(1975). The effects on subsequent sleep of an acute restriction of sleep length. *Psychophysiology* 12:367–370.

Weitzman ED, Nogeire C, Perlow M, Fukushima D, Sassin J, McGregor P, Gallagher T, Hellman L (1974). Effects of a prolonged 3-hour sleep-wakefulness cycle on sleep stages, plasma cortisol, growth hormone and body temperature in man. *Journal of Clinical Endocrinology and Metabolism* 38:1018–1030.

White L, Hahn PM, Mitler MM (1980). Sleep questionnaire in adolescents. *Sleep Research* 9:108.

Williams HL, Hammack JT, Daly RL, Dement WC, Lubin A (1964). Responses to auditory stimulation, sleep loss and the EEG stages of sleep. *Electroencephalography and Clinical Neurophysiology* 16:269–279.

Wilson ME, Lackey S, Chikazawa K, Gordon TP (1993). The amplitude of nocturnal melatonin concentrations is not decreased by oestradiol and does not alter reproductive function in adolescent or adult female rhesus monkeys. *Journal of Endocrinology* 137(2):299–309.

Wolfson A, Carskadon MA (1998). Sleep schedules and daytime functioning in adolescents. *Child Development* 69(4):875–887.

Zepelin H, Hamilton P, Wanzie FJ (1977). Sleep disturbance in early adolescence. *Sleep Research* 6:183.

Zulley J (1980). Distribution of REM sleep in entrained 24 hour and free-running sleep-wake cycles. *Sleep* 2(4):377–389.

Zulley J, Wever R, Aschoff J (1981). The dependence of onset and duration of sleep on the circadian rhythm of rectal temperature. *Pflügers Archiv. European Journal of Physiology* 391:314–318.

3. Endocrine Changes Associated with Puberty and Adolescence

GARY S. RICHARDSON AND BARBARA A. TATE

Endocrine Changes in Puberty

In humans, puberty is defined as the interval between first signs of disinhibition of the central neuroendocrine systems controlling pituitary-gonadal function and the completion of sexual development and achievement of reproductive competence. The morphologic correlates of puberty include rapid physical growth (the adolescent "growth spurt") and development of secondary sexual characteristics. These, in turn, are the result of the interdependent maturation of several endocrine systems, most prominently the secretion of sex steroids from the gonads.

Less well defined are the psychological and behavioral changes that accompany puberty. Alterations in sleep-wake behavior, while prominent, remain unexplained and may reflect a complex interaction between social changes in the pubertal child's environment and the changing internal neuroendocrine milieu. Neurophysiologic changes also occur during puberty, some of which appear to be steroid-dependent. The wide distribution throughout the brain of specific steroid receptors suggests a mechanism to correlate neurological, psychological, and behavioral changes; however, not all changes in structure and function of the nervous system during the pubertal transition are consequences of changing influences. While sex steroids have important effects on nervous system development, both during the initial prenatal exposure and during puberty, other maturational events are independent of sex steroids (Ojeda, 1991).

Animal models of puberty are clearly necessary to a systematic exploration of the physiology of the process of sexual maturation. Current models are characterized using definitions of analogous changes in sexual morphology and endocrine markers. In considering the utility of these models, it is important to realize that puberty occurs against a developmental background, aspects of which are independent of puberty itself, and comparison of the timing of puberty in various aspects indicates that it occurs at very different points in this developmental sequence. The manifestation of some behavioral changes associated with puberty in humans may not be present in all animal models if the expression of the affected behavior itself is subject to ongoing puberty-independent maturation.

In this chapter, we summarize the neuroendocrine and morphologic changes of puberty in humans, drawing on animal models where appropriate. The intent is to provide a framework for consideration of behavioral changes and alterations in sleep-wake behavior in adolescents. We consider, in turn, morphologic, neurophysiologic, and endocrine correlates of the pubertal transition, summarize what is known about the mechanisms, and consider how each could impact sleep-wake behavior in children.

From the endocrine perspective, puberty is defined as the period between the onset of secretion of pituitary gonadotropins and the attainment of reproductive competence (fertility). Studying effects of puberty on behavior requires examination of all manifestations of puberty including morphological changes (i.e., development of secondary sex characteristics), neuroendocrine changes, and alterations in neural systems modulating the endocrine axis.

Morphology of Puberty

Puberty is associated with two major physical changes: increased somatic growth (the pubertal "growth spurt") is accompanied by maturation of secondary sexual characteristics – pubic hair, genital development, and, in girls, breast growth. The remarkably consistent sequence in the appearance of these physical features allows their use as markers of sexual maturation. Tanner (Marshall & Tanner, 1968) synthesized individual markers into stages of sexual maturation ("Tanner stages") that have greatly simplified objective quantification of the process of sexual maturation (Figure 3.1).

Somatic growth accelerates shortly after the onset of sexual maturation. Reflecting differences in the age of sex steroid secretion, the growth spurt occurs earlier on average in girls (ages 10–12 years) than in boys (ages 12–14 years). Somatic growth includes rapid increases in

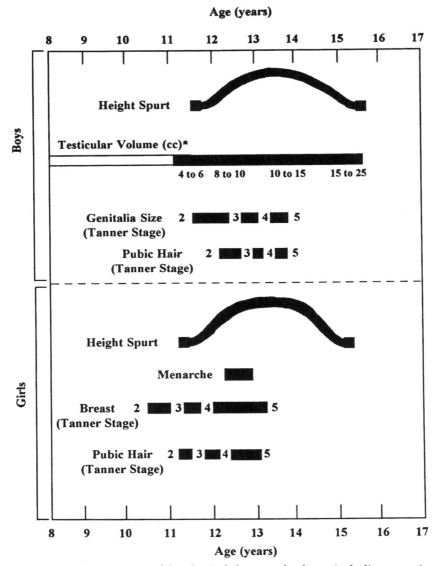

Figure 3.1. The sequences of the physical changes of puberty, including somatic growth, genital maturation, and development of secondary sexual characteristics, for boys (upper panel) and girls (lower panel). Adapted from Wheeler, 1991.

muscle mass and bone growth, particularly long bone length. This process proceeds until epiphyseal plates in long bones close and terminate long bone growth.

The endocrine regulation of these physical changes involves gonadal steroids and growth hormone (GH), which have both additive and independent effects on the adolescent growth spurt. Both GH and sex steroids augment growth during puberty. The increased secretion of sex steroids initiates the pubertal growth spurt in both sexes, with sex steroids modulating the secretion and synthesis of GH (Brook & Hindmarsh, 1992). Gonadal steroids also have the effect of limiting final height via their effects on skeletal maturation and epiphyseal growth plate closure (Brook & Hindmarsh, 1992).

The mechanisms that underlie the interaction of somatic growth and timing of puberty are unknown, but it has been proposed that metabolic signals can influence release of gonadotropin releasing hormone (GnRH). For instance, in the female rat, initiation of puberty is associated with increases in mRNA for insulin-like growth factor I (IGF-I) in liver, with consequent elevations in levels in the blood, but no increase in hypothalamic message. Intraventricular injections of IGF-I advanced the onset of puberty, however, suggesting that peripheral levels of IGF-I may influence development (Hiney, Srivastava, Nyberg, Ojeda, & Dees, 1996). Similar mechanisms may play a role in the influence of somatic development on regulation of the timing of sexual maturation.

Neuroendocrine Changes

The morphologic changes associated with puberty reflect the effects of underlying changes in neuroendocrine function. The center of this process is the pulsatile release of GnRH from neurons in the arcuate nucleus of the hypothalmus. Like other hypothalmic releasing functions, GnRH is transported to target cells (gonadotropes) in the anterior pituitary gland via the hypothalmic-hypophyseal portal circulation in the pituitary stalk (infundibulum). Direct measurements of plasma taken from this portal vasculature confirm that GnRH-positive neurons in the arcuate nucleus collectively comprise the neural oscillator, the firing pattern of which corresponds to the pulsatile GnRH release. A variety of neural inputs, as well as feedback influences of sex steroids, has been shown to alter systematically the frequency of the GnRH pulse generator.

GnRH pulses act on the gonadotropes in the anterior pituitary to produce corresponding pulses of the gonadotropins, luteinizing hormone

(LH), and follicle stimulating hormone (FSH). The precise frequency of the pulsatile GnRH stimulation determines the relative amplitude of LH and FSH release. The amplitude and pattern of pulsatile GnRH release, in concert with sex steroid levels, regulates gonadotropin gene expression. The importance of frequency in the hypothalmic-pituitary-gonadal (HPG) communication is apparent in studies of gonadotropin response to exogenous stimulation with GnRH in patients with congenital GnRH deficiency. Both continuous (nonpulsatile) and high-frequency (supraphysiololgic) administration of GnRH results in attenuation of the gonadotropin response.

The pulsatile release of LH and FSH from the pituitary stimulates testosterone production and spermatogenesis in the testis in the male and estradiol and folliculogenesis in the ovary in the female. As with the interaction between the hypothalmus and the pituitary, pulsatile stimulation is necessary to optimize the gonadal response to gonadotropins. The earliest assayable sign of puberty is pulsatile LH secretion during sleep. At an early age, when morphologic measures are still prepubertal (Tanner stage I), LH levels increase at night, eventually stimulating sleep-related secretion of sex steroids. This relationship appears to represent an effect of sleep per se, rather than a circadian rhythm in LH production, as limited data have demonstrated that acute reversal of the sleep-wake cycle in early pubertal children is associated with a reversal of sleep-dependent LH secretion as well. This suggests that some aspect of the neurophysiology of sleep relationship between sleep processes and neural components of the HPG axis seems unlikely because of the transient relationship between sleep and LH in puberty. In adults, sleep is not associated with augmentation of LH release. Indeed, sleep in the early follicular phase of the menstrual cycle in women is associated with slowing of GnRH pulses and decreased average LH concentrations. Naloxone administration during sleep restores waking pulse frequency, indicating that opiate systems are involved in sleep-related inhibition in this specific setting. Similar pharmacological dissection of the sleep-related augmentation of LH secretion early in puberty has not been performed.

Sex steroid hormones have widespread effects and are proximally responsible for most of the physiologic and morphologic changes associated with the pubertal transition. In addition, steroids in concert with other gonadal hormonal products (e.g., inhibin) feed back on higher levels in the HPG axis to modulate ongoing secretion. In the male, testosterone acts at the GnRH pulse generator to slow and attenuate

GnRH pulses, and at the pituitary to limit the amplitude of LH pulses. In females, feedback effects of estradiol are more complex. Inhibitory at low concentrations, the effects of estradiol on higher centers reverse at high concentrations. This stimulatory effect of estradiol is central to the crescendo increase in LH and estradiol across the mid to late follicular phase of the menstrual cycle, culminating in the LH surge and ovulation. Progesterone from the corpus luteum reverses the feedback effect, restoring inhibition and reducing LH levels back to baseline.

Neurophysiologic Correlates of Puberty

The third major category of changes associated with puberty involves changes in the central nervous system, both anatomic and functional. These changes can be divided into neural changes that are primary to the pubertal process (i.e., those involved in the onset of the pubertal sequence) and neural changes that are secondary to the changing endocrine environment of puberty.

As increases in pulsatile GnRH release precipitate the manifestation of puberty (i.e., gonadal maturation), the factors that regulate GnRH release constitute the neurophysiological events primary to the onset of puberty. A number of neurotransmitter systems modulate GnRH secretion (2-2). These include norepinephrine, epinephrine, dopamine, serotonin, gamma-aminobutyric acid (GABA), neuropeptide Y, acetylcholine, prostaglandins, and the opioid peptides (South, Yankov, & Evans, 1993). The sum effect of these systems regulating GnRH neurons appears to be both stimulatory and inhibitory. The stimulatory influences include noradrenergic, neuropeptide Y (Sutton, Mitsugi, Plotsky, & Sarkar, 1998), and glutamatergic neurons; all have been demonstrated to show increased input to GnRH neurons prior to the onset of puberty. In addition, in both monkeys and rats, the onset of puberty can be advanced by pulsatile administration with n-methyl-D-asparatate (NMDA) (Urbanski & Ojeda, 1987; Plant, Gay, Marshall, & Arslan, 1989), and an increase in NMDA-R1 receptors on GnRH neurons has been demonstrated in the pubertal rat brain (Gore, Wu, Rosenberg, & Roberts, 1996).

In adults, neurotransmitters that inhibit GnRH release include opioid peptides and GABA. The action of opioids appears to depend on the presence of significant sex steroid levels (Reyes-Fuentes & Veldhuis, 1993). While alterations in opioid tone do not appear to be important regulators of the timing of increased GnRH secretion at puberty, studies do suggest that a reduction of GABA inhibition is an important mechanism for stimulating GnRH release at puberty (Mitsushima et al., 1996). GnRH also appears to regulate its own release. In vitro studies of hypothalamic explants from pubertal male rats show an increased frequency of pulsatile GnRH secretion and a reduced sensitivity to GnRH autoregulation when compared with prepubertal tissue (Bourguignon, Gerard, Fawe, Alvarez-Gonzalez, & Franchimont, 1991).

With regard to secondary central nervous system (CNS) changes, an extensive literature has demonstrated that sex steroids have widespread actions within the CNS. Estradiol and testosterone receptors are distributed throughout the CNS, and sex-steroid dependent alterations and other CNS functions are well described. In addition, sex steroids play a role in the continuing maturation of the CNS, affecting the differentiation of nuclei (Arnold & Schlinger, 1993; Mortaud & Degrelle, 1996), dendritic growth, and synaptic foundation (Matsumoto, 1991; McCarthy, 1994). Here, definitive assignment of many of these changes to the pubertal sex steroid exposure (as opposed to antenatal sex steroid effects) is difficult because of reliance on animal models in which these developmental stages are not as distinct as they are in the human.

Control of Pubertal Onset

Identification of pubertal CNS changes that anticipate the onset of puberty requires delineation of CNS processes controlling the timing of pubertal onset. Here, several models have been proposed. Some of these and the supporting studies will be considered here by way of review. A more complete summary of these issues can be found in reviews by Ojeda (1991) and Reiter and Grumbach (1998).

Human puberty actually represents a reactivation of the HPG axis after a period of dormancy. Prior to birth, the fetal HPG axis is activated, producing steroid hormones that are important in the sexual differentiation of the fetus and the maturation of sex-hormone dependent structures and functions. At birth, the HPG axis is dormant, with suppressed levels of GnRH, gonadotropins, and sex steroids. Studies during this juvenile (prepubertal) period have shown that the arrest occurs at the level of GnRH pulse generator. Exogenous override of the inhibition with either gonadotropins or GnRH results in normal response of the lower levels of the sequence, demonstrating that these systems are lacking descending stimulation but are not independently arrested.

The precise nature of the "brake" mechanisms by which the GnRH system is restrained remains unclear. Broadly, two possibilities exist: increased activity of an inhibitory influence on the GnRH pulse generator or decreased stimulatory input. Several observations would seem to support the existence of both factors. First, a variety of neuropathologic processes is associated with precocious puberty in children, and this effect can be reproduced with hypothalamic lesions in experimental animal models (Ojeda, 1991). These findings are most consistent with loss of an inhibitory restraint on the pubertal process.

Second, experiments examining putative excitatory influences on GnRH neurons (e.g., NMDA projections) show that facilitation of this input is sufficient to activate the entire HPG axis. Further, in the rat, transient stimulation with NMDA agonists is sufficient to initiate the pubertal sequence, which is then sustained even after the exogenous stimulation is removed (Ojeda, 1991). This finding is most consistent with a primary role of diminished stimulatory influence. In view of support for both factors, and the variation across animal models, Ojeda (1991) suggests that both decreased stimulation and enhanced inhibition may be working to restrain GnRH release until the onset of puberty.

Melatonin and Control of Pubertal Onset

One intriguing hypothesis is that melatonin from the pineal gland serves as an inhibitory regulator of pubertal onset. Several lines of evidence support this hypothesis. Some types of pineal tumors have been associated with the delayed onset of puberty (Hochman, Judge, & Reichlin, 1981) and elevated levels of melatonin (Puig-Domingo et al., 1992). Children with destruction of the pineal gland, however, either as a consequence of a pineal region tumor or its treatment, show reduced nocturnal melatonin and advanced sexual maturation. An association between pineal tumors and premature sexual maturation, first described by Heubner in 1898 and appearing more often in boys than in girls (Kitay, 1954), is apparently due to secretion of chorionic gonadotropin by cells of the tumor and is unrelated to melatonin levels.

Melatonin has been shown to exert a hypogonadal effect either via direct inhibition of the GnRH pulse generator or by facilitating the feedback inhibition of circulating sex steroids (Figure 3.2). Decreases in melatonin levels were found in association with puberty (Waldhauser et al., 1984; Waldhauser & Dietzel, 1985), although not all investigators saw this relationship (Ehrenkranz et al., 1982; Penny, 1985). Daytime levels

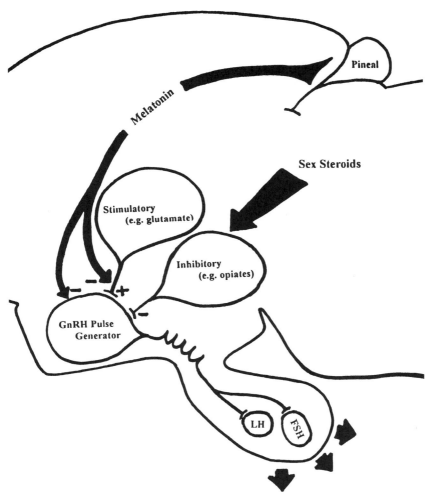

Figure 3.2. A schematic representation of the mammalian brain illustrating the relationship between the pineal, the hypothalamus, and the pituitary in the regulation of gonadotropin release. Adapted from Glass, 1988.

of melatonin do not appear to be related to stage of sexual maturation (Ehrenkranz et al., 1982; Penny, 1985), whereas nighttime levels show a negative correlation with pubertal stage (Waldhauser et al., 1984; Waldhauser & Dietzel, 1985). A similar finding was reported in rhesus monkeys, where nocturnal melatonin levels were inversely correlated with sexual maturation (Wilson & Gordon, 1989). Finally, nocturnal LH levels have also been reported to be inversely related to melatonin levels in children throughout the pubertal period (Waldhauser et al., 1984). Silman (1991) has argued, based on these findings, that somatic growth results in progressively reduced nocturnal melatonin concentrations (through increased volume of distribution for a constant pineal output). When melatonin levels fall below a critical threshold, the GnRH pulse generator escapes from the inhibitory constrains and the pubertal sequence begins.

The Silman hypothesis has the important advantage of incorporating an explanation for the secular trend of earlier age of pubertal onset over the past 200 years, a trend that is generally attributed to improved childhood nutrition and increased fat stores. There are, however, several concerns about a hypothetical role for melatonin as a regulator of pubertal onset. First, the available data are correlative. Direct manipulation of melatonin levels has not been possible in children, but attempts to manipulate the adult HPG axis in adults have not provided consistent evidence of an inhibitory effect of physiological concentrations of melatonin on HPG function. Second, attempts to confirm that pubertal onset is associated with falling melatonin levels in longitudinal intrasubject measurements have not been consistent with the Silman hypothesis (Cavallo, 1991).

Recent work characterizing the melatonin receptor (Weaver, Stehle, Stopa, & Reppert, 1993; Reppert, Weaver, & Ebisawa, 1994) has provided the basis for an alternative formulation. Data suggest that melatonin receptor expression in the brain and anterior pituitary decreases with age in the rat (Vanecek, 1988). The largest decrease in pituitary melatonin receptors occurs at the age of sexual maturation. Should this prove to be true in humans, it would provide an alternate mechanism for decreased inhibitory effects, independent of melatonin concentration.

Puberty and Timing of Sleep-Wake Behavior

Several aspects of the pubertal transition may affect circadian organization in general and the timing of sleep-wake behaviors in particular. Most of the available data have focused on the effects of sex steroids on circadian rhythms of motor activity and sleep-wake state. This reflects the widespread CNS distribution of sex steroid receptors including localization to neurons of the suprachiasmatic nucleus.

Available studies suggest that estrogen is associated with increased consolidation of motor activity and phase advance of activity onset. In female hamsters, for example, the elevated estrogen levels at proestrous are associated with an earlier onset of wheel running than on other days of the estrus cycle, producing a characteristic "scalloping" in the activity rhythm. Castration-replacement studies have shown a small effect on clock function with shortening of free running period. There appear to be important species differences, and there is not yet direct evidence to support an important effect in humans.

Summary

Puberty is a complex phenomenon associated with dramatic changes in morphology and in endocrine and neural systems. The potential input of each of these systems on sleep-wake organization is complex and extensive and includes both the widespread effects of sex steroids on the brain and the potential effects of activated neural systems that may be involved in the timing of pubertal onset. Demonstrated interactions between sleep and pubertal process also work in the opposite direction, with sleep facilitating the activation of the HPG axis early in puberty.

REFERENCES

Arnold AP, Schlinger BA (1993). Sexual differentiation of brain and behavior; the zebra finch is not just a flying rat. *Brain Behav Evol* 42:231–241.
Bourguignon JP, Gerard A, Fawe L, Alvarez-Gonzalez ML, Franchimont P (1991). Neuroendocrine control of the onset of puberty: Secretion of gonadotrophin-releasing hormone from rat hypothalamic explants. *Acta Paediatr Scand Suppl* 372:19–25.
Brook CG, Hindmarsh PC (1992). The somatotropic axis in puberty. *Endocrinol Metab Clin North Am* 21(4):767–782.
Cavallo A (1991). Plasma melatonin rhythm in disorders of puberty: Interactions of age and pubertal stages. *Horm Res* 36:16–21.
Ehrenkranz JR, Tamarkin L, Comite F, Johnsonbaugh RE, Bybee DE, Loriaux DL, Cutler GB Jr (1982). Daily rhythm of plasma melatonin in normal and precocious puberty. *J Clin Endocrinol Metab* 55:307–310.
Glass JD (1988). Neuroendocrine regulation of seasonal reproduction by the pineal gland and melatonin. *Pineal Res Rev* 6:219–259.
Gore AC, Wu TJ, Rosenberg JJ, Roberts JL (1996). Gonadotropin-releasing hormone and NMDA receptor gene expression and colocalization change during puberty in female rats. *J Neurosci* 16:5281–5289.
Hiney JK, Srivastava V, Nyberg CL, Ojeda SR, Dees WL (1996). Insulin-like growth factor I of peripheral origin acts centrally to accelerate the initiation of female puberty. *Endocrinology* 137:3717–3728.
Hochman HI, Judge DM, Reichlin S (1981). Precocious puberty and hypothalamic hamartoma. *Pediatrics* 67:236–244.

Kitay, JI (1954). Pineal lesions and precocious puberty: A review. *J Clin Endocrinol Metab* 14:622–625.

Marshall WA, Tanner JM (1968). Growth and physiological development during adolescence. *Ann Rev Med* 19:283–300.

Matsumoto A (1991). Synaptogenic action of sex steroids in developing and adult neuroendocrine brain. *Psychoneuroendocrinology* 16:25–40.

McCarthy MM (1994). Molecular aspects of sexual differentiation of the rodent brain. *Psychoneuroendocrinology* 19:415–427.

Mitsushima D, Marzban F, Luchansky LL, Burich AJ, Keen KL, Durning M, Golos TG, Terasawa E (1996). Role of glutamic acid decarboxylase in the pre-pubertal inhibition of the luteinizing hormone releasing hormone release in female rhesus monkeys. *J Neurosci* 16:2563–2573.

Mortaud S, Degrelle H (1996). Steroid control of higher brain function and be-havior. *Behav Genet* 26:367–372.

Ojeda SR (1991). The mystery of mammalian puberty: How much more do we know? *Perspect Biological Med* 34:365–383.

Ojeda SR, Andrews WW, Advis JP, Smith SS (1980). Recent advances in the endocrinology of puberty. *Endocr Rev* 1:228–257.

Penny R (1985). Episodic secretion of melatonin in pre- and postpubertal girls and boys. *J Clin Endocrinol Metab* 60:751–766.

Plant TM, Gay VL, Marshall GR, Arslan M (1989). Puberty in monkey is trig-gered by chemical stimulation of the hypothalamus. *Proc Natl Acad Sci USA* 86:2506–2510.

Puig-Domingo M, Webb SM, Serrano J, Peinado MA, Corcoy R, Ruscalleda J, Re-iter RJ, de Leiva A (1992). Brief report: Melatonin-related hypogonadotropic hypogonadism [see comments]. *N Engl J Med* 327:1356–1359.

Reiter EO, Grumbrach MM (1988). Neuroendocrine control mechanisms and the onset of puberty. *Ann Rev Physiol* 44:595–613.

Reppert SM, Weaver DR, Ebisawa T (1994). Cloning and characterization of a mammalian melatonin receptor that mediates reproductive and circadian responses. *Neuron* 13:1177–1185.

Reyes-Fuentes A, Veldhuis JD (1993). Neuroendocrine physiology of the normal male gonadal axis. *Endocrinol Metab Clin North Am* 22:93–124.

Silman R (1991). Melatonin and the human gonadotrophin-releasing hormone pulse generator. *J Endocrin* 128:7–11.

South SA, Yankov VI, Evans WS (1993). Normal reproductive neuroendocrinol-ogy in the female. *Endocrinol Metab Clin North Am* 22(1):1–28.

Sutton SW, Mitsugi N, Plotsky PM, Sarkar DK (1988). Neuropeptide Y (NPY): A possible role in the initiation of puberty. *Endocrinology* 123:2152–2154.

Urbanski HF, Ojeda SR (1987). Activation of luteinizing hormone-releasing hor-mone release advances the onset of female puberty. *Neuroendocrinology* 46:273–276.

Vanecek J (1988). The melatonin receptors in rat ontogenesis. *Neuroendocrinology* 48:201–203.

Waldhauser F, Dietzel M (1985). Daily and annual rhythms in human melatonin secretion: Role in puberty control. *Ann N Y Acad Sci* 453:205–214.

Waldhauser F, Weiszenbacher G, Frisch H, Zeitlhuber U, Waldhauser M, Wurtman RJ (1984). Fall in nocturnal serum melatonin during prepuberty and pubescence. *Lancet* 1:362–365.

Weaver DR, Stehle JH, Stopa EG, Reppert SM (1993). Melatonin receptors in human hypothalamus and pituitary: Implications for circadian and reproductive responses to melatonin. *J Clin Endocrinol Metab* 76:295–301.

Wheeler MD (1991). Physical changes of puberty. *Endocrin Metabol Clinics of North America* 20:1–14.

Wilson ME, Gordon TP (1989). Nocturnal changes in serum melatonin during female puberty in rhesus monkeys: A longitudinal study. *J Endocrinol* 121:553–562.

4. Maturational Changes in Sleep-Wake Timing: Longitudinal Studies of the Circadian Activity Rhythm of a Diurnal Rodent

BARBARA A. TATE, GARY S. RICHARDSON,
AND MARY A. CARSKADON

In addition to the maturation of endocrine and reproductive systems, puberty in human adolescents is associated with changes in the temporal patterns of several physiological and behavioral events. One of the most prominent behavioral changes is an alteration in sleep organization, specifically a delay in the timing of nocturnal sleep (Strauch & Meier, 1988; Carskadon, Vieira, & Acebo, 1993). Epidemiologic data demonstrate that length of nocturnal sleep declines across adolescence. Most older teenagers report that their sleep patterns on weekdays have an increasingly delayed time of sleep onset, yet they are constrained to wake up early due to school demands. On weekends, when school constraints are not present, sleep onset and sleep offset are delayed. This adolescent delay of the sleep-wake schedule is also associated with a more evening-type preference (Andrade, Benedito-Silva, & Menna-Barreto, 1992; Carskadon et al., 1993).

Although social factors are clearly important in the evolving sleep-wake pattern of adolescents, available evidence implicates peripubertal changes in physiologic mechanisms controlling the timing of sleep. Current models of these mechanisms allow two broad hypotheses: either the circadian system regulating sleep timing is altered to produce a delayed entrained phase position, or homeostatic processes are changed to delay sleep times relative to the circadian oscillator (Borbely, Achermann, Trachsel, & Tobler, 1989). This latter hypothesis remains largely unexplored and is not addressed here. By contrast, age-dependent changes

The work discussed in this chapter was supported by the Donald B. Lindsley Trustee Grant of the Grass Foundation, a grant from the Department of Psychiatry and Human Behavior, Brown Medical School, and grant MH52415 from the National Institute of Mental Health (NIMH).

in circadian organization have been the focus of extensive research, and it is now clear that ontogenetic changes in the circadian system occur in both animals and humans (Richardson, 1990). The emphasis of research on the ontogenesis of the circadian timing system has been on very early development (prenatal and early postnatal) and late in the ontogenetic process. The latter studies have tested the hypothesis that age-related changes in circadian organization underlie sleep disruption in the elderly. Neither animal nor human studies have focused on puberty, and very little is known about the biology of the circadian system in adolescent humans.

From an endocrine perspective, the pubertal transition is associated with changes in secretion and ambient concentration of hormones that provide a plausible foundation for alterations in circadian timing at this developmental transition (see Chapter 3). Primary among these changes is the onset of sleep-related luteinizing hormone (LH) secretion, with consequent induction of gonadal steroid synthesis and progressive increases in the concentration of estradiol in females and testosterone in males. Sex steroids have important effects throughout the brain and have been shown to affect directly the suprachiasmatic nucleus (Takahashi & Menaker, 1980; Albers, 1981; Morin, Fitzgerald, & Zucker, 1982; Moline & Albers, 1988). In addition, increased activity of several hypothalamic neurotransmitter systems associated with the pubertal disinhibition of LH release may directly affect neural control of circadian oscillations and/or sleep-wake homeostatic systems (Moore & Card, 1990; Miller, Morin, Schwartz, & Moore, 1996).

Several lines of evidence provide preliminary support for the hypothesis that changes in circadian function underlie the delay in sleep timing at the pubertal transition. Previous studies in children and adolescents have demonstrated a pubertal delay in the diurnal rhythm of objectively measured alertness (Carskadon, Harvey, Duke, Anders, Litt, & Dement, 1980). In addition, Cavallo (1991) demonstrated that normal pubertal development is associated with a delay in nocturnal melatonin secretion, although these data failed to achieve statistical significance. More recently, Carskadon, Acebo, Richardson, Tate, and Seifer (1997) used a unique experimental paradigm to assess circadian parameters in adolescents and showed that the phase of melatonin secretory offset is correlated with pubertal stage. Thus, it appears that changes in circadian organization may occur coincident with human puberty. Their nature, however, remains unclear and may reflect changes in the circadian oscillator itself or in other factors, exogenous or endogenous, that regulate oscillator phase. Distinction among these possibilities would be greatly facilitated by availability of an animal model that included endocrine and neurological maturational changes analogous to those of puberty in humans. This chapter presents preliminary data examining circadian parameters during puberty in an animal model, the *Octodon degus*.

Puberty has been studied in a number of mammalian species. Much work has been done in domestic animals, especially sheep, where a number of groundbreaking studies have been carried out examining the role of alterations in steroid feedback in the initiation of pulsatile gonadotropin release (Foster, Karsch, Olster, Ryan, & Yellon, 1986). The monkeys are an especially faithful model of the pubertal process in the human, because like humans, these animals have a long lag time between birth and attainment of sexual competence. That lag period is not present in most other mammalian species, particularly those commonly used for circadian studies. For instance, in general, rodents grow very rapidly after birth and become sexually competent within weeks (Ojeda, Urbanski, & Ahmed, 1986).

Another model system that has been studied is the decline in reproductive function and its subsequent activation in the seasonally breeding rodents. This process has been proposed as a model for the events that occur during puberty (Foster, Ryan, Goodman, Legan, Karsch, & Yellon, 1986). From the study of seasonal reproductive decline and recrudescence, a role of the pineal in regulation of reproductive function became apparent, although the role of the pineal in the human reproductive system is still unclear (see Chapter 3 for review). Therefore, extensive work on the events, timing, and mechanisms that regulate the onset of puberty has been published. To date, however, no comprehensive study of development and interaction of the circadian and sleep systems during puberty has been carried out.

We have chosen an animal with several characteristics that enhance its value as a model system for examining the interplay between the reproductive system, the circadian system, and the sleep-wake regulatory system during puberty. *Octodon degus* is a hystricomorph rodent native to Chile and Peru. Adult degus weigh approximately 250 to 400 grams and have a life-span of 6 to 7 years. The degu has a 90-day gestation, and although newborns are precocious, sexual maturation appears to be delayed until approximately 2 months of age. The degu breeds seasonally in the wild but appears to be neither photoperiodic nor to have a circannual reproductive rhythm, as it continues in the laboratory. Finally, the degu has diurnal patterns of sleep-wake and activity, and a stereotaxic atlas of the degu brain has been published (Wright & Kern, 1992).

We present here preliminary studies on the phase of the circadian wheel-running activity rhythm throughout the juvenile period of the degu as an initial test of the usefulness of this animal model for examining relationships between the circadian timing system and maturation.

Methods

Animals

Degus were born in our laboratory and maintained from birth on light-dark cycles for 12 hours of light and 12 hours of darkness (LD12:12, lights on 7:00 A.M.) in constant temperature conditions. Subjects were weaned at 5 weeks of age, ear tagged, and individually housed. The animals were provided guinea pig chow and water ad libitum. Animals were weighed approximately biweekly, and weekly average body weights were calculated for each subject from 5 through 25 weeks of age. In males, testes were palpated and rated for size; in females, the presence of vaginal opening was noted at the time of weighing. Phase of activity onset was calculated from running-wheel records for 16 (9 male and 7 female) degus from five litters.

Running-Wheel Activity Data Collection and Analysis

Each cage was equipped with a stainless steel running wheel. Running-wheel activity was continuously recorded by a computer-assisted data collection system (DataQuest, DataSciences, Inc., St. Paul, MN). The data were plotted and analyzed using the Circadia data analysis program (Behavioral Cybernetics, Cambridge, MA). Criteria for determining onset of activity phase were at least 20 wheel revolutions per 10-minute bin, bounded by at least 1 hour of inactivity and not recurring within 23 hours of the previous onset. An average of 7 days was used to calculate activity-onset phase each week.

Results

Figure 4.1 shows mean body weight for male and female degus from weaning through 21 weeks of age. An increase in body weight in both sexes occurs between 4 and 9 weeks of age, with the increase in body

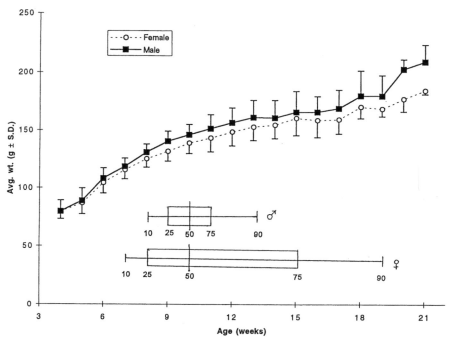

Figure 4.1. Average body weight in grams for degus from post weaning through 21 weeks of age. Data are mean ±SD; males (solid line) and females (dotted line) are shown separately. The percentage of males at each age showing detectable testis growth are shown below the weight data. The percentage of females at each age that have undergone first vaginal opening are also shown.

weight slowing between 9 and 16 weeks of age. A second increase in body weight appears to occur at 20 weeks of age.

Evidence of vaginal opening was not detected in any female subject prior to 5 weeks of age. Approximately 50% of the females showed vaginal opening at 9 weeks of age (Figure 4.1). An increase in testis size, detectable by palpation, was present in 50% of the males at 9 weeks of age (Figure 4.1). Maximum testes size was reached in 50% of the males by 16 weeks of age (data not shown).

Representative actograms from a male and a female degu are shown in Figure 4.2A and 4.2B respectively. Both males and females show a diurnal pattern of activity, with a consolidated bout of activity during the light phase and a period of relative quiescence during the dark phase.

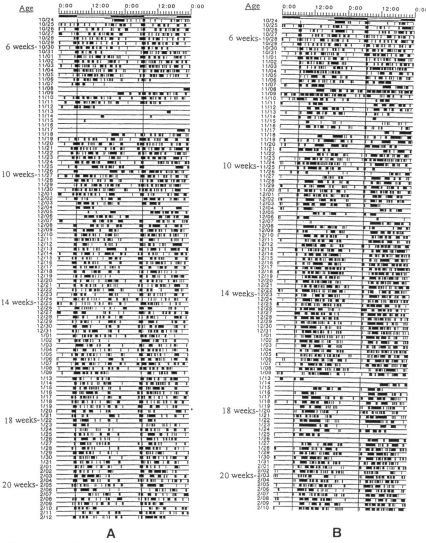

Figure 4.2. Actograms of running-wheel activity data from representative juvenile degus from weaning through 21 weeks of age. The lighting schedule is shown in the top horizontal bar. The vertical line connects the time of lights on throughout the record. These animals were exposed to a LD12:12 schedule (lights were on from 7:00 A.M. to 7:00 P.M.). Note the diurnal pattern of activity. Panel A is a juvenile male; panel B is a juvenile female. Data are double plotted. Gaps in the data are due to technical failures.

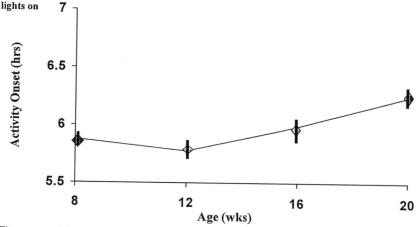

Figure 4.3. Mean running wheel activity onset time at 8, 12, 16, and 20 weeks of age. Activity onset shows a trend toward a later onset as degus age, which may reflect a delay in the phase of this circadian rhythm.

Mean activity onset time for ages 8, 12, 16, and 20 weeks is shown in Figure 4.3. As degus age, activity onset shows a trend toward a later onset, suggesting a phase delay in this circadian rhythm accompanying maturation.

Figure 4.4 shows the distribution of activity onset times within litters. Littermates show similar times of activity onset, which may reflect a genetic component to the timing of the phase of this circadian rhythm.

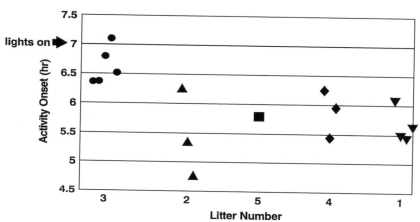

Figure 4.4. Activity onset at 20 weeks of age for each subject, grouped according to litter. Animals tend to show similar phase of activity onset within a litter, suggesting a genetic component to the timing of activity onset.

Discussion

The degu has a number of important features that make it a model worth examining in the context of the aims of our studies. Its size, with a maximum weight of 200 to 400 grams, and easy husbandry (Najecki & Tate, 1999) provide an economical experimental model. In addition, the precocial pups are easy to sex shortly after birth (Weir, 1970). Another advantage of the degu is the relatively long delay until reproductive maturation. Unlike the rat, for example, in which the onset of puberty occurs between 20 and 25 days of age, the onset of puberty in the degu does not appear to occur before 8 weeks of age. Hence, adolescent alteration of circadian parameters that require a number of days to assess is facilitated by a model with an extended developmental course. Finally, the degu has a clearly diurnal pattern of activity (Figure 4.2; Weir, 1970; Labyak & Lee, 1997), and we have successfully recorded sleep from adult animals (data not shown). Thus, this animal appears to provide a unique opportunity to investigate the relationships among the circadian, reproductive, and sleep-wake systems.

Our preliminary data showing clustering among littermates suggest that the phase relationship of activity onset and lights-on may be genetically determined in an individual degu. Furthermore, the onset phase of activity appears to show an age-related delay during this developmental stage. The precise relationships among stage of sexual maturation, the influence of sex steroid hormones, and alteration in the circadian activity rhythm are unclear without the results of further study.

Data from human adolescents suggest that sexual maturation may be associated with the initiation of a phase delay in sleep (Carskadon et al., 1993). Because the relationship of an overt rhythm to the environmental lighting cycle reflects the characteristics of the underlying circadian oscillator, we have hypothesized that the phase delay at sexual maturation is related to a fundamental change in the intrinsic circadian oscillator, with a predicted change in phase angle of overt rhythms. An alternative explanation for the delay in phase simultaneously with sexual maturation, however, is a direct effect of gonadal steroids on the period of the circadian oscillator or on the coupling of the oscillator to overt rhythms. In adult female hamsters, for example, estradiol has been demonstrated to shorten the period of the circadian oscillator and to reduce splitting of the activity rhythm (Morin et al., 1977; Morin & Cummings, 1982). In male hamsters, however, no effects of sex steroids on activity rhythms were seen (Morin & Cummings, 1982), and data from other species, especially the degu, suggest that the effects of sex steroids in the female hamster are not universal. In the degu, estrogen and progesterone do not appear to act directly on the circadian oscillator (Labyak & Lee, 1995).

Sexual maturation in the degu is associated with a phase delay in the activity due to developmental alterations in the circadian oscillator or to downstream effects of steroids on overt rhythms. We have begun to test these alternatives by carrying out the studies described here. The establishment of this animal model provides an opportunity to examine more intensively the links among sleep, circadian rhythms, and sexual maturation, using experimental techniques less available to human investigation. Our plans for future studies include examination of sleep and circadian rhythms under conditions of exogenous manipulation of pubertal events, whether by surgical intervention (e.g., castration), manipulation of photoperiod, or administration of receptor agonists and antagonists, as well as an examination of the neuroanatomical substrates of the circadian system (e.g., suprachiasmatic nucleus and its input and output pathways). In conclusion, we intend to develop a systematic series of studies to examine the mechanisms underlying this system and its relationship to the timing of sleep.

REFERENCES

Albers HE (1981). Gonadal hormones organize and modulate the circadian system of the rat. *Am J Physiol* 241:R62–R66.
Andrade MM, Benedito-Silva AA, Menna-Barreto L (1992). Correlations between morningness-eveningness character, sleep habits and temperature rhythm in adolescents. *Braz J Med Biol Res* 25:835–839.
Borbely AA, Achermann P, Trachsel L, Tobler I (1989). Sleep initiation and initial sleep intensity: Interactions of homeostatic and circadian mechanisms. *J Bio Rhythms* 4:149–160.
Carskadon MA, Acebo C, Richardson GS, Tate BA, Seifer R (1997). An approach to studying circadian rhythms of adolescent humans. *J Biol Rhythms* 12: 278–289.
Carskadon MA, Harvey K, Duke P, Anders TF, Litt IF, Dement WC (1980). Pubertal changes in daytime sleepiness. *Sleep* 2:453–460.
Carskadon MA, Vieira C, Acebo C (1993). Association between puberty and a circadian phase delay. *Sleep* 16:258–262.
Cavallo A (1991). Plasma melatonin rhythm in disorders of puberty: Interactions of age and pubertal stages. *Hormone Research* 36:16–21.
Foster DL, Karsch FJ, Olster DH, Ryan KD, Yellon SM (1986). Determinants of puberty in a seasonal breeder. *Recent Prog Horm Res* 42:331–384.
Foster DL, Ryan KD, Goodman RL, Legan J, Karsch FJ, Yellon SM (1986). Delayed puberty in lambs chronically treated with oestradiol. *J Reprod Fertil* 78:111–117.

Labyak SE, Lee TM (1995). Estrus- and steroid-induced changes in circadian rhythms in a diurnal rodent, *Octodon degus*. *Physiol Behav* 58(3):573–585.

——— (1997). Individual variation in reentrainment after phase shifts of light-dark cycle in a diurnal rodent, *Octodon degus*. *Am J Physiol* 273:R739–R746.

Miller JD, Morin LP, Schwartz WJ, Moore RY (1996). New insights into the mammalian circadian clock. *Sleep* 19(8):641–667.

Moline ML, Albers HE (1988). Response of circadian locomotor activity and the proestrous luteinizing hormone surge to phase shifts of the light-dark cycle in the hamster. *Physiol Behav* 43:435–440.

Moore RY, Card JP (1990). Neuropeptide Y in the circadian timing system. *Annals of New York Academy of Science* 611:227–257.

Morin LP, Cummings LA (1982). Splitting of wheelrunning rhythms by castrated or steroid treated male and female hamsters. *Physiol Behav* 29:665–675.

Morin LP, Fitzgerald KM, Zucker I (1977). Estradiol shortens the period of hamster circadian rhythms. *Science* 196:305–307.

Najecki D & Tate B (1999). Husbandry and management of the degu (*Octodon degus*). A new research model. *Lab Animal Medicine* 23:54–57.

Ojeda SR, Urbanski HF, Ahmed CE (1986). The onset of female puberty: Studies in the rat. *Recent Progress in Hormone Research* 42:385–442.

Richardson GS (1990). Circadian rhythms and aging. In E. L. Schneider & J. W. Rowe, eds., *Handbook of the Biology of Aging* (3d ed.), pp. 275–295. San Diego, Harcourt Brace Jovanovich.

Strauch I, Meier B (1988). Sleep need in adolescents: A longitudinal approach. *Sleep* 11:378–386.

Takahashi JS, Menaker M (1980). Interaction of estradiol and progesterone: Effects on circadian locomotor rhythm of female golden hamsters. *Am J Physiol* 239:R497–R504.

Weir BJ (1970). The management and breeding of some more hystricomorph rodents. *Laboratory Animals* 4:83–97.

Wright JW, Kern MD (1992). Stereotaxic atlas of the brain of *Octodon degus*. *J Morphol* 214:299–320.

5. Nutrition and Circadian Activity Offset in Adolescent Rhesus Monkeys

MARI S. GOLUB, PETER T. TAKEUCHI, AND TANA M. HOBAN-HIGGINS

Data have been presented by several investigators demonstrating a shift toward later bedtimes in teenagers. These data have practical implications for sleep deprivation, daytime sleepiness, school performance, and driving safety. However, it is not entirely clear from the human data to what extent later bedtimes are a consequence of changes in life-style (such as release from parental bedtime regulations, peer socialization activities, and part-time jobs) and to what extent they reflect a biologically driven maturation process. If biological maturation leads to the ability to stay up late or the ability to adhere to earlier bedtimes, then we can hypothesize that developmental trends in circadian activity are tied to other aspects of maturation during adolescence and will be disrupted by interventions that generally interfere with adolescent maturation. Data in this chapter suggest that adolescent trends in later sleep onset occur in nonhuman primates and can be disrupted by zinc deprivation, a nutritional intervention that leads to retardation of adolescent growth, skeletal, and sexual maturation. This is a new piece of information supporting the biological origin of altered bedtimes during adolescence. The background for the study is first presented, followed by data indicating that shift in the offset of daily activity normally occurs in rhesus monkeys during the period of adolescent maturation and that it can be prevented by zinc deprivation.

The authors acknowledge and thank the collaborators on the adolescent rhesus monkeys studies: Eric Gershwin, Carl Keen, Dennis Styne, Francesca Ontell, Bill Lasley, Robert Walters, and Andrew Hendrickx. This research was supported by the National Institute of Child Health and Human Development (HD14388 and HD43209) and the National Center for Research Resources (RR00169).

Nutrition in Adolescence

The adolescent growth spurt, a phenomenon familiar to all parents, has been quantified in detail on a population basis (Marshall & Tanner, 1969; Marshall & Tanner, 1970; Tanner & Davies, 1985). The rate of height growth increases 30% to 50% over a 2-year period in the preteen and early teen years and then drops to near zero. Less documented but equally impressive is the increase in food intake that accompanies the growth spurt. Clearly, the need for energy and protein for growth makes adolescence a vulnerable period for malnutrition. In addition to the demands of growth, maturation of specific organ systems leads to increases in specific nutritional needs. The onset of menstrual cycles in girls places an added strain on iron availability (Cai & Yan, 1990; Bergstrom, Hernell, Lonnerdal, & Perrson, 1995). Bone mineralization, which peaks in adolescence (Theintz et al., 1992), results in high requirements for calcium, magnesium, and other minerals. In response to the particular needs of adolescents, the National Research Council has established specific Recommended Dietary Allowances (RDAs) for this age group (National Research Council, 1989). The RDAs for iron, calcium, phosphorous, magnesium, riboflavin, and niacin are higher for adolescents than for adults. In U.S. teenagers, protein-calorie deficiency is not common, but surveys show that few teenagers eat the recommended amounts of many essential vitamins and minerals, including calcium, magnesium, zinc, vitamin A, vitamin E and, in girls, iron and phosphorus (Johnson, Johnson, Wang, Smiciklas-Wright, & Guthrie, 1994).

Nonhuman Primate Models of Adolescence

Rhesus monkeys provide a unique, well-characterized model for adolescence. Primates are the only species that show "true" adolescence (Watts & Gavan, 1982), a growth spurt followed by puberty (onset of ovarian cycling or sperm production), development of morphologic secondary sex characteristics, onset of fertility, and epiphyseal closure and cessation of linear growth. Additionally, the bulk of bone mineralization takes place prior to achievement of full growth in nonhuman primates (Pope, Gould, Anderson, & Mann, 1989), as is the case in humans but not in other laboratory animal models. Other relevant characteristics of primate adolescent maturation exhibited by both humans and rhesus monkeys are a prolonged juvenile period after infancy and prior to sexual maturation (Pereira & Fairbanks, 1993) and, in females, a period of "adolescent sterility" subsequent to onset of mature ovarian cyclicity (Lemarchand-Beraud, Zufferey, Reymond, & Rey, 1982; Resko, Goy, Robinson, & Norman, 1982; Talbert, Hammond, Groff, & Udry, 1985). The timing and sequencing of all these events depends on a coordinated production of hormones and growth factors under regulation of the hypothalamus that is more complex and prolonged in primates than in other species. Characterization of the role of the hypothalamus in pubertal events is a major current focus of research in both male and female rhesus macaques (Perera & Plant, 1992; Terasawa, 1995). Gradually, the role of gonadotropin releasing hormones, neurotransmitters, and growth factors modulating electrical input from other brain areas and feedback via systemic circulation is coming to be understood. There is also a considerable literature available in monkeys on growth during adolescence, and the roles of growth hormone, IGF-I, and steroid hormones (Wilson, Gordon, & Collins, 1986; Wilson, 1989; Tanner, Wilson, & Rudman, 1990). These research programs provide a valuable background for studies of adolescent behavioral development.

It is important to point out some of the parallels in life events and interpersonal milestones in the adolescence of humans and monkeys (Savin-Williams & Weisfeld, 1989; Steinberg, 1989). During adolescence, monkeys establish their individual social status in the group and begin to participate in adult activities, such as vigilance for predators and foraging for food, that require more advanced motor and cognitive skills (Caine, 1986; Pereira & Fairbanks, 1993). Female adolescents begin acting as caregivers to infants in the troop and participating in female social grooming bouts. It is interesting to note that mortality in young male monkeys shows a peak during adolescent years that declines as adult status is reached. In some species, males leave their natal group to join a geographically distinct group. There are also important differences from humans, however, such as the matrilineal family group of rhesus monkeys, in which fathers have no particular role in the raising of their biological offspring, and seasonal breeding, which synchronizes sexual maturation as well as reproduction.

Our studies of circadian activity in adolescence used female rhesus monkeys. The events of adolescence in female rhesus monkeys take place during a 2-year period prior to sexual maturation, which occurs at about 4 years of age (see Figure 5.1). The growth spurt in females occurs between 27 and 30 months of age in our colony (Blackwelder & Golub, 1996). In general a ratio of 1 to 4 can be used to compare maturation

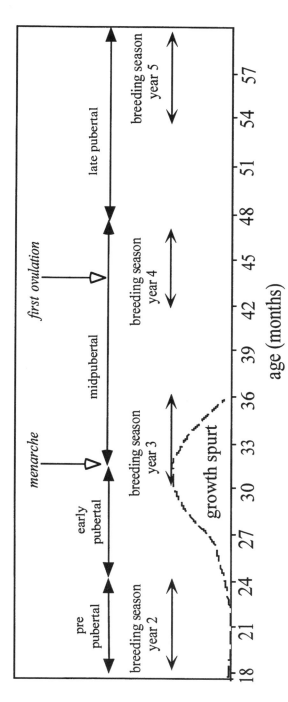

Figure 5.1. Diagram of major landmarks of adolescence in the female rhesus monkey. The maturation rate of rhesus relative to humans is approximately 1:4 (1 year in rhesus = 4 years in humans).

in rhesus monkeys with that in humans (a 1-year-old rhesus monkey is approximately equivalent in maturation to a 4-year-old child). This makes it possible to perform sequential maturational measures relevant to adolescence over a 2.5-year period in monkeys that would require 10 years in humans.

The Biology of Brain Development in Primate Adolescence

Surprisingly little information on anatomical and functional changes in the brain is specific to adolescence. Some classic anatomical studies of human and rhesus monkey brain development have included the adolescent period. These studies found that the processes of synaptic pruning and myelination that dominate postinfancy brain development continue during adolescence, targeting primarily the late maturing, frontal areas of the brain (Yakovlev & Lecours, 1967; Benes, 1989; Zecevic, Bourgeois, & Rakic, 1989). For instance, intracortical myelination is prominent as seen by increases in size of the corpus callosum and anterior commissure (Pujol, Vendrell, Junque, Marti-Vilalta, & Capdevila, 1993). In addition, a decrease in size of some frontal cortical areas (as detected by magnetic resonance imaging, or MRI) (Jernigan, Trauner, Hesselink, & Tallal, 1991) is presumably secondary to elimination of extraneous connections. Changes in neurotransmitter receptor distribution have been demonstrated in adolescent monkeys (Lidow & Rakic, 1992).

There is considerable information from electroencephalographic (EEG) measures in humans. Maturational patterns of EEG activity are consistent with the interpretation of greater synchrony and coherence; distinct changes are detected at 12–13 years of age (Hudspeth & Pribram, 1990, 1992). Sensory-evoked potentials show a shorter latency, presumably reflecting decreased processing time (Courchesne, 1990). Consistent with this, reaction times also decline during the adolescent years (Kail, 1993). There is a decrease in amplitude and duration of various frequency bands of sleep EEG throughout development (Feinberg, 1974; Feinberg, March, Fein, Floyd, Walker, & Price, 1978), with the delta frequency band in the frontal and temporal areas showing the latest changes (Buchsbaum, Mansour, Teng, Zia, Siegel, & Rice, 1992; Hudspeth & Pribram, 1992). Nonlinear models of maturation time courses of delta are similar to those for cortical metabolic rate and synaptic density (Feinberg, 1990; Keshavan, Anderson, & Pettegrew, 1994). Although not unique to the adolescent period, the change in sleep EEG, particularly delta frequency in frontal areas, may be effective markers of adolescent brain maturation.

Although there are descriptions of qualitative advances in cognitive function in adolescence, we were not able to find quantitative data addressing age-dependent patterns of change. Emotional and interpersonal characteristics of adolescent development have perhaps been most explored and attempts have been made to relate them to the general biology of adolescent development through correlation with events of sexual maturation or levels of gonadal hormones (Nottelmann, Susman, Inoff-Germain, Cutler, Loriaux, & Chrousos, 1987; Warren & Brooks-Gunn, 1989).

Sex differentiation of brain function is thought to be established during earlier ontogenetic periods but to emerge during adolescence. For instance, gender differences in event-related potentials (ERPs) occur in adolescence (Shibasaki & Miyazaki, 1992; Hill & Steinhauer, 1993). Estrogen receptors that appear in cortical areas after puberty (McLusky, Naftolin, & Goldman-Rakic, 1986) may be relevant, but very little is known about the biological basis of sexual differentiation of the cortex in adolescence.

Effect of Zinc Deprivation on Adolescent Development

Zinc deprivation in adolescence is a particularly interesting topic because of a series of studies conducted in the Middle East in the 1960s (Prasad, Miale, Farid, Sandstead, & Schulert, 1963; Carter et al., 1969; Halsted, Ronaghy et al., 1972). A syndrome of severe growth retardation ("nutritional dwarfism"), lack of sexual development, and absence of epiphyseal closure was described in young Iranian and Egyptian men 19–20 years of age. This syndrome was reversed by a diet containing zinc supplements, whereas an otherwise adequate diet lacking the supplement was not effective. Zinc is an important essential trace element that is associated with protein in the diet (Walsh, Sandstead, Prasad, Newberne, & Fraker, 1994). It is an active constituent of over 200 enzymes and also has a major structural role ("zinc fingers") in proteins. Although the exact etiology of the Mideast adolescent syndrome could not be established, the response to zinc emphasized the potential importance of this essential trace element in adolescent development.

For a number of years, we have studied the influence of zinc deprivation in the development and behavior of rhesus monkeys (Golub,

Keen, Gershwin, & Hendrickx, 1995). These studies focused on periods of most rapid growth: late gestation (Golub, Gershwin, Hurley, Baly, & Hendrickx, 1984), early infancy (Golub, Gershwin, Hurley, Saito, & Hendrickx, 1984), and, more recently, adolescence. Two levels of zinc deprivation have been used. *Marginal* zinc deprivation (4 micrograms of zinc per gram of diet) does not influence growth or health of adult monkeys except during late gestation when a significant decline in plasma zinc concentration occurs along with some changes in hematological and clinical chemistry and immune function measures. Offspring show a small amount of growth retardation at birth and a transient period of growth retardation after weaning. *Moderate* zinc deprivation (2 micrograms of zinc per gram of diet) leads to clear signs of zinc deficiency in late pregnant dams and a more serious set of consequences in their infants (Keen et al., 1993). We did not include *severe* zinc deficiency in these studies.

Our initial study of adolescence was of male monkeys given marginal zinc deprivation from conception and extending throughout adolescence. They demonstrated reversal task (Golub, Gershwin, Hurley, & Hendrickx, 1988). Subsequently, we conducted a study to determine whether some of the effects of zinc deprivation on behavior were concurrent and reversible (rather than a permanent consequence of zinc deprivation effects at an earlier period of development). This study (Golub, Takeuchi, Keen, Gershwin, Hendrickx, & Lonnerdal, 1994) used a crossover design with one group fed a zinc-adequate diet for 15 weeks followed by a moderately zinc deficient diet and then the zinc adequate diet. Data analysis indicated that performance of behavioral tests of attention and memory were better when the monkeys were eating the zinc-adequate diet than when they were eating the zinc-deficient diet. Further, the level of spontaneous activity during the testing sessions was lower during the zinc-deficient diet period. This suggested that a short-term zinc deprivation during adolescence could influence behavior in a reversible manner.

A detailed study of adolescent maturation in zinc-deprived female rhesus monkeys was then undertaken (Golub, Keen et al., 1996). Moderate zinc deprivation was begun in the late juvenile period, prior to the adolescent growth spurt. End points related to growth, sexual maturation, and bone maturation were measured. During the adolescent growth spurt, zinc-deficient monkeys showed a deficit in weight gain and linear growth and exhibited depressed plasma zinc concentrations relative to controls (Figure 5.2). After menarche, there was a deficit in bone growth, mineralization, and maturation. Some effects on sexual maturation were noted, but all monkeys reached menarche and began menstrual cycles. Our studies of diurnal rest-activity cycles were conducted in this same group of zinc-deprived female rhesus monkeys and their controls (Golub, Takeuchi, Keen, Hendrickx, & Gershwin, 1996).

Zinc Deprivation and Circadian Rest-Activity Cycles

Environmental Conditions of the Experiment

In an animal experiment, it is possible to provide a highly controlled environment that prevents the influence of confounding factors and reduces individual variability. The female adolescent monkeys in this study were all born in outdoor half-acre cages at the California Regional Primate Research Center, and they lived there in multiaged groups of 80–100 animals until they were 16 months of age. At that time, they were transferred to an indoor room and housed with a like-age cage mate. The indoor cage room was one of two located in a separate building on the grounds of the Primate Center. The rooms were automatically controlled for light (fluorescent lights on from 7:00 A.M to 7:00 P.M.) and temperature. There were no windows in the room. Light intensity at the front of the cage was 9.6 ± 1.2 foot candles (depending on the location of the cage) during "lights on"; no light was detectable during "lights off." Cages were washed at 2-week intervals. Water was available ad libitum from an automatic watering system and food was provided twice daily. All monkeys participated in behavioral testing using operant methodology (food reinforcer) 2 days per week. On behavior testing days, the daily feeding was withheld until after testing.

The study population consisted of two cohorts, cohort 1 and cohort 2, balanced for group, that entered the experiment in successive years. Because rhesus monkeys are seasonal breeders (infants are born in May, June, and July each year), it was possible to obtain 16 females each year all of whom were born within a 2-month period. After adaptation to indoor caging and to the experimental diet, the animals began behavioral testing, trimonthly physical exams, and activity monitoring.

Dietary Zinc Deprivation

Monkeys were fed a diet made from purified components, with egg white as the protein source. Commercial animal diets contain varying

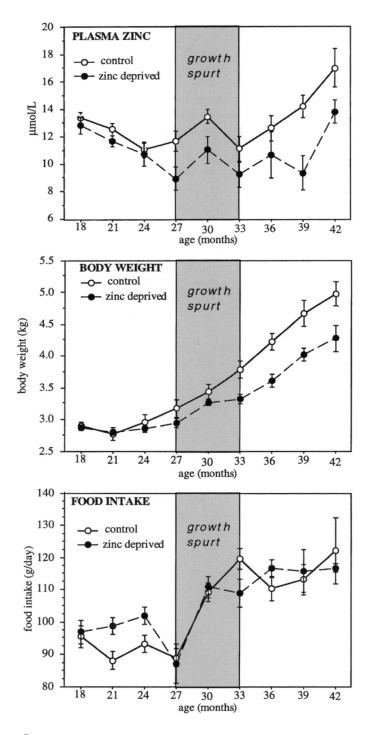

58

amounts of trace elements, depending on the source of the ingredients used for each particular lot. Purified diets are necessary to control precisely the trace element content of the diet. Our basal diet contained exactly the recommended amounts of all nutrients for monkeys, with the exception of zinc. Without added zinc, the basal diet contained about 2 micrograms of zinc per gram of diet; this was used as the *zinc-deprived diet*. Zinc carbonate was added to the *control diet* to reach a concentration of 50 micrograms of zinc.

Actimeters

Actimeters designed for use in humans were obtained from Individual Monitoring Systems (Baltimore, MD). In children, the actimeters are typically strapped to the wrist or ankle; in monkeys, the monitors were placed in a pouch and attached with cable ties to the back of a harness that was worn by the animals throughout the experiment. In this location, the monkeys could not reach the monitor; monkeys were separated from their cage mates during monitoring sessions to prevent manipulation or damage to the monitors.

A mercury switch in the monitor recorded trunk movement in two directions (side to side, backward and forward), and all switch closures occurring over a 1-minute period were recorded and stored by a microchip in the monitor. At the conclusion of a weekend monitoring session, these data could be transferred by cable to a computer for processing.

Procedures for Activity Monitoring

Activity monitoring was carried out on weekends when only cage cleaning and feeding were scheduled in the cage room. Each monkey was monitored every other week until the age of menarche (30 months of age). In a subgroup of the first cohort (N = 4/group) monitoring

---

Figure 5.2. Time course of changes in plasma zinc, weight gain, and food intake in zinc-deprived female adolescent monkeys. Plasma zinc and growth rate began to fall off from controls during the premenarchal adolescent growth spurt (menarche occurred on the average at 30 months of age). Food intake data demonstrate that changes in appetite were not responsible for the reduction in growth rate. Group differences were significant for body weight at 30, 33, and 36 months of age and for plasma zinc at 30 and 39 months of age. Food intake was also significantly higher in the zinc deprived group than in controls early in the experiment from 21 to 24 months of age. (See Golub, Keen, et al., 1996.)

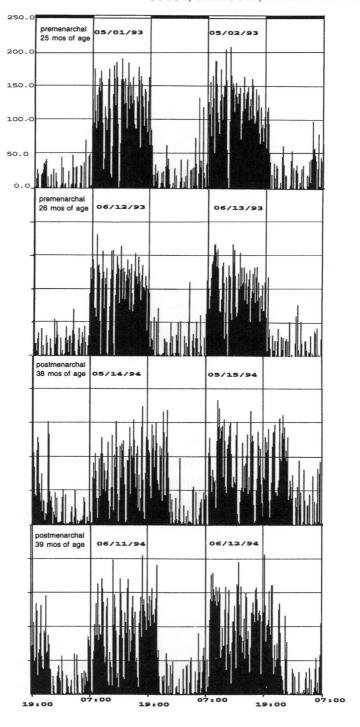

continued on a monthly basis for an additional year. The actimeters were attached on Friday afternoon and removed on Monday. Data from 7:00 A.M. Saturday to 7:00 A.M. Monday were used for diurnal activity summaries.

Circadian Activity Patterns in Adolescent Rhesus Monkeys

Plots of minute-by-minute activity over 48 hours demonstrated very distinct diurnal rest-activity cycles in premenarchal monkeys (see Figure 5.3). Animals become active immediately at "lights on" at 7:00 A.M. Although there was considerable interanimal variability, they averaged about 60 activity counts per minute during the day and 7 counts per minute at night. Another variable we looked at was periods of inactivity during the day. The longest periods during the day when no activity occurred were about 8 minutes long. These could be considered "breaks" and typically occurred around midday. We also examined delay in circadian activity offset, measured as the time between "lights out" and the onset of rest phase. The onset of the rest phase occurred on the average 20 minutes before "lights out" in the youngest animals at the beginning of the experiment.

Changes in Delay in Circadian Activity Onset over Adolescence

Delay in circadian activity offset appeared to demonstrate maturational changes in individual animals and in the group as a whole. Figure 5.3 shows the weekend actigraphs of an individual control monkey in cohort 1 in the spring of the year (May–June) before and after menarche (which occurred in October). Whereas the onset of the rest

←—————————————————————————————

Figure 5.3. Actigraphs from one adolescent female rhesus monkey demonstrating increased delay in circadian activity offset after menarche. Recording was done for a 48-hour period over a weekend. The lights were on from 7:00 A.M. to 7:00 P.M. Graphs are included from the spring of the premenarchal year and the spring of the postmenarchal year (this monkey reached menarche October 12, 1993 at the age of 30.6 months). Comparisons are made by time of year because circadian activity offset displays a seasonal as well as a maturational pattern in rhesus. The graphs demonstrate an onset of the rest phase very close to "lights out" (7:00 P.M.) before menarche, but a continuation of the daytime activity pattern after "lights out" in the postmenarchal year. The postmenarchal data also seem to display more frequent "breaks" or rest periods during the activity phase than during the premenarchal period.

phase was close to "lights out" in the premenarchal year (first two actigraphs), activity extended well beyond light offset later in adolescence
(last two actigraphs). In the actigraph for the weekend of May 14, 1994,
this monkey was awake and active past midnight on both Saturday and
Sunday. While the experimental paradigm does not provide us with any
indication of the types of activity she was engaging in, it is important to
keep in mind that she was located in a room with 15 like-aged monkeys
with whom she was very familiar, and that while visual communication
was limited, auditory communication, both in terms of vocalizations and
of auditory cues for typical behavior patterns, was available.

Figure 5.4 shows the group data for circadian activity offset for the
control monkeys of cohort 1 in their pre- and postmenarchal year. Data
are plotted by time of year, because circadian activity offset appeared
to demonstrate seasonal as well as maturational changes. Prior to the
breeding season (September) the delay in activity offset was significantly longer than during the breeding season (December). It is unclear whether the increase in this delay from March to September was
due to maturation or to seasonal influences. Data from adult monkeys
are unfortunately not available to determine whether seasonal changes
in circadian activity occur in mature animals. However, the difference

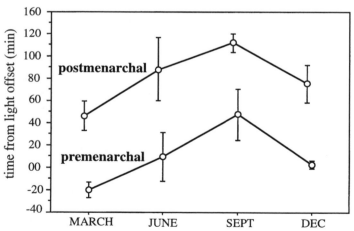

Figure 5.4. Group data for four control female rhesus monkeys during their
premenarchal and postmenarchal year. Comparisons are made by time of year
because delay in circadian activity offset displays a seasonal as well as a maturational pattern in rhesus. Delays in circadian activity offset were significantly
higher in March, June, and December of the postmenarchal year as compared
with the premenarchal year.

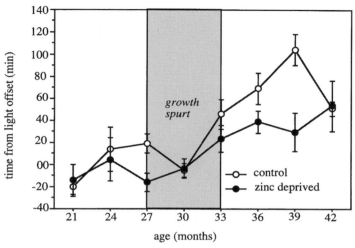

Figure 5.5. Comparison of maturational changes in delay in circadian activity offset in control and zinc-deprived female rhesus monkeys. Data from both cohorts is combined in the graph. (See Golub, Takeuchi, et al., 1996.)

between the premenarchal and postmenarchal data at the same time of year can be interpreted as a maturational change.

There are other possible explanations for the increase in time to circadian activity offset during adolescence. Although environmental factors (light, temperature, cage location, maintenance routines) were tightly controlled, there may have been other environmental changes unknown to us that influenced the animals' diurnal rhythms. This explanation is unlikely because cohort 2 animals, who were a year younger during this same time period and were housed in the same room, demonstrated the premenarchal pattern of early onset of the rest phase at the same time that older cohort 1 animals were demonstrating later onset of rest (see Figure 5.5, which plots combined data from cohort 1 and cohort 2). It is also possible that time from entry into the experiment, rather than chronological age, was the important factor, perhaps in disrupting normal circadian control. This explanation also seems unlikely, because no significant trend in phase duration (as determined from cosinor analysis) was seen across the experiment for cohort 1. However, definitive examination of this possibility would require another experiment in which monkeys began to be studied after menarche. Finally, maturational changes in activity parameters other than circadian activity were also seen in the study (Golub, Takeuchi, et al., 1996), indicating a more general developmental pattern.

Effect of Zinc Deprivation on Delay in Circadian Activity Offset

Figure 5.5 compares data on delay in circadian activity offset in control and zinc-deprived groups. The graph combines data from cohort 1 and cohort 2. Cohort 1 (n = 4/group) entered the experiment one year before cohort 2 and was studied through 42 months of age. Cohort 2 (10/group) was studied through 33 months of age. Repeated measures ANOVA with age and dietary zinc as independent variables was used to evaluate the data. Data from cohorts 1 and 2 were analyzed separately. There was a significant effect of age on delay in circadian activity offset in both cohorts. There was also a significant effect of dietary zinc on delay in circadian activity in cohort 1 (18–45 months of age, p = .017) but not in cohort 2 (18–33 months of age). For details of the statistical analysis, see Golub, Takeuchi, et al., 1996b. In general, the zinc-deprived group did not appear to show the same pattern in increase in delay in circadian activity offset over the course of the experiment that was shown by controls. These data are preliminary but suggest that maturational changes in delay in circadian activity offset, like other aspects of adolescent maturation, are impaired by zinc deprivation.

Conclusions and Future Directions

The experiment indicated that there are maturational patterns in circadian activity during adolescence. We are currently performing a similar study using combined iron and zinc deprivation, and a very common pattern of undernutrition in adolescent girls. We hope to undertake more extensive studies of brain maturation in adolescence, including EEG, evoked potentials, cognitive testing, and diurnal rest-activity cycle measures to provide a more integrated view of adolescent brain development that includes data relevant to sleep-waking patterns. Understanding the mechanism of nutritional effects on adolescent growth and development may also provide clues to the origin of delay in circadian activity offset in adolescent rhesus monkeys, which resembles later bedtimes seen in teenagers.

REFERENCES

Benes FM (1989). Myelination of cortical-hippocampal relays during late adolescence. *Schizophrenia Bull* 15:585–593.
Bergstrom E, Hernell O, Lonnerdal B, Perrson LA (1995). Sex differences in iron stores of adolescents: What is normal? *J Pediatr Gastrenterol Nutr* 20:215–224.

Blackwelder T, Golub MS (1996). Premenarchial weight gain in rhesus macaques. *Am J Physiol Anthropol* 99:449–454.

Buchsbaum MS, Mansour CS, Teng DG, Zia AD, Siegel BV Jr, Rice DM (1992). Adolescent developmental change in topography of EEG amplitude. *Schizophrenia Res* 7:101–107.

Cai MQ, Yan WY (1990). Study on iron nutritional status in adolescence. *Biochem Environ Sci* 3:113–119.

Cain N (1986). Behavior during puberty and adolescence. In G. Mitchell & J. Erwin, eds., *Comparative Primate Biology*, vol. 2A, *Behavior, Conservation and Ecology*, pp. 327–361. New York: Alan R. Liss.

Carter JP, Grivetti LE, Davis JT, Nasiff S, Mansour A, Mousa WA, Atta AE, Patwardhan VN, Abdel Moneim M, Abdou IA, Darby WJ (1969). Growth and sexual development of adolescent Egyptian village boys: Effects of zinc iron and placebo supplementation. *Am J Clin Nutr* 22:59–78.

Courchesne E (1990). Chronology of postnatal human brain development: Event-related potential, positron emission tomography, myelinogenesis and synaptogenesis studies. In J. Rohrbaugh, R. Parasuraman, & H. Johnson, eds., *Issues in Event-Related Potential Research: Basic Issues and Applications*, pp. 210–241. New York: Oxford University Press.

Feinberg I (1974). Changes in sleep cycle patterns with age. *J Psychiat Res* 10:283–306.

 (1990). Gamma distribution model describes maturational curves for delta wave amplitude, cortical metabolic rate and synaptic density. *J Theor Biol* 142:149–161.

Feinberg I, March JD, Fein G, Floyd RC, Walker JM, Price L (1978). Period and amplitude analysis of 0.5–3 c/sec activity in NREM sleep in young adults. *Electroenceph Clin Neurophysiol* 44:202–213.

Golub MS, Gershwin ME, Hurley LS, Baly DL, Hendrickx AG (1984). Studies of marginal zinc deprivation in rhesus monkeys: I. Influence on pregnant dams. *Am J Clin Nutr* 39:265–280.

Golub MS, Gershwin ME, Hurley LS, Hendrickx AG (1988). Studies of marginal zinc deprivation in rhesus monkeys: VIII. Effects on early adolescence. *Am J Clin Nutr* 47:1046–1051.

Golub MS, Gershwin ME, Hurley LS, Saito WY, Hendrickx AG (1984). Studies of marginal zinc deprivation in rhesus monkeys: IV. Growth of infants in the first year. *Am J Clin Nutr* 40:1192–1202.

Golub MS, Keen CL, Gershwin ME, Hendrickx AG (1995). Developmental zinc deficiency and behavior. *J Nutr* 125:2263S–2271S.

Golub MS, Keen CL, Gershwin ME, Styne DM, Takeuchi PT, Ontell F, Walter RM, Hendrickx AG (1996). Adolescent growth maturation in zinc deprived rhesus monkeys. *Am J Clin Nutr* 64:274–282.

Golub MS, Takeuchi PT, Keen CL, Gershwin ME, Hendrickx AG, Lonnerdal B (1994). Modulation of behavioral performance of prepubertal monkeys by moderate dietary zinc deprivation. *Am J Clin Nutr* 60:238–243.

Golub MS, Takeuchi PT, Keen CL, Hendrickx AG, Gershwin ME (1996). Activity and attention in zinc deprived adolescent monkeys. *Am J Clin Nutr* 4:908–915.

Halsted JA, Ronaghy HA, Abadi P, Haghshenass M, Amirhakimi GH, Barakat RM, Reinhold JG (1972). Zinc deficiency in man: The Shiraz experiment. *Am J Med* 53:277–284.

Hill SY, Steinhauer S (1993). Assessment of prepubertal and postpubertal boys and girls at risk for developing alcoholism with P300 from a visual discrimination task. *J Stud Alcohol* 54:350–358.

Hudspeth WJ, Pribram KH (1990). Stages of brain and cognitive maturation. *J Educ Psychol* 82:881–884.

(1992). Psychophysiological indices of cerebral maturation. *Int J Psychophysiol* 12:19–29.

Jernigan TL, Trauner DA, Hesselink JR, Tallal PA (1991). Maturation of the human cerebrum observed in vivo during adolescence. *Brain* 114:2037–2049.

Johnson RK, Johnson DG, Wang MQ, Smiciklas-Wright H, Guthrie HA (1994). Characterizing nutrient intakes of adolescents by sociodemographic factors. *J Adolesc Health* 15:149–154.

Kail R (1993). Processing time decreases globally at an exponential rate during childhood and adolescence. *J Exp Child Psychol* 56:254–265.

Keen CL, Lonnerdal B, Golub MS, Olin KL, Graham TW, Uriu-Hare J, Hendrickx AG, Gershwin ME (1993). Effect of the severity of maternal zinc deficiency on pregnancy outcome and infant zinc status in rhesus monkeys. *Pediatr Res* 33:233–241.

Keshavan MS, Anderson S, Pettegrew JW (1994). Is schizophrenia due to excessive synaptic pruning in the prefrontal cortex? The Feinberg Hypothesis revisited. *J Psychiat Res* 28:239–265.

Lemarchand-Beraud T, Zufferey M, Reymond M, Rey I (1982). Maturation of the hypothalamo-pituitary-ovarian axis in adolescent girls. *J Clin Endocrinol Metab* 54:241–246.

Lidow MS, Rakic P (1992). Scheduling of monoaminergic neurotransmitter receptor expression in the primate. *Cerebral Cortex* 2:410–416.

Marshall WA, Tanner JM (1969). Variations in pattern of pubertal changes in girls. *Arch Disorder Childhood* 44:291–303.

(1970). Variations in the pattern of pubertal changes in boys. *Arch Dis Childhood* 45:13–23.

McLusky N. Naftolin G, Goldman-Rakic P (1986). Estrogen formation and binding in the cerebral cortex of the developing rhesus monkey. *Proc Natl Academy Sci USA* 83:513–516.

National Research Council (1989). *Recommended Dietary Allowances*. Washington, DC: National Academy Press.

Nottlemann ED, Susman EJ, Inoff-Germain G, Cutler GB Jr, Loriaux DL, Chrousos GP (1987). Developmental processes in early adolescence: Relationships between adolescent adjustment problems and chronologic age, pubertal stage and puberty-related serum hormone levels. *J Pediatr* 110:473–480.

Pereira ME, Fairbanks LA (1993). *Juvenile Primates*. New York: Oxford University Press.

Pereira AD, Plant TM (1992). The neurobiology of primate puberty. *CIBA Found Symp* 168:252–262.

Pope NS, Gould KG, Anderson DC, Mann DR (1989). Effects of age and sex on bone density in the rhesus monkey. *Bone* 10:109–112.

Prasad AS, Miale A Jr, Farid Z, Sandstead HH, Schulert AR (1963). Zinc metabolism in patients with a syndrome of iron deficiency anemia, hepatosplenomegaly, dwarfism and hypogonadism. *J Lab Clin Med* 61:537–549.

Pujol J, Vendrell P, Junque C, Marti-Vilalta JL, Capdevila A (1993). When does human brain development end? Evidence of corpus callosum growth up to adulthood. *Ann Neurol* 34:71–75.

Resko JA, Goy RW, Robinson JA, Norman RL (1982). The pubescent rhesus monkey: Some characteristics of the menstrual cycle. *Biol Reprod* 27:354–361.

Savin-Williams R, Weisfeld G (1989). An ethological perspective on adolescence. In G. Adams, R. Montemayor, & T. Gullotta, eds., *Biology of Adolescent Behavior and Development*, pp. 249–274. Newbury Park, CA: Sage Publications.

Shibasaki H, Miyazaki M (1992). Event-related potential studies in infants and children. *J Clin Neurophysiol* 9:408–418.

Steinberg L (1989). Pubertal maturation and parent-adolescent distance: An evolutionary prespective. In G. Adams, R. Montemayor, & T. Gullotta, eds., *Biology of Adolescent Behavior and Development*, pp. 71–97. Newbury Park, CA: Sage Publications.

Talbert L, Hammond M, Groff T, Udry J (1985). Relationship of age and pubertal development to ovulation in adolescent girls. *Obstet Gynecol* 66:542–545.

Tanner J, Davies P (1985). Clinical longitudinal standards for height and height velocity for North American children. *J Pediatr* 107:317–329.

Tanner JM, Wilson ME, Rudman CG (1990). Pubertal growth spurt in the female rhesus monkey: Relation to menarche and skeletal maturation. *Am J Hum Biol* 2:101–106.

Terasawa E (1995). Control of luteinizing hormone-releasing hormone pulse generation in nonhuman primates. *Cell Mol Neurobiol* 15:141–164.

Theintz G, Buchs B, Rissoli R, Slosman D, Clavien H, Sizonenko PC, Bonjour JP (1992). Longitudinal monitoring of bone mass accumulation in healthy adolescents: Evidence for a marked reduction after 16 years of age at the levels of lumbar spine and femoral neck in female subjects. *J Clin Endocrinol Metab* 75:1060–1065.

Walsh CT, Sandstead HH, Prasad AS, Newberne PM, Fraker PJ (1994). Zinc: Health effects and research priorities for the 1990s. *Env Health Perspect* 102 (suppl. 2):5–46.

Warren MP, Brooks-Gunn J (1989). Mood and behavior at adolescence: Evidence for hormonal factors. *J Clin Endocrinol Metab* 69:77–83.

Watts ES, Gavan, JA (1982). Postnatal growth of nonhuman primates: The problem of the adolescent spurt. *Hum Biol* 54:53–70.

Wilson ME (1989). Relationship between growth and puberty in the rhesus monkey. In D. de Waal, ed., *Control of the Onset of Puberty II*, pp. 137–149. New York: Elsevier Science Publishers.

Wilson ME, Gordon TP, Collins DC (1986). Ontogeny of luteinizing hormone secretion and first ovulation in seasonal breeding rhesus monkeys. *Endocrinology* 118:293–301.

Yakovlev PI, Lecours A (1967). The myelogenetic cycles of regional maturation of the brain. In A. Minkowski, ed., *Regional Development of the Brain in Early Life*, pp. 3–70. Oxford: Blackwell.

Zecevic M, Bourgeois J-P, Rakic P (1989). Changes in synaptic density in motor cortex of rhesus monkey during fetal and postnatal life. *Developmental Brain Research* 50:11–32.

6. Toward a Comparative Developmental Ecology of Human Sleep

CAROL M. WORTHMAN AND MELISSA K. MELBY

This exploratory comparative survey of the ecology of human sleep arises from a question posed by a pediatrician who studies mood disorders and sleep (Dahl, 1996; Dahl et al., 1996). In an attempt to gain insights into sleep regulation from ecological theory and research, he questioned what anthropologists know about sleep. The bald, if somewhat overstated, answer was: zero. Sleep, in its ubiquity, seeming nonsociality, apparent universality, and presumed biologically driven uniformity, has been overlooked as a background variable. Amazingly, it has not engaged a discipline dedicated to the study of human behavior, human diversity, and their cultural biological bases. A notable exception is the evolutionary-ethologically informed approach to the anthropological study of sleep pioneered by the work of McKenna and colleagues on sleep arrangements, infant state regulation, and risk for sudden infant death syndrome or SIDS (McKenna, 1991, 1992, 1996; Mosko, McKenna, Dickel, & Hunt, 1993). Harkness and Super have also documented cultural variation in infant sleep in relation to their studies of child care practices (Harkness & Super, 1996; Super, Harkness, van Tijen, van der Vlugt, Fintelman, & Kijksta, 1996), and scattered reports document sleep behavior (Ferreira de Souza Aguiar, Pereira da Sliva, & Margues, 1991).

Sleeping arrangements (who sleeps by whom) have been closely documented and subjected to cross-cultural analysis because of interests in incest taboo, psychoanalytic views of culture and personality, and emphases on family structure, child care practices, gender, and personality (Barry & Paxson, 1971; Whiting & Whiting, 1975; Whiting, 1981; Herdt, 1989; Morelli, Oppenheim, Rogoff, & Goldsmith, 1992; Schweder, Jenson & Goldstein, 1995; Wolf, Lozoff, Latz, & Paludetto, 1996). Sleep scarcely figures in the literature on human evolution, barring speculation about the survival challenges for secure sleep faced by a ground-dwelling, naked large ape and the possible coevolution of these features with sociality, tool use, and fire. But the paleoanthropological record consists of material remains, and, as the ironic truism notes, behavior fossilizes poorly. Whereas much can be gleaned from floral-faunal associations, tool sources and distribution, and analysis of living sites to reconstruct ecological parameters and infer behavior patterns (Potts, 1996a,b), sleep, like gathering and child care, is low-tech and unrepresented until dwelling sites of the neolithic.

Recognition of the paucity of anthropological work on sleep is galvanizing: a significant domain of human behavior that claims a third of daily life remains largely overlooked by a discipline dedicated to the holistic study of the human condition. The question initially posed to us was clearly motivated by the possible value to existing research on sleep, state regulation, and chronobiology of comparative data concerning the evolutionary-ecological bases of sleep and the expectable range of variation in sleep behavior. Several circumstances support this expectation. First, sleep research has characterized the ontogeny and physiology of human sleep and sleep architecture, as well as extensively documented sleep-rest behavior and biology across animal taxa, especially mammals (reviewed in Allison & Van Twyver, 1970; Allison & Cicchetti, 1976; Meddis, 1983; Anderson, 1984; Campbell & Tobler, 1984; Siegel, 1995; Tobler, 1995). Nevertheless, despite recognition of the minimal sample size and limited ecological range represented in the taxonomic comparative literature (Tobler, 1995), the comparative study of sleep has not extended to population variation in humans.

Second, although sleep deprivation and chronobiological experiments have monitored acute and midrange effects of manipulated sleep ecologies (Mitler, Carskadon, Czeisler, Dement, Dinges, & Graeber, 1988; Walsh, Shweitzer, Anch, Muehlbach, Jenkins, & Dickins, 1994; Berger & Phillips, 1995; Drucker-Colín, 1995; Salzarulo & Fagioli, 1995), the developmental and lifetime ecologies of sleep normative among Western populations studied so far appear to the anthropologist as scarcely representative of the extant and expectable range of human sleep ecologies. Specifically, patterns of solitary sleep on heavily cushioned substrates, consolidated in a single daily time block, and housed in roofed and solidly walled space, contrast with the variety of sleep conditions among traditional societies. These conditions include multiple and multi-age sleeping partners; frequent proximity of animals; embeddedness of sleep in ongoing social interaction; fluid bedtimes and wake times; use of nighttime for ritual, sociality, and information exchange; and relatively exposed sleeping locations that require fire maintenance and sustained vigilance.

The present analysis represents a preliminary attempt to address these issues substantively, by considering the micro, macro, developmental, and evolutionary ecology of human sleep. To this end, we draw upon the thin extant cross-cultural anthropological literature that pertains to the ecology of human sleep, heavily augmented by data from in-depth interviews of contemporary ethnographers concerning sleep conditions and patterns across a worldwide range of traditional forager, pastoralist, horticulturist, and agriculturalist communities. Although scarcely definitive, this survey provides sufficient evidence to suggest that the sleep pattern, architecture, and ontogeny of Western postindustrial populations may be grounded in a distinctive sleep ecology, from infancy on, and that a comparative, cross-cultural investigation is required for a more complete understanding of sleep, its developmental and regulatory neurobiological substrates, and its chronobiological correlates. Consonant with the focus of this volume on adolescents, the distribution of sleep deprivation for ritual or agonistic purposes, including for adolescent rites of passage, is also noted.

Components of Human Sleep Ecology

Sleep behavior and architecture clearly have strong biological determinants. Yet consider Henri Rousseau's famous picture, *Sleeping Gypsy*, in which a rigidly prostrate, colorfully clad dusky figure, clutching a stick, lies asleep on bare earth amid a barren landscape beneath a blank full moon, under the alert gaze of an adjacent lion. The impact of the painting relies largely on what is missing, namely the usual social and material contexts of sleep, and the sense of danger aroused when these contexts are absent. A solitary, unprotected, and unequipped sleeper is an aberration; for humans, sleep is embedded in behaviorally, socially, and culturally constituted environments enabling safe sleep. Safety concerns not only macropredators such as lions or human enemies, but also buffering elements, protection from micropredators such as mosquitoes, and general reduction of external disturbance and predation risk. Safety also inheres in membership in a well-functioning social group that frames and

populates the context for sleep. Shelter for and accoutrements of sleep
define its physical microenvironment. Moreover, the diurnal patterning
of sleep is influenced by a set of structural and cultural features operating variably across the life course, including labor demands, schedules
of social and ritual activity, status and role differentiation, and beliefs
about the nature and functions of sleep.

The following sections outline the constituent factors defining sleep
ecology, proximal to distal, and illustrate them with examples from published and new ethnographic material. The new material is drawn from
interviews on sleep of ethnographers with intimate knowledge of one
or more societies. The societies, locations, and sources, arranged by subsistence type, are as follows:

1. Foragers: Ache (Paraguay, Magdalena Hurtado) (Hill & Hurtado,
   1996), Efe (Zaire, Robert Bailey) (Bailey & DeVore, 1989), !Kung
   (northwest Botswana, Melvin Konner) (Lee & DeVore, 1976;
   Marshall 1976; Lee, 1984), Hiwi (southern Venezuela, Magdalena
   Hurtado) (Hurtado & Hill, 1987, 1990).
2. Pastoralists: Gabra (northern Kenya, John Wood) (Prussin,
   1995; Wood, n.d.); mixed agriculturalist Swat Pathan (Pakistan,
   Frederik Barth) (Barth, 1965, 1981, 1985).
3. Horticulturalists: Baktaman (highland Papua New Guinea,
   Frederik Barth) (Barth, 1975); Gebusi (highland Papua New
   Guinea, Bruce Knauft) (Knauft 1985a,b); Lese (Zaire, Robert
   Bailey) (Bailey & DeVore, 1989).
4. Agriculturalists: Balinese (Singaraja, Buleleng Province, northern
   Bali, Frederik Barth) (Wikan, 1990; Barth, 1993).

Ours is a sample of convenience, selected on the basis of accessibil-
ity and knowledge of the ethnographer, roughly drawn across conti-
nents, climates, and subsistence types. The aim was to apply an analytic
framework concerning determinants of sleep ecology to glean an initial
impression of the constituents and variability in that ecology across a
range of settings, rather than to establish a definitive comparative ethnographic account. Such an account must be drawn from future primary
ethnographic and comparative cross-cultural analytic work. We hope
that the present discussion will alert others to the need for research in
this area, provide a framework for comparative data collection and analysis, and suggest the value of an ecological approach for augmenting
existing sleep research paradigms.

Microecology of Human Sleep

A set of physical, cultural, and biotic factors defines the proxemics of sleep ecology, that is, the actual conditions under which people sleep. Humans sleep under remarkably diverse customary circumstances.

Proximate Physical Ecology of Sleep

Bedding includes substrate, covering on substrate, covers, pillow, and sleep garments. Except during infancy or illness, humans everywhere habitually sleep in a recumbent position, although the specifics of the position (e.g., prone, supine) may vary individually or be constrained by bedding. By contrast, the appurtenances of sleep, both substrates and covers, vary widely. Foragers inhabiting tropical or mild climates who move regularly do not sleep on platforms, but directly on the ground, which may or may not be prepared. !Kung sleep on a skin, a blanket, or nothing, over conforming sandy surfaces; Efe sleep on thinly strewn leaves, or perched between two logs, on rather hard, irregular ground; Ache lie on mats; and Hiwi use hammocks. None customarily uses pillowing materials, though individual Efe may use a pillow of bound leaves, and !Kung may use a wad of clothing. Nor does any group in our forager sample regularly use covering. Indeed, Efe remove clothing to reduce the danger of ignition from the fire kept going in the hut at night. !Kung may rarely use a blanket. All other groups in our sample, even the nomadic herders, the Gabra, sleep on platforms a foot or more off the ground. Sleeping platforms or beds are made of solid (wood strips [Gebusi], narrow sticks [Gabra], split black palm [Baktaman]) or webbed (leather strips [Swat Pathan], palm fronds [Lese]) surfaces on which bark and a mat (Gebusi), skin (Gabra, Pathan), or blanket (Pathan) may be placed. Covering among these nonforaging groups varies from occasional use of bark cloth capes over the torso (Gebusi), to a thin cotton cloth (Lese), which may be that used for clothing during the day (Gabra), to a thin sheet in summer and heavy blankets in winter (Pathan). Among the nonforaging societies in our sample, pillows are used only by Swat Pathan, who sleep with large cotton-stuffed, muslin-covered bolsters as pillows, and men cover their face and upper torso with the thin cloth they also carry by day.

Minimization of bedding, compared with the plethora of mattresses, sheets, pillows, duvets, and blankets of Westerners, may have to do not only with technology, resources, and climate but also with avoidance of undesirable concomitants of profuse bedding. Besides providing padding, thermal protection, or physical barriers, bedding may harbor parasites (fleas, bedbugs, lice) or producers of allergens (mites) and thus promote disease transmission or respiratory distress or illness. For instance, introduction of blankets among Fore in highland Papua New Guinea was paralleled by dramatic increases in rates of asthma among adults, apparently mediated by high levels of house mites in the blankets (Dowse, Turner, Stewart, Alpers, & Woolcock, 1985; Turner, Stewart, Woolcock, Green, & Alpers, 1988). At the least, bedding may be minimized because people find bites (or rather the immunologic responses to bites) uncomfortable, the activities of ectoparasites may disturb sleep, and the maintenance of sanitary bedding may be onerous. Swat Pathan prefer to lie on blankets rather than skins because the latter become flea-ridden more rapidly. Because beds become quickly bedbug-infested, the well-to-do cover the blankets with silk sheets to keep them off. Infested bedding is washed in cold water and/or hung in intense sun. Absent among our sample groups, but not infrequent in Africa or Asia, is the use of headrests, of variable shape and construction, which support the head but do not harbor ectoparasites.

Presence of Fire

Fire is a source of light (predator protection), heat (thermal protection), smoke (fumigant but irritant), unpredictable noise, and visual stimulation. It may also require tending during the night and thus enhance vigilance and increase periodic wakings. Presence of fire provides protection from predators, particularly among peoples without solid-walled domiciles, including all foragers sampled and the nomadic Gabra. Thus, it promotes a feeling of security. Further, heat generated by fire offers thermal protection and lowers humidity levels to enhance sleep comfort. Fires also have important fumigant properties. Dwellings, particularly those with thatch or shingle roofs, can harbor large populations of insects and rodents that are unpleasant or even dangerous to the human inhabitants. Smoke from fires plays the important and well-recognized role of controlling such pests, and perhaps even of damping ectoparasites. Fires are often built up for cooking the evening beverage and meal, and unventilated cooking fires fill the upper reaches of the space with smoke which filters through the roof and walls and gradually clears as the fire burns down (e.g., Gabra, Gebusi, Lese, Baktaman). In the aforementioned groups, fires are not replenished in the night, but burn down to smouldering embers by morning. Degree of particulate air pollution in the sleeping space may thus be variable but high at times. Smoky fires also deter nocturnal flying insects, such as mosquitoes, that are vectors for disease. For instance, mosquito bite rates among inhabitants of the lower Sepik River basin, a region holoendemic for malaria, correlate inversely with smoke levels and are highest among young men who live in youths' houses and are unused to tending fires (personal communication, B. Genton, July 24, 1992; for specific cases illustrating interactions of human host with mosquito vector circadian behaviors in lowland Papua New Guinea, see Genton et al., 1995; Nakazawa et al., 1995; Bockarie, Alexander, Bockarie, Obam, Barnish, & Alpers, 1996).

In groups for which the protective and thermal functions of fire are important, such as the foragers in our sample who have no or insubstantial dwellings (Ache, Hiwi, Efe, !Kung), sleepers rouse frequently in the night to monitor the fire and replenish it as necessary. Fire also produces steady, irregular (in volume, frequency, and quality) noise that some ethnographers report as being subliminally monitored in sleep: continual small noises are reassuring, loud pops are arousing, and the absence of sound wakes the sleeper concerned with fire maintenance. The presence of the flicker and the faint glow from the fire is reported as comforting and soothing or hypnotic, conducive to sleep during periods of nighttime insomnia, and facilitative of reassuring visual scans of the sleeping space. Finally, where there is no barrier between fireplace and sleeper (e.g., Ache, Efe, !Kung), risk of burns is high and sleepers apparently learn to regulate or monitor movements to avoid contact with the fire. Where sleeping spaces are restricted and densely populated or sleepers stay close to the fire for dryness and warmth, virtually every member of the group may have scars from burns that may be localized and minor or more extensive and severe. Parents may be particularly anxious about risk to infants and small children, a concern that increases vigilance even in sleep.

Finally, presence of fire in the sleeping space alters air quality and composition, not only through particulate components of smoke, but also via direct effects on gas composition. Fuel type (e.g., dung, wood) and quality (wet, dry, resinous) along with type of fire and fireplace construction determine smoke quantity and quality. In addition, fires consume oxygen and produce gases, including carbon monoxide, whose amount and composition again depend on fire dynamics (heat, ventilation). Thus, fires in sleeping spaces may strongly influence air quality, particularly in spaces that are closely sealed for insulation (Swat Pathan in winter) or to exclude malignant spirits (Lese). Incense burners may also be used in sleeping spaces to deter insects (Bali), disguise human odors (Gabra), or invoke spiritual protection.

Sleep Space or Structure

The construction and layout of dwellings determines properties of sleeping spaces regarding degree of social separation, protection from elements, thermal insulation, and physical security. Building size, layout, and materials heavily influence degree of physical, acoustic, or visual separation from others, awake or asleep. The two-meter-round huts of Efe and !Kung, constructed of stick frames covered with leaves or grass, respectively, present no physical barrier among sleepers in the hut, and little visual or acoustic separation from the outside (see related examples in Eibl-Eibesfeldt, 1989, pp. 632–633). Physical security from predator or enemy assault is minimal and protection from rain is reasonably good, but insulative value is low. These contrast with the mud and mud-stone walls of Lese and Swat Pathan, respectively, which provide high visual, acoustic, social, and climate barriers, but vary in degree of internal partitioning. Lese dwellings have internal partitions of sticks that do not extend to the ceiling and provide solely visual separation, whereas Swat Pathan houses have two or three rooms around a courtyard, separated by solid walls. By further contrast, Gebusi and other communal long-house dwellers of the Pacific and Asia sleep in large (60- to 100-feet long) structures with internal partitions that provide visual and physical but not acoustic separation from other residents, who may number from 20 to 100 (Eibl-Eibesfeldt, 1989, pp. 635–638). Among Gebusi, the longhouse contains a communal cooking area and sex-segregated living space, comprising a long central room (about 17×34 feet) with sleeping platforms on either side for men, and a narrow windowless sleeping space (about 7×34 feet) partitioned off along one side and with a separate interior entrance for women (Knauft, 1985a, p. 23). In general, gender, age, and status differentials influence size and quality of sleeping areas used by individuals. Gebusi again exemplify this point, for women's sleeping areas are literally peripheralized to a narrow outer side of the longhouse. The pattern of smaller and peripheral sleeping spaces for women and children, with large central spaces reserved for men, characterizes all the ethnographically documented groups of the Strickland-Bosavi region in which Gebusi reside, and these groups practice gender inequality to varying degrees (Kelly, 1993, pp. 40–41). Accordingly, the spaces used for sleeping both reflect and influence not only the proximal physical environments of sleep but also their social context.

Proximate Social Ecology of Sleep

Consonant with any human behavior, sleep has social meaning articulated with other aspects of social life and work, although the degree of its sociality differs across societies. This variation arises from two sources: sleeping arrangements and social partitioning of sleep-wake states. As noted earlier, sleeping arrangements have long interested anthropologists, who have linked the cross-cultural variation in such arrangements with diverse factors, from climate (Whiting, 1981), to sex roles or gender inequity (Whiting & Whiting, 1975; Paige & Paige, 1981; Herdt, 1989), to moral economy (Schweder et al., 1995). Consequently, anthropologists have been concerned with sleeping arrangements as expressions or determinants of social relationships and the social order, rather than with their implications for the biology or experiential quality of sleep itself.

Sleeping Arrangements

The number, sex, age, and proximity of others in sleep varies widely across and even within societies. For instance, the number and composition of sleepers in the small (about 2 meters in diameter) leaf huts of Efe foragers vary, but virtually no one sleeps alone, and one may routinely find two adults, a baby, another child, a grandparent, and perhaps a visitor sleeping together in the small space. Two or three sleep along the back of the hut, one on either side of the fire, and another one or two around the edges. Degree of physical contact is high, with full body contact and frequent entwining of appendages of two or three sleepers, along with periodic arousals associated with rearrangement movement of others, noises (cries, sniffs, snores, etc.), and traffic associated with staggered bedtimes and occasional elimination. Hammock sleeping among Hiwi foragers is associated with even higher levels of kinesthetic sensation and mutual disturbance or accommodation. Gebusi women sleep in a narrow (about 2.3 meters) space, packed like sardines along with infants and children of various ages, whereas men and boys lie on sleeping platforms segregated in an adjacent space. Sexes differ, then, in habitual degrees of physical contact in sleep, but all experience periodic arousal associated with movements of others on the mats, waking or sleeping.

These societies do not have beds per se, whereas groups using beds (Swat Pathan, Bali) or bedlike sleeping platforms (Gabra, Lese) differ in the number and sex-age composition of bed-sharing partners. Among Gabra, husband and wife use separate beds in the sleeping portion of the tent: women sleep with infants and small children, fathers sleep with sons. Lese couples sleep together and with infants; one or two children may sleep in another space on a bed with a visiting child or two, though adult or child may also sleep on mats on the floor. Finally, the Swat Pathan allocate a bed to each person, preferentially, but the beds are in shared spaces. Men often sleep on a bed in the men's house along with a variable number of other men in separate beds. Couples should have their own bed, used by the mother, whether the father is there or not, and accommodating the smallest child or children. Young women and children sleep in the same room, on separate beds or not, depending on family resources; elder persons sleep separately, and female visitors sleep with age-appropriate family members. Sleeping alone in a house is regarded as completely undesirable; sleeping alone in a room is possible though unlikely. Similarly, for Balinese, sociality pervades sleeping and waking states: being alone for even five minutes is undesirable, even when asleep, so widows and widowers who sleep alone are viewed as unfortunate and even sociospiritually vulnerable.

Thus, sleep in traditional societies is rarely solitary; however, the degree of cosleeping varies from shared sleeping locations to separate locations within shared spaces to separate spaces within buildings with low internal acoustic separation. Besides creating varying degrees of physical contact and stimulation, such social sleeping practices create possibilities for socially entrained nighttime arousal or disturbance linked to the activities of others. Insofar as the amount, pattern, and architecture of sleep varies with age, age composition of cosleepers affects the probability of arousals due to awakenings and activities (crying of infants, pain cries of the ill or afflicted, nightmare cries of children, frequency of urination, and even differences in absolute need for sleep with concomitant amounts of insomnia). Moreover, the presence of cosleepers affects temperature and air quality, along with background levels of noise and activity, including breathing, which all create gradients defining the microenvironments of sleep.

Separation of Sleep-Wake States

The degree of definition between sleeping and waking behavior varies widely and is strongly linked to housing construction patterns of social and ritual activity. Particularly among societies with insubstantial housing and low demands for work scheduling, such as foragers, the boundaries of sleep and waking are very fluid. Neither !Kung nor Efe have bedtimes, so time of falling asleep varies widely within and among individuals. People stay up as long as something interesting – a conversation, music, dance – is happening and they participate; then they go to sleep when they feel like it. Indeed, someone may go to sleep and get up later because they hear something going on and wish to participate. Moreover, a member of either society who wakes up any hour of the night may begin to hum, or go out and play the thumb piano; others may join in, and music or even a dance may get going, depending on the willingness of others to join in. Virtually no one is told to be quiet because others are sleeping, though people avoid unnecessary disturbance of sleepers. Additionally, no one, including children, is told to go to bed, and individuals of any age may nod off amid ongoing social intercourse and fade in and out of sleep during nighttime social activities. Thus, as in many other aspects of social life, foragers show high fluidity in sleep-wake patterns.

Among both foragers and our other sample groups, inclusion of the young from infancy in group activities socializes them into culturally appropriate sleep-wake patterns. Differential needs of individuals or the young are usually accommodated, which may increase the impact when for ritual purposes they are not accommodated, as in the case of some initiation rituals. Balinese, who engage in extensive nighttime ritual activity, bring children along with them to all rituals, where they may fall asleep at will, although in this case they must learn to stay awake as adults. In other words, bedtimes are not fixed and sleep-wake boundaries are rather fluid in our sample population, even for the young. Nevertheless, bedtimes in particular, and sleep-wake patterns in general, may be constrained by a host of structural and cultural factors addressed later in our discussion of the macroecology of sleep.

In sum, sleep in these traditional societies is collective, and it occurs in social space; yet, at the same time, it is usually conventional to leave the sleeper alone, spared of undue disturbance, as the boundary of wake and sleep is fluid.

Biotic Microecology of Sleep

Human life and sleep are populated not only with people but also with other creatures, some domesticated and present by design, others intrusive and unwanted. In either case, the presence and activity of fauna influence human sleep patterns.

Presence of Animals

Larger domesticated animals frequently coreside with humans, who keep them for protection or subsistence purposes. Efe, for instance, keep dogs used in hunting in the hut with the rest. A sleeper discomfited by a sleeping hound may pound on it to drive it, howling, away (it creeps back later), but the specific breed of dog (the relatively "barkless" bisinje) barks rarely, at intruders only, and seldom disturbs sleepers with night-time barking. Dogs kept by !Kung, Baktaman, and Gebusi are also reported to bark seldom and feebly, being kept for assistance in hunting and treated very poorly. By contrast, dogs run loose in packs in the streets of Swat Pathan villages, and their fights, barks, and mating activities can create disturbance, particularly on hot summer nights when people sleep out on their roofs. Gabra herders keep watchdogs to drive off predators and raise the alarm over stock raiders. Dogs set up a clamor on average once or twice a night, and only rarely is a night undisturbed by a major outbreak of barking. Gabra, however, appear to determine whether to get up or not by the urgency of the tumult.

Humans often sleep near their domesticated animals, usually to guard them and at times to take advantage of their warmth. Nearby animals can also be noisy. Gabra keep camels, goats, and sheep in enclosures (*bomas*) on either side of the line of tents in the encampment. Thus, they are surrounded by constant animal noises, notably the baaing and bleating of the sheep and goats kept on one side, though the noise level declines after 2:00 to 3:00 A.M. Boys and young men sleep on skins on the ground in *bomas* to provide close protection, so the sleepers in tents nearby need not be as vigilant. Domestic animals are kept by Swat Pathan in the gated courtyard of the house and locked in at night. Their heavy breathing and continuous munching are reported as pleasant, reassuring sounds. Roosters, however, can be very raucous, and may begin to crow at 3:00 A.M. Ethnographers report that people appear to habituate to these routine, albeit periodic and unpredictable noises, although it remains unknown whether this is true, and whether level of arousability or vigilance in sleep is conditioned by level of danger or insecurity.

Macropredators: Humans and Large Carnivores

Urbanized Western peoples are prone to forget that large predators represented a major mortality hazard in the past and continue to remain so for some populations today. Fear of predators can constrain nighttime activity and keep people indoors, and maintenance of fires through the night, especially among tropical peoples, is as much a matter of warding off predators as of staying warm. Vigilance against predators, such as wolves in the northern steppes or large cats in low latitudes around the globe, generally promotes sleeping with others, indoors and/or close to a fire. Stories of spectacular bouts of predation, by large cats or wolves, occur in most if not all societies where such predators are present. Predator tales haunt the imaginations of inhabitants, constrain their behaviors, and maintain wariness or anxiety about vulnerable situations such as nighttime and sleep. A dramatic instance of this phenomenon is documented in our ethnographic sample among the Ache. A small band was stalked for days by a panther, three adults were attacked and two were killed, and the band stayed on the move and built brush corrals nightly until the panther was ambushed by a vigilant lookout while it raided the camp late one night. Hill and Hurtado have heard the story retold repeatedly, in great detail, throughout the time that they have worked with the Ache, up to 32 years after the event. They note that: "The average Ache man or woman does not get eaten by a jaguar. Nonetheless, these things do happen occasionally and have important influences on many other aspects of Ache life, from foraging tactics to marriage patterns to mythology" (Hill & Hurtado, 1996).

Similarly, both fear and practice of raiding and warfare tend to disrupt activity patterns and constrain living and sleeping sites. Responses to threat of human predation include congregation in more compact, and hence defensible, living and sleeping areas and construction of barriers or structures. Belief in other human or spiritual predators such as witches or malevolent spirits is also linked to practices to ensure safe sleep and avoid isolation. Such practices tend to change the psychology (in terms of fear or security), patterning, and microecology of sleep.

Moreover, rituals to detect witches or attract or repel spirits are often held at night and can keep participants up for long, regular periods.

Parasites and Nighttime Pests

The discussions of bedding and fire have also touched on human concerns about ectoparasites and nighttime pests such as mosquitoes. Practices aimed at reducing exposure to such pests not only have the effect of abating transient discomfort caused to the host but also diminish the risk of insect-borne disease. Ectoparasites can be a source of nighttime unease and discomfort for the human host, largely through the itching or stinging caused by their movement and bites. The scratching and other movement occasioned by their activity can further rouse other sleepers. Efe often groom each other before sleep, taking each other's heads in hand to scratch and remove ectoparasites. Activity of internal parasites, such as filarial worms, are frequently entrained to specific times of day, and these may disturb sleep if their activity occurs at night. Lastly, flying insects active at night, most prominently mosquitoes, can be not only a source of irritation, through buzzing and biting, but also a major vector for disease, the most prevalent and significant of which is malaria. Cultural practices that minimize or exacerbate exposure to bites and, thus, risk of malaria directly influence not merely transient comfort, but also health (Brown, 1981, 1986). Such practices related to sleep include repelling by fire, use of incense, type and care of clothing and coverings, and housing design. The potential efficacy of these practices is indicated by Hurtado's finding that mites, fleas, and lice were absent in the dirt sampled from Hiwi sleeping hammocks. Hiwi frequently shake and wash their hammocks so that, although fleas and lice are present on dogs and people, they are not harbored in the bedding. Widespread practices of changing and/or airing and beating bedding materials likely play similar parasite- and mite-reducing roles.

Beliefs that organize parasite-avoidant behaviors are thus adaptive (Hart 1990). For instance, Lese hold strong fears of nighttime witchcraft and spirit activity. This fear keeps them in their houses at night with doors and windows tightly closed and locked, and strongly discourages casual nighttime activity outside; a village where bedtime averages around 8:00 P.M. is usually silent by 9:00 P.M. Such behavior concurrently reduces rates of mosquito bite and, thus, risk of malaria. Conversely, practices designed to reduce exposure to parasites, such as use of smoky fires or tightly closed sleeping spaces, also alter ventilation and air quality and thence may also influence sleep regulation and health risk by other routes.

Macroecology of Human Sleep

The previous sections have outlined factors shaping the microecology of sleep settings; however, the distribution of sleep over the day is driven by several structural and cultural features that shape overall activity patterns. These factors include patterns of labor and leisure, ritual practices and religious beliefs, demography and settlement patterns, climate and physical ecology, concomitants of statuses such as social rank or gender, and the social organization of the life cycle. Life-cycle status cuts across all the other dimensions so that very different activity patterns and sleep ecologies may be experienced at different points of the life-span.

Labor Demands

Unsurprisingly, labor demands may strongly determine sleep and wake patterns, either directly by constraining work schedules or indirectly by affecting degree of tiredness and need for sleep versus energy for other activities. Division of labor within a society, by age, gender, trade, or caste-class furthermore shapes the distribution of workloads and creates heterogeneity in activity patterns within communities. Direct effects of subsistence activity on sleep-wake schedule are particularly evident among pastoralists. For Gabra, because midday heat stress on animals is high and suppresses optimal grazing, the ideal daily schedule is to milk the animals and take them out to graze at 4:00 A.M., return around 8:00 A.M. to rest the herds in the heat of the day, go out again midafternoon, and return for the night around 8:00 P.M. This they seldom do except when it is very hot, reportedly for fear of early morning stock raids. Generally, herders depart around 9:00 A.M., but routinely nap during midday, when animals are fairly inactive and unlikely to wander. Upon herders' return at dusk (6:00–7:00 P.M.), there remain milking, evening mealtime, and all other community social activities. Thus, Gabra average bedtimes of 11:00 to 11:30 P.M. are the latest of the groups in our sample. Similarly, during the cultivation season Swat Pathan farmers may go out at dawn to work for 1–2 hours, then return for breakfast, then later go out at varied, scheduled nighttime hours to open and close irrigation channels during the times allotted to them. Contrastingly, foragers such as !Kung or horticulturalists such as Gebusi confine

subsistence labor to daylight hours, and their degree of nighttime activity is driven by other, social factors. Differential workloads can support
intrapopulation differences in work and sleep patterns. Lese women's
subsistence work is so onerous that they quickly go to sleep soon after
the evening meal, whereas men often stay up longer to socialize at the
men's community gathering place (*baraza*). Similar reasons may underlie Gebusi patterns of women's retiring after dark for 10 hours' sleep-rest
in a separate space, contrasted with men's frequently remaining up for
rituals and séances. In general, a combination of energetic demand and
caloric restriction, or even micronutrient deficiency,[1] may induce a tolerance or desire for inactivity or somnolence, if not increased absolute
amount of sleep.

Seasonal labor demands, particularly among horticulturalists and
agriculturalists, are often associated with distinctive sleep-wake patterns, field clearing, planting, crop guarding, and harvesting as being
periods of intensified demand and reduced rest. Unless foragers can
engage in significant food storage, daily workload is rarely seasonal
and varies less than among other subsistence types. On the other hand,
diurnal activity patterns may be shaped by specific foraging opportunities available at discrete times and seasons (e.g., collection of turtle eggs
as they are laid at night). Many pastoralist and agropastoralist groups
have seasonal or permanent satellite camps to take advantage of remote
foraging opportunities for the herds. Routines of daily life are often
shifted and less regularized in herd camps. Gabra, for example, send
young men out with camel, goat, or sheep herds in search of pasturage,
which is patchy and unpredictable due to rains. Tents are not used, and
herders sleep on the ground. Visiting occurs between the main and satellite camps; the latter have more resident young people, who stay up to
talk, sing, and dance into the night. Daily routines are more fluid and
sleep schedules are erratic, punctuated by lots of visiting among camps.
Travel occurs at night to avoid daytime heat, so visitors may arrive at
1:00 or 2:00 A.M., whereupon hosts get up and prepare food, usually
killing a goat.

Ecological parameters, including thermal load and water stress, can
also affect activity patterns. In our small sample of societies, midday
naps are associated with heat and water stress among Gabra herders
and their animals, and with summer heat stress among Swat Pathan

---

[1] Micronutrient deficiencies associated with lassitude include iron-deficient anemia and
iodine-deficient hypothyroidism.

farmers. Customary siesta taking is well recognized and widespread, and usually is associated with increased nighttime activity so that sleep is rather more distributed around the clock.

Social Activity

Conversation

Patterns of social activity also influence amount of nighttime activity, and thus patterns of sleep. Expectations for nighttime conversation, and gender-graded participation in nighttime activity, vary widely across societies. !Kung, for instance, are intensely conversational; night talk functions to entertain, pass time, address conflicts and disputes, and work through and solidify relationships. Charges of stinginess in food sharing (especially of meat), accusations of adultery, or other marital problems stimulate hours of conversation that may extend far into the night and include not only the immediate issue, but the airing of various other general and personal concerns as well. The extensive talk is crucial to formation and maintenance of social relationships and thus to patterns of group coherence or fission, and marital formation and dissolution. Talk, both by day and by night, acts as a means for addressing social-political issues essential to foraging agreements and managing disputes. Individual participation in these conversations is voluntary and variable. Efe exhibit similar behavior, so that individual times for falling asleep or waking and reengaging vary on a daily basis contingent on what is happening.

Notably, sleep or the appearance of sleep offers one way to "check out" of interminable, slow-moving circular, or frustrating debates. Because the boundary demarcating sleep and wake is fuzzy in the culture settings under discussion, where both sleeping and waking are viewed as social behaviors, a retreat into sleep can represent an acceptable way to withdraw from active social engagement.[2] Such withdrawals feature in men's meetings and houses. Thus, a Gabra man in the midst of a meeting or extended discussion may simply pull his cloth over his head and roll over to "sleep." "Check-out" sleep behavior may occur by day as well as night.

---

[2] We owe this observation to Frederick Barth (personal communication, March 14, 1997), whose unparalleled lifetime of ethnographic fieldwork across a wide range of settings lends confidence to his generalization.

Festivities and Dances

Nighttime social activity or preparations for such activity can alter sleep-wake patterns; hence, cultural patterns of sociality influence circadian activity schedules. Dances and other social activities can shade into informal ritual as well, as in the case of the great cycle of nighttime shadow puppet plays among Balinese, or the trance dancing of !Kung. Celebratory dance among !Kung is stimulated by such occasions as rainfall, a large haul of game, or the arrival of another group that swells the numbers to critical mass for dance. Groups differ in frequency of dance, from once or twice a week, to only once a month. Dance duration varies as well, lasting until midnight or, more often in the case of celebratory dance, into the small hours or all night. Participation is voluntary, and people leave and reenter, with sleep or napping between. Sleep catch-up (sleeping in, napping, and earlier bedtime) usually occurs the next day. About once a month (25 times in 22 months in field observation, Knauft, 1985a,b) Gebusi hold dances or feasts that go on all night.[3] Again, catch-up sleep may occur the next day: a photograph by Eileen Cantrell captures a Gebusi woman, in full dance array (paint, feather headdress, nose bone), asleep under her barkcloth cape on a woodpile in full sun, following an all-night dance. Contrastingly, Baktaman break the evening sleep routine with dances only about six times a year. Torches are made with difficulty, so dances are coordinated with the full moon; if it is overcast as usual, then the event is canceled. Dances last only two or three hours, after which participants feel they have been up quite late.

Visiting and Traveling

Travel and visitors disrupt daily routines. Travel may entail early departures, late arrivals, or even night travel, as noted for Gabra. Herders and foragers who move routinely, even daily, generally do not travel far, but migration among groups who move less frequently and have more complex materials for camp setup can be considerably more disruptive of sleep-wake schedules. Visitors also bring novelty, enhance sociality, and extend conversations or entertainment into the night. In Swat Pathan men's houses, bedtime may very between 8:00 and 11:00 P.M.,

---

[3] All-night ritual with costume, dance, and song is found throughout documented Strickland-Bosavi peoples and represents the principal occasion for intercommunity gatherings (Schieffelin, 1976; Knauft, 1985a; Kelly, 1993).

but the presence of visitors prompts staying up later. !Kung stay up and may even hold a dance when visitors or another band are in camp. Both in Gabra main and satellite herd camps, habitual nighttime arrival of visitors and rules of hospitality prolong social activity far into the night.

Ritual Practices

Rituals frequently take place at night, perhaps in part to minimize conflict with routine daytime activity, and largely to take advantage of the special features of associations with night. Ritual practices can alter sleeping patterns both directly by occurring at night or indirectly by entailing prior preparations or travel. It is worth noting again that the line between ritual and nonritual social activity may be blurred, as in the distinction of the !Kung trance dance for ritual healing or social celebration. Injuries or acute illness necessitate immediate performance by the !Kung of a trance dance (Katz, 1982), which when held for healing purposes is highly intense and is shorter than the more relaxed celebratory dances. In general, rituals involving trance and altered mental states tend to be preferentially held at night, perhaps to harness neurobiological features of chronobiology, including sleepiness, sleep onset, and the effects of mild sleep deprivation. Practices that combine cognitive demand or load with sleep deprivation may potentiate dissociated states. For instance, on average every 11 days Gebusi men hold séances in which spirits must be kept awake all night through the intercession of a medium who in the course of the night, in dialogue with and supported by all the other men of the community, may sing from memory through the text of a hundred songs about complex matters. During the course of the night, even the spirit medium may doze lightly, sitting erect and cross-legged, while keeping things "simmering." In this context, the line between social engagement and somnolescent semi- or quasi-engagement is a fluid one, and Gebusi actively socialize men for ability to stay awake while on the edge of consciousness. Although all men phase in and out of somnolence during the séance, anyone falling really deeply asleep can be subject to hazing.[4] Fostering sociality in somnolence might involve socialization of the neurophysiology of sleep in

---

[4] A favorite "joke" on someone who succumbs to sleep consists of dressing in warfare gear, taking up weapons, and screaming at the sleeper. If he starts out of sleep with horrified alarm, convinced he is about to be killed in a raid, the joke is viewed as hilarious, an unqualified success.

states in which the transition from somnolent-sociable to trance-sociable is facilitated. Spirit mediums could simply be the most adept at this: communicative dreaming or waking visions as cultivated by them may entail using the sleep drive to fuel the spirit visions and verbal performances of the séance.

Balinese have highly developed nocturnal ritual and spiritual pursuits: night is a ritual time, a time of spirit activity, tuned to moon phases and astrological periods. Virtually all rituals (weddings, funerals, meditation, shadow play), including the elaborate collective ritual performances, occur at night. In dedication to the gods, Balinese purposely stay up for two or three nights to participate in these events, in large part because they are important communal activities, but eager in part for trance and the dissociative states induced by sleep deprivation. Here, the goal is to attain an inner detached spiritual state, rather than a vision or visitation, though the latter is valued and heavily discussed if it occurs. In these various communal, ritual pursuits, Balinese remain up about seven nights a month, 1–2 days a week. Rather than deplore lack of sleep, they cultivate radical deprivation as a desideratum. Senior men emphasize their chronic sleep shortage and claim or boast of sleeping only 2–3 hours per night. These assertions, while unfounded, constitute claims to social importance, responsibility, and competence. It is a discourse of male responsibility, not employed by women, who nonetheless participate fully in ritual and spiritual life.

Cultural-specific religious observances may be required at early or late hours on a regular or seasonal basis and can strongly influence activity pattern. Perhaps the most widespread institutionalized example is the Islamic observance of Ramadan, a month during which food and drink may be consumed only between sundown and around 2:30 to 4:00 A.M. Daytime fasting sharply skews activity patterns toward evening with delayed sleep onsets so far as occupation allows, so that the wealthy as well as women and children stay up through the early hours and then sleep well into the morning. Among the Swat Pathan in our ethnographic sample, observance of Ramadan occasions a near reversal of circadian activity, to nighttime wake and daytime sleep. Men, however, involved in labor requiring daylight are forced to be active through the day, also. Richard Burton provides a vivid description of Ramadan in Cairo a century ago, and notes the impact of this radical inversion of schedule on mood and behavior: "the chief effect of the 'blessed month' upon True Believers is to darken their tempers into positive gloom" (Burton, 1893, p. 74).

Rites of passage often alter sleep patterns. Gabra, for example, stay awake all night before a wedding: men stand in front of the bridal tent awaiting the bride, and women sing at the bride's place. Many initiation rituals or ritual cycles involve sleep deprivation that likely serves dual purposes as a test of endurance or control, and as an inducer of cognitive states that amplify the impact of the rituals. Among the Baktaman, the trials undergone in ritual initiation and grade promotion for boys and men include staying or being kept awake. Senior men oversee initiates and prevent sleep with prods or harangues, but the ideal is to remain awake oneself to demonstrate capacity to meet the trial. Sleeplessness is compounded by sensory overloading from verbal hazing, overheating with large bonfires, or beatings with nettles. Similar practices are widespread across Papua New Guinea (see examples in Herdt, 1982), and common in other traditions, including the spirit quests of North American peoples and the initiation cycles of the age-set societies of sub-Saharan Africa.

Although initiates are seldom kept awake for more than one day-night-day sequence, they may experience chronic sleep disruption induced by periodic, unpredictable loud and/or terrifying night noises made by initiators with, for instance, spirit whistles, spirit flutes, or bull roarers. The usual targets of such initiation rituals are adolescent and male, though female initiation is also practiced, frequently with different rituals and less harsh treatment (Paige & Paige, 1981). Other chapters in this volume provide evidence for distinctive features of chronobiology at adolescence that likely present specific demands and opportunities for socialization into the late evening and early morning hours. The initiates described here, however, are not the only ones to experience sleep disturbance or deprivation: preparations for, management of, and festivities associated with initiation engage many members of the community and can entail round-the-clock involvement.

In sum, several common features of ritual suggest that aspects of chronobiology may be exploited, cognitive-neuroendocrine states may be manipulated, and/or sensitive developmental periods may be targeted as mediators or moderators of ritual efficacy (see also d'Aquili & Laughlin, 1979; Lex, 1979). First, many rituals are performed at a specific time of day. Second, some rituals involve sleep deprivation or disruptions of diurnal schedule and may combine these with other forms of hazing and with social isolation. Third, adolescents are a common target for rituals and practices requiring or allowing sleep deprivation and phase-shifted activity patterns. In addition, the previous features are sometimes also combined with consumption of specific foods or with fasting, which would also alter physiologic state.

Settlement Pattern, Arrangement

Both social and physical ecology affect the pattern and arrangement of settlements, which, in turn, influence the degree of security in and potential disruption of sleep. Small, widely dispersed settlements, such as those of most foragers (here, !Kung, Efe, Ache, Hiwi) and many pastoralists (here, Gabra) provide less protection from predators and enemies, albeit also less potential for sleep disruption. As described earlier, Hill and Hurtado (1996) recount a particularly harrowing instance, in which a small band of Ache were stalked and terrorized by a predatory jaguar for days before they could reach another, larger group: their sleep was heavily disrupted during and after this time. Demography (population size, structure by age and sex) and population density determine margins of vulnerability and defensibility, as well as overall activity levels and patterns.

Constraining Beliefs

Beliefs – about function and meaning of sleep, night danger, ghosts, dreams – establish explanatory models and emotional-interpretive frameworks that influence not only sleep behaviors but also sleep quality. For instance, beliefs about developmental needs and vulnerabilities inform parenting and child care practices, including naps and bedtimes (Super & Harkness, 1994), sleeping arrangements (solitary vs. cosleep, McKenna, 1992), and carrying-sleeping devices (cradle, cradleboard, etc., Chisholm, 1983). Sleep can be seen as a necessary mental and physical restorative, or a time of significant spiritual work. It can also be viewed as risky: Gebusi believe that, in sleep, the spirit departs and socializes in the world of spirits. The spirit or double wanders only in sleep, thus becoming vulnerable to predation by witches and malign spirits of the head (see also the excellent description for a related group, the Etoro, in Kelly, 1976). In dreaming, spiritual life is activated, and spirits come to the dreamer who also enters their world. Deep sleep is considered risky because the sleeper's spirit may wander off too far and partially or wholly fail to return. Indeed, morning bird calls are thought to summon a sleeper's spirits to return. As described earlier, the spiritual vulnerability of a sleeper enforces the notion that sleep is social, never solitary. Thus, sleep socialization and practices among Gebusi may aim to mitigate against habitual deep sleep, given its high perceived risks (all deaths are attributed to sorcery).

Concerns about exposure to ghosts, spirits, and witchcraft during sleep and, particularly, dreaming are reported in many societies and influence evening activities, bedtimes, and sleeping arrangements. Thus, Lese tightly lock up their houses and go to bed around 8:00 P.M. to avoid witchcraft, whereas Balinese often stay up very late to participate in the important nighttime world of ritual and spiritual life. Similar to Gebusi, they also believe that loss of soul (*atma*, vital spirit) occurs nearly nightly in dreaming (Wikan, 1990, p. 173) and that sleeping with others mitigates the dangers of soul loss.

Beliefs and practices are frequently grounded on cultural models directly associating sleep quality and sleeping conditions with physical well-being. For instance, Lese may attribute a case of jaundice to leaving a door or window ajar at night and allowing a malignant spirit to enter, whereas Gebusi may blame themselves if an unattended ill or elderly person dies, on the grounds that they were left alone, open to attack by spirits.

Effects of Status

Social statuses, based on age, class or social standing, and gender, define many aspects of daily experience, including those of sleep. Status influences most dimensions of the micro- and macroecology of sleep, including workload, activity patterns, sleeping companions, and sleeping conditions. Women, for instance, almost universally sleep with infants and often with children, while men and boys are more likely to sleep in exposed or risky conditions. Poor or socially marginal individuals frequently sleep in more crowded, disrupted, and insecure situations, whereas the powerful or affluent generally repose in less populated and more controlled conditions. By illustration, membership of men's houses in Swat villages varies considerably, from 10–20 up to 30–40 men, but some of the craftsmen castes, shopkeepers, and religious leaders sleep in their own small *betak* guest rooms. Further, some statuses are viewed as particularly vulnerable, polluting, or dangerous and are vigilantly coddled or systematically segregated. For instance, Baktaman women remove to a menstrual hut for childbirth or menses, where they usually have several women companions but are separated from children, except young nurslings. In general, the young, ill, or elderly are attended and accorded special sleeping situations, as well as exempted from early rising and strenuous work. Adolescents, and particularly unmarried young men, often sleep separately from family units, in the open (Gabra, !Kung),[5] in sex-segregated quarters (Gebusi), in a separate hut (Efe, Lese), in a men's house (Baktaman, Swat), or in separate camps with herds (Gabra, pastoralist Swat).

Physical Ecology

Defined by climate, season, access to heat and light sources, and technology, physical ecology drives activity patterns and living conditions and thus shapes sleep ecology. Climate comprises circannual and circadian temperature, rainfall, and humidity patterns, while seasons also entrain alterations in day length and incident light. Nearly all of our ethnographic sample live in mild climates near the equator, but among circumpolar peoples variation in daylength has dramatic effects on activity patterns that have been heavily studied (Condon, 1983; see Condon, 1987, for an ethnograhic example relating to adolescents).

Throughout human history, distribution and availability of fuel sources and technological limitations on use of fuels for heat or sources of light have influenced patterns of activity and habitation. Notably, the human need for sleep in hours per day is exceeded by the number of hours of dark in the day for all (in the case of equatorial peoples) or part (in the case of higher latitudes) of the year. Hence, humans are awake and active during the dark as well as daylight hours, but limited capacity for nighttime illumination has historically constrained the range of activities that can safely, effectively, or efficiently be pursued at night. Depending on the kinds and availabilies of fuel sources and lighting technology, the problem of lighting may be very large, and the liberation through electricity from the tyranny of night boredom inestimably exciting and valuable. Barth (1975) noted of Baktaman that, particularly during wet nights spent on hunts and away from the longhouse, the longing for day, waiting for the sun so that one could get up again, can be intense and the night can seem endless. The tyranny of dark and the chaining of activity to day length can produce perdurable human

---

[5] For closely related /Gwi, see camp map indicating separate sleeping spot used by young men (Eibl-Eibesfeldt, 1989, p. 633).

preoccupations that are reflected in widespread myth, magic, and ritual, as well as technology. Furthermore, the human use of fuel sources (for cooking and heat, as well as light and protection) contributes to a high ecological impact by the species.

Daytime Napping

A robust extant literature documents a human tendency to be biphasic, with a preponderance of sleep behavior at night and a midafternoon trough in alertness coinciding with elevated drowsiness (Mitler et al., 1988; Tobler, 1995). Here, the ethnographic literature becomes impressionistic at best. Because none of the societies included in the present report practices fixed bedtimes, the absence of demarcated napping periods is unsurprising. Nevertheless, we have the impression that societies do differ in the extent of napping behavior, and that specific physical and cultural ecologies may discourage or encourage napping. Sun exposure and pressure of heat and/or desiccation appear to promote midday napping. The Gabra, for example, live in dry regions with seasonally high midday temperatures. Midday is a slow period for animals and people, when all seek shade and converse desultorily, perform small handwork, or nap. Napping occurs anywhere, in the shade, on cloth. Gabra were observed to nap in small blocks (15–30 minutes) at any time throughout the day; old men may even sleep longer, up to 2 hours at a time. Similarly, among Swat agriculturalists who must work in summer, men return at around noon to eat and drowse before returning to the fields around 2:30 P.M. Women, who do not work much in the fields, routinely nap after the bustle of morning chores and midday meal preparation and serving are completed. Balinese also commonly nap, as they feel like it, usually between 1:00 and 3:00 P.M.

Napping, dozing, or resting have causes other than intrinsic chronobiological ones (Lubin, Hord, Tracy, & Johnson, 1976). Hiwi baffled ethnographers because they live in a relatively rich environment where caloric returns for foraging are high, yet for much of the year they do not forage enough hours in the day to meet fully their caloric needs (Hurtado & Hill, 1990). Rather, they spend large blocks of the day, mainly the afternoon, in camp napping in their hammocks, chatting, or performing relatively sedentary tasks. They concluded that two factors mitigate against Hiwi extending the food quest: sun exposure and resultant heat load, and need to minimize exposure to enteric pathogens (specifically hookworm). Marginal nutrition with consequent low blood sugar levels and heavy parasite load, associated with iron-deficient anemia, both conduce directly to lassitude, weariness, and increased resting (Jenike, 1996). Additionally, illness powerfully affects sleep; the physiology of immunologic response to illness organizes "sick behavior," including rest, drowsiness, and sleep (Hart, 1990; Grazia de Simoni, Imeri, De Matteo, Perego, Simard, & Tarrazzino, 1995; Krueger & Majde, 1995). By illustration, the Efe were not observed to nap unless sick. In fact, anyone seen napping was presumed unwell due to the frequency of malaria. That societies exhibit differing degrees of napping behavior and degrees of institutionalization of napping (as in the cases of Spain or Italy) may be taken as symptomatic of the diverse ecological factors that drive sleep behavior and its patterning over the day.

Sexual Intercourse

Although sleeping arrangements are heavily influenced by culturally determined sexual mores and views of sexuality, patterns of sleep themselves are little influenced by sexual activity for most individuals over most of the life course in most societies. That sexual intercourse is private among humans enjoins a discreetness that mitigates against disruption of others' sleep by this behavior, but patterns of cosleeping may make unobtrusive sex difficult. Gabra couples engage in intercourse in the tent, in front of the children who are presumably but not always asleep. The same is true for !Kung (Shostak, 1981, p. 111). Contrastingly, many highland New Guinea societies such as the Gebusi do not allow intercourse in the longhouse, which precludes its being a nocturnal domestic activity. On the other hand, pursuit of sexual exploits can disturb sleep of the parties themselves. Even when liaisons are sanctioned, sexual partners may have to wait until others are asleep. As noted, sleeping arrangements are often designed to prevent clandestine night trysts, but where they are condoned among the young and unmarried, the idea as well as the act of seeking sexual liaisons may disrupt sleep considerably. Tahitians provide a vivid ethnographic instance of practices rather widespread in Polynesian traditional society in the behavior called *motoro*, or night crawling, in which a young man enters a girl's house at night when everyone is asleep and seeks to have sex or make an assignation with her (Levy, 1973, pp. 123–124). As traditionally practiced, *motoro* was a component of mate selection and courtship.

Developmental Ecology of Human Sleep

Sleep and the Life Course

The ethnographic data document wide variation in the ecologies of human sleep, while the embeddedness of sleep in social life has concurrently emerged as a cross-cutting theme. Comparative ethnographic analysis raises the intriguing possibility that these diverse sleep ecologies and behaviors exert organizational effects on state regulation, that is, on the neurobiological systems regulating cognitive arousal and attentional states. Most of the comparative data on sleep ecology focus on infants, because of the emphasis on early experience widespread among human developmentalists. Because the present volume focuses on adolescents, we will expand treatment of the scant literature on this developmental period. In addition, life history profiles of sleep ecology for Gabra and Gebusi men and women are outlined to underscore the need for a life-span approach to human sleep ecology and behavior.

Socialization of sleep and associated state regulation commences with the functional supports and demands presented by infant care practices (Trevathan & McKenna, 1994). Barry and Paxton (1971) reviewed ethnographic data from 173 societies and noted unusual uniformity: infants are reported to sleep at night with at least one person (mother) present in the same bed (43.9%) or room (24.3%, mother in separate bed; 31.8%, mother present, location unspecified). The father is present in 44.5% of these societies, and often other family members are as well.[6] In our small sample series, infants and small children virtually never sleep in a room alone. This circumstance reflects not only practical demands of prolonged breast feeding, but also a concern for welfare and protection of the young. That this concern may be intense is reflected among Ache mothers who hold their infants on their laps throughout the night until weaning at around age 4 years, to guard against cold and

---

[6] Exclusion of cases coded as having uncertain data (n = 45) did not influence our results. In this subset of 128 societies, mother slept in the same bed (43.8%) or room (21.9%, mother in separate bed; 34.4%, mother present, location unspecified) in all cases.

the dangerous creatures residing on the forest floor.[7] In accord with this observation, cross-cultural analysis has established that infant-carrying practices correlate with climatic factors (Whiting, 1981), and the cross-cultural sample used here revealed that young infants were customarily held or carried in 73.6% of the 61 cases where data were reliable (Barry & Paxton, 1971).[8]

Throughout the day, sleep of infants occurs in the context of ongoing everyday social intercourse in virtually all societies, as babies are carried or kept in close proximity to their mothers or care givers. Several anthropologists have studied the implications of social embeddedness for infant development (Whiting, Landauer, & Jones, 1968; Super & Harkness, 1994; Bakeman, Adamson, Konner, & Barr, 1997), although few have considered the consequences for sleep or state regulation (but see Super & Harkness, 1994). In her analysis of Balinese infant development incorporating Bateson's intensive ethological photographic study, Mead noted that: "Balinese children learn to sleep in almost any position." The ability to sleep nearly at will in the midst of ongoing activity carries forward to adulthood: "Actors, seated behind the curtains of an outdoor theater, in full view of the audience, take off their headdresses between scenes and sleep sitting, and members of an audience sleep standing up when the dialogue becomes dull" (Mead & Macgregor, 1951, p. 96). Infants learn not only to sleep and to be awake but also to move between these states in populated, sensorily dynamic social settings. After weaning, sleep settings become more culturally variable and often undergo age- and gender-graded changes across the life course.

Because the focus of this volume is adolescent sleep, this developmental period commands attention in the present treatment despite the dearth of ethnographic material on sleep conditions at this age. In general, adolescence emerges from the comparative literature as a period when culturally expected, tolerated, or enforced changes in behavior and residence patterns (Schlegel & Barry, 1991) occur in conjunction with altered activity and sleep patterns. Reorganization of residence, work roles, social status, degree of freedom or surveillance, and onset

[7] Barth also observed that Baktaman newborns are naked for the first 3 months, held next to the mother's skin for warmth, and cradled on the mother's lap at night. (Both ethnographers – Hurtado for Ache and Barth for Baktaman – note how strenuous lap cradling is for mothers).
[8] Exclusion of codings noted as uncertain did affect this analysis. Of the 121 cases coded as having usable data, infants were held or carried more than half the time in 57% of societies, and more than occasionally and up to half the time in 27.3%.

of reproductive career frequently occur at this time, and furthermore they tend to involve gender-specific forms and schedules that increase gender divergence in everyday life. Moreover, as noted in previous sections, late childhood or adolescence often is a period at which individuals are subjected to elaborate rites of passage or become central actors in ritual activity that involves wakefulness for preparation or performance. Functions may also be purely social, to facilitate adolescent acquisition of adult social persona and to promote mate selection. Examples include the exclusively nighttime dance cycles for youth of Kenyan Kikuyu (Leakey, 1977, pp. 392–438).

In many societies, adolescents experience exacerbation or emergence of gender-differentiated socialization practices aimed to promote gender-appropriate social, productive, and reproductive competencies. Daughter guarding (restriction of activity, control over sleep setting) occurs in societies exhibiting high concern for female premarital chastity or, even more commonly, a desire to control a daughter's mate choice to allow for kin-arranged marriage (Whiting, Burbank, & Ratner, 1986). But whereas adolescent daughters tend to experience regulation of activity and sleep, sons often are given greater freedom. They frequently are moved into boys' or men's quarters, and it is not unusual for young unmarried men to have their own living-sleeping areas or structures where their activity is fairly unregulated and gregariousness is marked. They are also more likely to spend long periods of time out of the home for activities such as transhumant herding, crop guarding, travel, trade, visiting, raiding, or warfare. Thus, the activity and sleep schedules and settings of male adolescents and unmarried young adults tend to be the most distinctive of any sex or age group. Concomitantly, cultural tolerance of disruptive, schedule-shifted behavior of young male adults and adolescents can be fairly high.

To generalize across the life course, sleep settings may or may not be heavily sex- and age-graded, but the intensely social sleep experiences of infancy are followed by sleep in either the same bed or close proximity with others throughout most of the life-span. The number and density of cosleepers tends to be greater for females than males across the life-span, related to child care practices and regulation of sexual access (e.g., daughter or mate guarding). Men are more likely to be placed in separated settings (from the unregulatedly convivial to the harsh boot camp–like) with other men in late adolescence and early adulthood. Solitary sleep may become more likely in late age and widow- or widowerhood. The following summaries drawn from our ethnographic minisample

illustrate both cross- and intracultural variation in sleep ecologies over
the life course.

Sleep Life History Case 1: Gabra

A Gabra infant sleeps with its mother, and often the next older sibling,
on her sleeping platform in the family tent, at least until weaning at
around 3 years. Children of both sexes sleep on either parental bed,
though boys begin to move out of the tent around ages 5–6 and have
completely moved out by ages 9–10 years. In the main encampment,
boys and young men sleep with the camels on skins on the ground
in the corral, or *boma*, often next to the pen for camel calves. As they
pass puberty, boys go out to satellite camps with increasing frequency,
where schedules are fluid and they sleep with the others on the ground
around a fire in the open. Young men may go with camels to dry camps
for many years, roughing it and living on camel milk and blood. Upon
his late marriage (at age 40 years, on average), a man returns to the main
camp to live with his wife in her tent, where he has a bed in the sleeping
area opposite his wife's. He continues to go herding until he has sons
old enough to do so, and they will travel out to camps to check on the
camels. Widowers remarry, so that they have access to a domestic tent
in the main camp through later life.

In contrast to a boy, a Gabra girl, until she reaches menarche and
is married, at around age 12–15 years, sleeps in the family tent and is
carefully guarded to ensure preservation of virginity. Loss of virginity
forfeits both eligibility for marriage and bride price to the family. With
the tent her mother gives her, a young married woman joins her husband's kingroup and sets up residence in their camp. Given the large
discrepancy in marriage age, relatively early widowhood is likely. Once
her own children are married or moved out, a widow sleeps alone unless
a young grandchild or older granddaughter joins her. Tent size reflects
the life course of the family: it grows as the family grows, and shrinks
as children depart and portions are given to them, until the widow may
be left with a tiny structure just barely big enough for her.

Sleep Life History Case 2: Gebusi

Gebusi infants are born into the world of women framed by gender
inequality. Carried in a sling net bag (*bilum*) when the mother is awake
and nursed for the first 3 years, infants sleep on mats with their mothers

in the women's section of the longhouse. At dark, women, infants, and children retire to this narrow windowless space, where they do not socialize but sleep closely packed until daybreak. The women's section is partitioned along its length from the central, men's space. In this area, using resin lamps and bamboo torches, men sleep, socialize, and stay up late into the night, or all night for frequent séances. Séances are secret from women, raucous and bawdy at times. Despite the flimsiness of the partition, an ethos of absolute division of the sexes enjoins the maintenance of apparent obliviousness among women toward men's night activity. By about age 3 or 4 years, boys begin to visit the men's section at night, where they may fall asleep on their fathers' laps early on or attend fitfully to men's conversation. When they become cranky, boys may be passed to the mother over the partition. Duration and frequency of boys' stay or sleep in the men's section increases with age until they no longer enter the women's section. Girls remain with their mothers and join other women in the husband's longhouse when they marry. Sleeping arrangements do not change in older age or widow- or widowerhood.

Socialization of State Regulation

One of the more tantalizing features emerging from our preliminary foray into comparative sleep ecology is the suggestion that culturally specific sleep ecologies across ontogeny are paralleled by variation in state regulation or management of attentional systems (alertness, arousability-soothability, sleep-wake, and other state transitions). Perhaps the most striking instance of this possibility in our sample concerns the Balinese. As detailed earlier, Balinese infants are carried and held continuously by a series of care givers and are able to sleep under any circumstances. Balinese retain and exhibit this capacity as adults. Also from an early age, Balinese exhibit fear sleep (*tadoet poeles*, Mead & Macgregor, 1951) or soul loss (*kesambet*, Wikan, 1990) – precipitously and heavily falling asleep under intense emotion, when they (or even, for children, their mother) are highly anxious, badly frightened, or upset. Mead describes it thus: "As children and later as adults, Balinese go to sleep in situations that are threatening or dangerous, and sleep so soundly that they have to be shaken awake. A thief falls asleep while his case is being decided; servants fall asleep if they have broken or lost something; a child at a delivery will sleep soundly on the platform bed on which the birth is taking place. The Balinese have the expression, *tadoet poeles*, literally, 'afraid sleep,' in which sleep is represented as the natural sequence of fear, where the expected American response to fear is wakefulness" (Mead & Macgregor, 1951, p. 96). The phenomenon has not been systematically studied, but photographic documentation of fear sleep or soul loss indicates its form and persistence. In his photodocumentary ethnological study of Balinese, Bateson (1942, pl. 68, nos. 3–6, and p. 191) recorded the case Mead mentioned about a thief falling asleep in the midst of heated discussion by angry villagers during his trial. From ethnographic work undertaken nearly 50 years later, a photograph recently published by Wikan (1990, pl. 8) provides evidence that *kesambet*, or *tadoet poles*, can be established early indeed. The image captures a baby girl slumped on her side on the ground just outside a doorway. The toddler's mother had been frightened, and the child had gone into fear sleep or soul loss; the unremarkable nature of her reaction is reflected in the apparent lack of attention to the collapsed child, despite the nearby presence of several adults and children in what is obviously a busy domestic scene.

On one level, fear sleep or soul loss would appear to constitute a particularly elaborated version of a pattern widely distributed across societies, in which sleep presents a means to "check out" social intercourse (personal communication, Fredrik Barth, March 14, 1997). Such a turnoff, however, involves a major shift in attentional state maintained by complex regulatory systems not readily invoked at will; as Mead notes, this behavior contrasts sharply with American models of coping with stress through increased arousal and vigilance. Neurobiological tuning of state regulatory systems must somehow be involved, although the ontogenetic bases are at present uncertain. Thus, the Balinese case of fear sleep would appear to suggest that the state regulatory processes governing sleep-wake transitions may be somewhat differently "tuned" or organized under different sociocultural conditions. Besides fear sleep, another culturally conditioned syndrome of state regulation is the well-documented culture-bound syndrome of *latah*, argued to be an elaboration of the startle reflex (Simons & Hughes, 1985). This behavior is provoked by unexpected, forceful events (e.g., a sudden "boo!" behind one's back) and becomes elaborated through habitual teasing. Furthermore, Bali is a society that engages in extensive nighttime ritual, including pursuit of altered consciousness. Infants and children attend rituals with their parents. Parents may assist them to attain a trance as children, but by the late teens young people may engage in their own in spiritual pursuits involving meditation and cultivation of sleep deprivation and altered consciousness.

On another level, then, the case of fear sleep or soul loss raises questions concerning the impact of socialization practices and developmental ecologies on the ontogeny of arousal-attention regulation. Two other observations, less well developed, lend additional support to the notion that state regulation can be socialized in part through sleep practices. First, as noted already, Gebusi men practice engaged, sociable somnolence during séances aimed to produce trance and engagement with spirits. They also appear to become conditioned to stay awake and socially involved while on the edge of consciousness: deep sleep is risky because the spirit departs to commune with other spirits and may wander off too far. On the other hand, Gebusi women must retire daily to their narrow, dark sleeping area and cope with 10-hour periods of enforced quiet and inactivity at night: shortly after dark, they retire to the women's area and remain there quietly until dawn. Given that they sleep with their children, and given the periodic rowdiness of the men next door, it is unlikely that their nights represent unbroken bouts of sleep. Sleep behavior is hypothesized to accomplish some biologically or cognitively crucial task (Drucker-Colín, 1995; Maquet, 1995; Marks, Shaffery, Oksenberg, Speciale, & Roffwarg, 1995; Siegel, 1995), yet complementary cognitive needs subserved by other forms of rest and somnolence have rarely been considered (Lubin et al., 1976). The high prevalence of low-arousal states in traditional societies indicates large, as yet unexplored territory concerning determinants of optimal cognitive loads, arousal regulation, and needs for and values of different forms of rest (such as sleep versus daydreaming).

A second phenomenon suggesting possible culture-specific population differences in stability of state regulation is the presence of sudden unexplained nocturnal death syndrome (SUNDS) in several southeast Asian countries and Japan (Tanchaiswad, 1995). SUNDS, which occurs primarily among young adult males, has claimed more attention as U.S. incidence has increased in parallel with an influx of Asian refugees into the country. Though poorly understood, both cultural-psychological and neurological factors have been raised as contributory causes of this syndrome (Adler, 1995; Tanchaiswad, 1995). It is likely that, analogous to SIDS, a combination of factors (e.g., developmental neurological vulnerability of state regulation, stress or anxiety, smoking, or drinking) operates to produce such deaths.

The Western model of sleep status as binary (awake-asleep) may actually represent a specific cultural model that highlights the poles and ignores or disparages the intervening gradations in what is essentially a continuum of alertness. This and related issues on consciousness and attention regulation are a concern to researchers (Hobson & Stickgold, 1996). In other societies, sleep behaviorally, and perhaps conceptually, may lie on a continuum of arousal where other modes (from, for instance, disengaged semialert, to somnolence or drowsing, to dozing, to napping) are more tolerated and perhaps more prevalent. Socialization for extended nocturnal inactivity such as Gebusi women experience could represent a noninfrequent instance of chronic surplus rest, as opposed to the more heavily studied sleep deficit situation. The architecture of states of arousal and sleep in extended nocturnally inactive periods among individuals who have grown up under such conditions (as, for instance, all Gebusi do because children sleep with their mothers) merits close study. Additionally, a variety of factors (e.g., heavy workloads, chronic morbidity or parasitization, poor nutrition) influence the need for and value of extended rest.

Evolutionary Ecology of Human Sleep

The evolution of sleep and state regulation are not of central concern for the present discussion, for here we are considering the contemporary range of human variation in sleep behavior, its possible consequences and sequelae. Rather, human evolutionary history is relevant to the issues at hand insofar as it defines the set of constitutional capacities, vulnerabilities, constraints, and plasticities that undergird and structure patterns of human variability in sleep behavior. Future comparative work on human sleep needs to take such factors into account and should contribute to our understanding of the evolutionary bases of not only universals but also variation in this behavior and the associated phenomena of state regulation and emotion. For instance, there may be ontogenetic and genetic bases for variation in sleep needs that have their evolutionary bases in the geographically wide range of physical and social ecologies inhabited throughout human evolution, for ability to exploit such a broad spectrum of ecologies has clearly been and remains of high selective advantage.

At present, we point merely to the evolutionary context of sleep requirements and life-span sleep behavior development. We noted that humans need fewer hours of sleep than the number of hours of dark available throughout the year in the periequatorial regions in which our species evolved. We also noted that dark has constrained human activity, depending on technological limitations. If sleep is so valuable and dark limits the utility of wakefulness, why have humans not evolved to need more hours of sleep per day? One answer may be that many aspects of sociality and information-sharing can proceed independent of illumination; our ethnographic survey suggests this is the case in virtually all societies, and that important, meaningful "social work" goes on at night when other forms of productive work are not possible.

An even more weighty reason may involve needs for nocturnal security. As ground-dwelling, group-living, and relatively defenseless apes, sleeping humans are especially vulnerable to a host of predators, which would have placed a high premium on vigilance and generated selection pressures for sleep efficiency and against expanded sleep need. Dahl (chapter 16 in this volume) has stressed the importance of a feeling of security for sound sleep and poses the question of an evolutionary basis for sleep disturbance when conditions are perceived as insecure. Perhaps the general amount of sleep that humans require, individual differences in sleep demand, requirement of perceived security to sleep well, and developmental changes in sleep need and pattern over the life course all conduce to meeting, in the context of a social group, the need for continual vigilance or at least relative alertness throughout the night. Infants, children, adolescents, adults, elderly, and even the two sexes have diversely organized chronobiologies (Kelly, 1991; Reyner, Horne, & Reyner, 1995), differing by sleep and wake timing, latency, and patterning, thereby ensuring that someone may be aware or readily rousable at all hours.

Observed changes in sleep patterns throughout the life cycle support this notion. Imagine a small group comprising members of diverse ages. Young infants, with their unconsolidated sleep pattern and frequent cycling through waking and sleeping, will periodically cry and move throughout the night (Armstrong, Quinn, & Dadds, 1994). Earlier sleep onset and offset in an elderly member will provide early morning wakefulness, whereas the phase shift in adolescents to later sleep onset and offset (Carskadon, 1990) will provide late night coverage (while giving opportunity for social activity outside direct adult supervision [Kelly, 1991]).[9] Developmental diversity in chronobiological organization of wakefulness provides advantage to individuals living in social groups. Cosleeping or sleeping in close proximity would compound these effects. Cosleepers have been found to

[9] Surprisingly, published cross-sectional or longitudinal actigraphic studies that have focused on developmental trends from early childhood to adulthood appear to be lacking, although extensive studies are in progress (Sadeh, Hauri, Kripke, & Lavie, 1995).

coordinate activity states, sleep less deeply, and/or exhibit more night-time arousals than solitary sleepers (Pankhurst & Horne, 1994; Mosko, Richard, McKenna, & Drummond, 1996; Mosko, Richard, & McKenna, 1997). Additionally, the architecture of sleep, with sleep cycles of average 90 minutes' duration, provides cyclical variation in level of arous-ability, which is maximal during REM sleep. In our small group scenario, arousals by one member can result in transient arousals in others and thereby reduce the probability that all group members will be deeply asleep at any given time. Facultative ability to adjust depth of sleep to level of perceived security would have allowed for setting levels of rousability as required to tend fires, monitor young, and maintain environmental security throughout the night. Sensitivity of sleep onset and quality to perceived physical and social security likely reflects the evolutionary importance of security demands in sleep and of the material and social ecological means by which those demands are met.

Finally, the fluid nature of sleep-wake boundaries, absence of strict bedtimes, and long periods of involuntary inactivity that we report for traditional human societies and which likely characterized human history, suggest the need to reconsider definitions of "normal" rest and sleep patterns, reassess the standard model of sleep architecture, and review the potential value of somnolent resting states.

Comparative Sleep Ecology

Based on the cross-cultural comparative survey outlined here, we may now turn to consider sleep behavior among Western industrial societies and evaluate the generalizability of the sleep research based in such settings. Several features of sleep among Westerners emerge as distinctive and may be characterized in terms of sleep practices, sleep ecology, and ontogeny. Sleep practices distinctive among Westerners include the following:

1. Solitary sleep from early infancy, supported by cultural norms and beliefs about risk of overlying need for infant independence of autonomy, and need for sexual decorum.
2. Consolidation of sleep into a single long bout.
3. Distinct bedtimes, enforced in childhood and reinforced by highly scheduled daytime hours, for work or school, and mechanized devices for waking.

Table 6.1. Characteristics of Western Sleep Settings

Secure	Minimal Sensory Information	Stable Sensory Properties
Low risk from pathogens, predators, elements, enemies	Solitary to single cosleeper; no to moderate body contact Climate-controlled Acoustically insulated Dark, odorless Padded bed and smooth bedding	Climate-controlled Dearth/absence of disturbance (noise, movement, light)

4. Housing design and construction that provide remarkably sequestered, quiet, controlled environments for sleep in visually and acoustically isolated spaces.

These practices combine with other ecological features to produce the characteristic conditions of sleep outlined in Table 6.1.

Settings for sleep are relatively secure, not only from the physical elements but also from threatening organisms including pathogen-bearing disease vectors such as mosquitoes, fleas or lice, predators, and human enemies. By design, they provide minimal sensory stimulation. Several cultural-ecological factors are conducive to such settings. One factor includes a cultural ideal of one person per bed per room, except for cosleeping married couples (Schweder et al., 1995), with a corollary minimization of body contact in sleep. Conflict of cultural goals for contact minimization with marital norms of cosleeping has been partially mitigated for Americans by the evolution of bed size, from twin, to double, to queen, to king. Housing insulation and climate control obviate a need for vigilance to sustain thermal comfort and even ensure that sleepers will not be assailed by exogenous odors, while window coverings ensure complete darkness. Padding and bedding are extraordinarily elaborated and ideally involve a double mattress substrate of various (sometimes impressively complex) design and up to 2 foot depth, covered by a pad with various degrees of padding, and a sheet; a pillow or pillows up to 26 inches square, enveloped in cover and case; and, over the sleeper, a sheet, blankets, and/or duvet, also enclosed in cover and case.[10] Finally,

---

[10] Extensive, heavy bedding has been identified as a health risk, in relation to thermal load and risk for sudden infant death syndrome (Sawczenko & Fleming, 1996).

Table 6.2. Comparison of Contexts for Sleep

Laboratory	Non-Western
Solitary	Social
Dark/dim	Dark/dim
Silent	Noise
Climate-controlled	No/human climate control
Mattress, pillow	No mattress, pillow
Absence of fire	Fire present
Stable	Dynamic
Physically secure	Socially secure
Bounded (temporally, physically)	Fuzzily bounded (temporally, physically)

sleep contexts have highly stable sensory properties, due not only to climate control to buffer temperature, noise, and odor from without, but also to a dearth of interior sources of disturbance from noise, movement, or light.

Because their goal is to study sleep and they are located in Westernized societies, sleep laboratories have provided a faithful reflection of the particular cultural ecology of Western sleep. As noted in Table 6.2, sleep research generally involves solitary sleepers who repose on densely padded substrates, with a pillow, in dark, silent, climate-controlled settings also characterized as sensorily muted and stable, physically secure, and devoid of a fire. Hence, parallel with the distinctiveness of Western sleep, sleep laboratories present environments that mimic these features while also allowing a number of variables to be controlled or manipulated to tease out causal functional pathways (Hobson & Steriade, 1986; Hobson, 1989). These settings, although successful research paradigms for elucidating dimensions of sleep patterning, physiology, regulation, and clinical correlates, may also of necessity and at times inadvertently eliminate variation that is crucial for understanding the full potential range of "normal" sleep, as well as the causes and consequences of individual variability, normal and pathological.

The limited cross-cultural survey presented here has nonetheless amply documented that humans can and do sleep routinely under a wide variety of conditions. Standing out from this diversity, several features can be roughly generalized as contrasting with Western domestic and laboratory sleep settings (Table 6.1). It should be stressed that these are crude generalizations advanced for the sake of preliminary comparison and require empirical examination. With these caveats, "non-Western" settings may be posed as populated or social, possibly including not only people of various ages but also animals. Settings are usually dark or dim, but are less reliably quiet, vulnerable to interior and exterior sources of noise. Climate control may be absent, inherent in housing construction, or mediated by human regulation of heat sources or air circulation. Although sleep substrates generally are sufficiently elastic or padded to accommodate the body's curves and angularities, the use of heavy padding is rare and pillows or abundant coverings are uncommon. Fire is usually present in some form. Hence, non-Western sleep settings tend to be sensorily dynamic. They are also less bounded in temporal, social, or physical terms. Sleep security is generated as much or more by its social as by its merely physical features.

Recent technological innovations have taken the study of sleep and dreaming out of the laboratory and into natural settings (Mamelak & Hobson, 1989; Stickgold, Page-Schott, & Hobson, 1994; Ajilore, Stickgold, Rittenhouse, & Hobson, 1995; Sadeh & Gruber, chapter 14 in this volume), which doubtless will expand our understanding of sleep "in the wild." Notwithstanding such advances, a paradigmatic constraint remains. Our current scientific understanding of sleep reflects not only characteristics of the contexts in which it has been studied but also the properties of the people who have been studied, namely relatively wellnourished Westerners who have grown up in and are habituated to a specific set of sleep ecologies. Again, distinctive features of these ecologies may influence the sleep behavior, physiology, and architecture of the subjects and thereby mediate subject-based population-specific effects on data yielded by basic research and the models derived by them.

Table 6.3 contrasts sleepers represented in existing literature (Hobson, Spagna, & Malenka, 1978) to non-Western sleepers. Available sleep data generally are drawn from subjects who habitually sleep alone or with one other person and who have a developmental history of chronic solitary sleep. Western sleepers practice routinized bed- and wake-times strongly entrained to work or school, and again have done so throughout development. Hence, their sleep is highly bounded and consolidated, frequently restricted or curtailed by scheduling constraints, and preferably ungarnished by other forms of somnolence. Sleep is achieved

Table 6.3. Comparison of Sleep Subjects

Laboratory	Non-Western
Habitual solitary sleep/limited cosleep	Habitual social sleep, cosleep
Developmental history of chronic solitary sleep	Developmental history of chronic social sleep
"Lie down and die" model of sleep in restricted intervals; few, brief transitions	Need-bases, opportunistic, transitive model of sleep; more frequent, graduated transitions
Lifetime habituation to conditions as in lab	Lifetime habituation to dynamic sleep settings

and maintained in sensorily static and deprived (but potentially cognitively dense) conditions. In other words, the Western sleepers have lifetime habituation to many of the sleep conditions represented in the laboratory, and they tend to practice a "lie down and die" model of sleep.

By contrast, non-Western sleepers habitually engage in cosleep in shared beds and/or spaces, and they have a developmental history of chronic social sleep. Moreover, they experience fluid sleep schedules entrained to less rigid work schedules and have done so throughout development. Consequently, throughout life, their sleep is less highly temporally or ecologically bounded and consolidated, they move through sleep-wake states more often, and these transitions are more likely to be framed by periods of somnolence. Sleep onset and maintenance are achieved under sensorily dynamic settings. Depending on the society, they are more likely than are contemporary Westerners to have experienced an excess rather than restriction of available downtime, or sleep and somnolence.

To summarize, humans exhibit substantial cross-cultural diversity in sleep patterns and sleep ecologies. Age-, gender-, and status-graded practices can generate divergent sleep patterns and contexts within populations. Social, temporal, and behavioral boundaries of sleeping and waking are fluid and variably actuated; sleep is often integrated in sociality. Daily variability of sleep and activity patterns differs cross-culturally. Amount, kind, and predictability of sensory loads in sleep vary, as do the physical spaces and bedding in which sleep occurs. Nonetheless, in most of these dimensions, current Western sleep settings and behaviors appear distinctive from the dynamic settings and fluid behavior of "traditional" societies.

Sleep Ecology and Biology: Implications and Speculations

The degree of human diversity in sleep and sleep regulation remains largely undocumented, but the available evidence suggests systematic variation in distribution, length, and variability in sleep episodes. Effects of the dynamic properties of sleep settings remain to be systematically elucidated, but the possibility remains that physical, social, and temporal factors generating variation in human sleep ecology, as reviewed here, may be paralleled by variation not only in sleep behavior but also its physiology. This question deserves direct investigation in future sleep research. Possible behavioral corollaries of cross-cultural variation in sleep could include: number, duration, and pattern of sleep arousals; patterning, duration, and architecture of sleep episodes (if not the absolute amount of sleep); and variation in sleep quality and latency. Furthermore, such variation may be associated with facultative adjustment of chronobiology that is differentially patterned for sleep-entrained systems. Differences in habitual sleep behavior and ecology may either reflect or drive differentially organized state regulation – that is, regulation of states of arousal and attention. This possibility further suggests that the particularities of Western sleep ecologies may contribute to the patterns and prevalence of sleep disorders observed in those settings. More generally stated, specific cultural settings and practices may be associated with specific, distinctive risks for disorders of sleep and state regulation. Impact of sleep ecology on state regulatory systems may be both acute and long-term, mediated through ontogenetic effects. Additional comparative studies of sleep patterns and physiology across the life-span are needed to characterize whether and how such effects are produced.

Even more speculative is the possibility that variation in state regulation reflected in sleep, along dimensions such as arousability or soothability, or in latency and speed of state transitions in arousal, intercalates with variation in emotional regulatory systems. Emotion regulation is integral to intelligent, motivated, and meaningful experience and behavior (Leder, 1990; Damasio, 1994; LeDoux, 1996; Worthman, 1999). If present, such associations of cultural ecologies of sleep to such "basic" physiologic regulatory systems as sleep biology, chronobiology, state regulation, and emotion regulation would imply that these systems are partially influenced or organized through cultural ecologies operating developmentally and across the life-span. Further, these associations may argue the need for attention to cultural ecology in the explanation, prevention, and possible treatment of disorders of these systems.

For instance, the practice of solitary sleep for infants leads, among other things, to an absence of exogenous stimuli that influence breathing, cardiovascular function, and sleep architecture in the sleeping infant (McKenna et al., 1994; Mosko et al., 1996; Mosko et al., 1997). Sleep and waking states and state transitions are apparently produced by suites of state regulatory mechanisms that function as a dynamical system. Modeling of dynamical systems has demonstrated that they are organized, or "tweaked" by episodic, irregular inputs. Some investigators (Mosko et al., 1993; McKenna, 1996) have argued that cosleeping provides infants with stimuli that organize their immature systems and thereby buffer them from risk for regulatory failures in sleep over a developmentally vulnerable postnatal period. The same logic may apply to difficulties in state regulation at other times of life, including risk for mood and behavior disorders in adolescence (Dahl, Chapter 16 in this volume) or risk for sleep-associated stroke or sleep apneas in aging. Another consequence of early and chronic solitary sleep is that state regulatory systems are deprived of many opportunities to learn to achieve and maintain sleep under sensorily dynamic settings with variable, unpredictable sensory inputs. Such a developmental deficit could have two consequences. First, it may potentiate greater difficulty in state regulation (including maintenance of attention) over the day; that is, it may impede development of ability to identify, achieve, and maintain optimal states of arousal in the face of dynamic sensory loads and shifting demands for attention. Put simply, American parents put their infants to sleep under conditions of minimal sensory load, but later expect their children to titrate arousal and focus attention appropriately in a world with high sensory loads and heavy competing demands for attention. Second, early sleep practices may lead to increased difficulty in effecting desired and appropriate state transitions, as in falling asleep, waking, concentrating, or relaxing. Thus, sleep practices and ecologies may contribute to risk for sleep disorder, as well as to other difficulties of state regulation, as in mood or learning disorder.

Finally, we stress the possible effects of socioeconomic status and subcultural variation as important intrapopulation sources of variation in sleep behavior and ecology. The previous section treated "Western" societies as generalized entities and ignored their internal diversities; so, largely, has sleep research. Yet class and economics play a major role in sleep ecology by influencing virtually all of the dimensions addressed in the present analysis; the "Western" characteristics outlined here represent cultural ideals largely achieved by the more affluent but less reliably attainable by the less affluent. The housing, demography, activity patterns, and social ecology that accompany conditions such as poverty and/or high-density living influence the likelihood and nature of cosleeping, degree of social and physical security, extent of sensory buffering or disturbance (in temperature, noise, touch, smell, light, or predictability, and degree of reliable scheduling), and hence the temporal, social, and sensory boundedness of sleep. Moreover, differences across and within Western societies result in variable sleep ecologies and practices that deserve exploration beyond the small literature on infant care practices and their consequences (Lozoff, Wolf, & Davis, 1984; Schachter, Fuches, Bijur, & Stone, 1989; Abbott, 1992; Morelli et al., 1992; Gantley, Davies, & Murcote, 1993; Harkness & Super, 1996).

Conclusions

In his compendious lifework on comparative human ethnology, Eibl-Eibesfeldt (1989) overlooked sleep behavior.[11] Neglect by a founder of the scientific study of behavior simply reflects the general neglect of sleep activity by the social and behavioral sciences. The present analysis takes a first step toward redressing this oversight by sketching an analytic framework for human sleep ecology. Integrating ecologically grounded comparative studies of sleep behavior with concomitant physiologic measures in individuals across the life-span is needed to reveal the natural history of sleep. Understanding the natural history of sleep will, in turn, provide a much stronger foundation for assessment and study of sleep needs and dysfunctions in specific contexts, such as in our own society. The wide diversity of observed sleep behaviors and ecologies suggests that humans will exhibit plasticity of associated sleep physiologies and chronobiology. More speculatively, study of variation in sleep behavior and ecology may provide fresh insight into ecological bases of variation in state regulation of attention and arousal, with implications for understanding regulatory disorders,

---

[11] There is a brief nod (Eibl-Eibesfeldt, 1989, pp. 70–74) to developmental chronobiology, with reference only to sleep patterns in free-running isolation or under continuous light.

in sleep, psychopathology, and learning problems. As rapid worldwide cultural and technological change transform sleep behavior and ecology, comparative studies that probe these questions are clearly needed.

REFERENCES

Abbott S (1992). Holding on and pushing away: Comparative perspectives on an eastern Kentucky child-rearing practice. *Ethos* 20:33–65.

Adler SR (1995). Refugee stress and folk belief: Hmong sudden deaths. *Social Science and Medicine* 40(12):1623–1629.

Ajilore O, Stickgold R, Rittenhouse C, Hobson J (1995). Nightcap: Laboratory and home-based evaluation of a portable sleep monitor. *Psychophysiology* 32:92–98.

Allison, T, Cicchetti DV (1976). Sleep in mammals: Ecological and constitutional correlates. *Science* 194:732–734.

Allison T, Van Twyver H (1970). The evolution of sleep. *Natural History* 79: 56–65.

Anderson J (1984). Ethology and ecology of sleep in monkeys and apes. *Advances in the Study of Behavior* 14:165–229.

Armstrong K L, Quinn RA, Dadds MR (1994). The sleep patterns of normal children. *Medical Journal of Australia* 161:202–206.

Bailey RC, Devore I (1989). Research on the Efe and Lese populations of the Ituri forest, Zaire. *American Journal of Physical Anthropology* 78:459–471.

Bakeman R, Adamson L, Konner M, Barr R (1997). Sequential analyses of !Kung infant communication: Inducing and recruiting. In E. Amsel & K. Renninger, eds., *Change and Development: Issues of Theory, Method, and Application*, pp. 173–192. Mahwah, NJ: Lawrence Erlbaum.

Barry HI, Paxson LM (1971). Infancy and early childhood: Cross-cultural codes 2. *Ethnology* 10:466–508.

Barth F (1965). *Political Leadership among Swat Pathans.* London School of Economics Monographs on Social Anthropology, vol. 19. London: Athlone Press, University of London.

  (1975). *Ritual and Knowledge among the Baktaman of New Guinea.* New Haven: Yale University Press.

  (1981). *Features of Person and Society in Swat. Collected Essays on Pathans: Selected Essays of Fredrick Barth.* vol. 2. London: Routledge and Kegan Paul.

  (1985). *The Last Wali of Swat.* New York: Columbia University Press.

  (1993). *Balinese Worlds.* Chicago: University of Chicago Press.

Bateson G, Mead M (1942). *Balinese Character: A Photographic Analysis.* New York: New York Academy of Sciences.

Berger R, Phillips N (1995). Energy conservation and sleep. *Behav Brain Res* 69:65–73.

Bockarie MJ, Alexander N, Bockarie F, Obam E, Barnish G, Alpers G (1996). The late biting habit of parous *Anopheles* mosquitoes and pre-bedtime exposure of humans to infective female mosquitoes. *Transactions of the Royal Society of Tropical Medicine and Hygiene* 90:23–25.

Brown PJ (1981). Cultural adaptations to endemic malaria in Sardinia. *Medical Anthropology* 5:311–339.

(1986). Cultural and genetic adaptations to malaria: Problems of comparison. *Human Ecology* 14:311–332.

Burton RF (1893). *Personal Narrative of a Pilgrimage to al-Madinah and Meccah.* vol. 1. London: Tylston and Edwards.

Campbell SS, Tobler I (1984). Animal sleep: A review of sleep duration across phylogeny. *Neuroscience and Biobehavioral Reviews* 8:269–300.

Carskadon MA (1990). Patterns of sleep and sleepiness in adolescents. *Pediatrician* 17:5–12.

Chisholm J (1983). *Navajo Infancy: An Ethological Study of Child Development.* Hawthorne, NY: Aldine.

Condon R (1983). *Inuit Behavior and Seasonal Change in the Canadian Arctic.* Ann Arbor: UMI Research Press.

(1987). *Inuit Youth: Growth and Change in the Canadian Arctic.* New Brunswick, NJ: Rutgers University Press.

Dahl RE (1996). The impact of inadequate sleep on children's daytime cognitive function. *Seminars in Pediatric Neurology* 3:44–50.

Dahl RE, Ryan ND, Matty MK, Birmaher B, al-Shabbout M, Williamson DE, Kupfer DJ (1996). Sleep onset abnormalities in depressed adolescents. *Biological Psychiatry* 39:400–410.

Damasio A (1994). *Descartes' Error: Emotion, Reason, and the Human Brain.* New York: Avon Books.

d'Aquili E, Laughlin C (1979). The neurobiology of myth and ritual. In E. d'Aquili, C. Laughlin, & J. McManus, eds., *The Spectrum of Ritual*, pp. 152–182. New York: Columbia University Press.

Dowse GK, Turner KJ, Stewart GA, Alpers MP, Woolcock AJ (1985). The association between *Dermatophagoides* mites and the increasing prevalence of asthma in village communities within the Papua New Guinea highlands. *Journal of Allergy & Clinical Immunology* 75:75–83.

Drucker-Colín R (1995). The function of sleep is to regulate brain excitability in order to satisfy the requirements imposed by waking. *Behav Brain Res* 69:117–124.

Eibl-Eibesfeldt I (1989). *Human Ethology: Foundations of Human Behavior.* New York: Aldine de Gruyter.

Ferreira de Souza Aguiar G, Pereira da Silva H, Marques N (1991). Patterns of daily allocation of sleep periods: A case study in an Amazonian riverine community. *Chronobiologia* 18:9–19.

Gantley M, Davies DP, Murcote A (1993). Sudden infant death syndrome: Links with infant care practices. *British Medical Journal* 306:16–20.

Genton B, al-Yaman F, Beck HP, Hii J, Mellor S, Narara A, Gibson N, Smith T, Alpers, MP (1995). The epidemiology of malaria in the Wosera area, East Sepik Province, Papua New Guinea, in preparation for vaccine trials. I. Malariometric indices and immunity. *Ann Trop Med Parasitol* 89(4):359–376.

Grazia de Simoni, M, Imeri L, De Matteo W, Perego C, Simard S, Tarrazzino S (1995). Sleep regulation: Interactions among cytokines and classical neurotransmitters. *Advances in Neuroimmunology* 5:189–200.

Harkness S, Super CM, eds. (1996). *Parents' Cultural Belief Systems: Their Origins, Expressions, and Consequences.* New York: Guilford Press.

Hart BL (1990). Behavioral adaptation to pathogens and parasites: Five strategies. *Neurosci Biobeh Rev* 14:273–294.

Herdt G (1989). Father presence and ritual homosexuality: Paternal deprivation and masculine development in Melanesia. *Ethos* 17:326–370.

—— ed. (1982). *Rituals of Manhood.* Berkeley: University of California Press.

Hill K, Hurtado AM (1996). *Ache Life History: The Ecology and Demography of a Foraging People.* Foundations of Human Behavior. New York: Aldine de Gruyter.

Hobson J (1989). *Sleep.* New York: Scientific American Library.

Hobson J, Spagna T, Malenka R (1978). Ethology of sleep studied with time-lapse photography: Postural immobility and sleep-cycle phase in humans. *Science* 201:1251–1253.

Hobson J, Steriade M (1986). The neuronal basis of behavioral state control. In V. Mountcastle, ed., *Intrinsic Regulatory Systems of the Brain*, vol. 4, *Handbook of Physiology*, pp. 701–823. Bethesda, MD: American Physiological Society.

Hobson J, Stickgold R (1996). The conscious state paradigm: A neurocognitive approach to waking, sleeping, and dreaming. In M. Gazzaniga, ed., *The Cognitive Neurosciences*, pp. 1373–1389. Cambridge, MA: MIT Press.

Hurtado AM, Hill KR (1987). Early dry season subsistence ecology of Cuiva (Hiwi) foragers of Venezuela. *Human Ecology* 15:163–187.

—— (1990). Seasonality in a foraging society: Variation in diet, work effort, fertility, and sexual division of labor among the Hiwi of Venezuela. *Journal of Anthropological Research* 46:293–346.

Jenike M (1996). Activity reduction as an adaptive response to seasonal hunger. *Am J Hum Biol* 4:517–534.

Katz R (1982). *Boiling Energy: Community Healing among the Kalahari !Kung.* Cambridge, MA: Harvard University Press.

Kelly DD (1991). Sleep and dreaming. In E. R. Kandel, J. H. Schwartz, & T. M. Jessell, eds., *Principles of Neural Science*, pp. 792–804. New York: Elsevier.

Kelly R (1976). Witchcraft and sexual relations. In P. Brown & G. Buchbinder, eds., *Man and Woman in the New Guinea Highlands*, pp. 36–53. Washington, DC: American Anthropological Association.

—— (1993). *Constructing Inequality.* Ann Arbor: University of Michigan Press.

Knauft BM (1985a). *Good Company and Violence: Sorcery and Social Action in a Lowland New Guinea Society.* Berkeley: University of California Press.

—— (1985b). Ritual form and permutation in New Guinea: Implications of symbolic process for socio-political evolution. *American Ethnologist* 12:321–340.

Krueger J, Majde J (1995). Cytokines and sleep. *International Archives of Allergy and Immunology* 106:97–100.

Leakey L (1977). *The Southern Kikuyu before 1903.* London: Academic Press.

Leder D (1990). *The Absent Body.* Chicago: Chicago University Press.

LeDoux J (1996). *The Emotional Brain: The Mysterious Underpinnings of Emotional Life.* New York: Simon and Schuster.

Lee R B (1984). *The Dobe !Kung. Case Studies in Cultural Anthropology.* New York: Holt, Rinehart, and Winston.

Lee RB, DeVore I, eds. (1976). *Kalahari Hunter-Gatherers: Studies of the !Kung San and Their Neighbors.* Cambridge, MA: Harvard University Press.

Levy R (1973). *Tahitians: Mind and Experience in the Society Islands.* Chicago: Chicago University Press.

Lex B (1979). The neurobiology of ritual trance. In E. d'Aquili, C. Laughlin, & J. McManus, eds., *The Spectrum of Ritual*, pp. 117–151. New York: Columbia University Press.

Lozoff B, Wolf AW, Davis MS (1984). Cosleeping in urban families with young children in the United States. *Pediatrics* 74:171–182.

Lubin A, Hord D, Tracy M, Johnson L (1976). Effects of exercise, bedrest and napping on performance decrement during 40 hours. *Psychophysiology* 13:334–339.

Mamelak A, Hobson J (1989). Nightcap: A home-based sleep monitoring system. *Sleep* 12:157–166.

Maquet P (1995). Sleep function(s) and cerebral metabolism. *Behav Brain Res* 69:75–83.

Marks G, Shaffery J, Oksenberg A, Speciale S, Roffwarg H (1995). A functional role for REM sleep in brain maturation. *Behav Brain Res* 69:1–11.

Marshall L (1976). *The !Kung of Nyae Nyae.* Cambridge, MA: Harvard University Press.

McKenna JJ (1991). *Researching the Sudden Infant Death Syndrome (SIDS): The Role of Ideology in Biomedical Science.* Stony Brook, NY: Research Foundation, SUNY.

McKenna JJ, Mosko S, Richard C, Drummond S, Hunt L, Cetel MB, Arpaia J (1994). Experimental studies of infant-parent co-sleeping: Mutual psychological and behavioral influences and their relevance to SIDS (sudden infant death syndrome). *Early Human Development* 38:187–201.

(1992). Co-sleeping. In M. Carskadon, ed., *Encyclopedia of Sleep and Dreaming*, pp. 143–148. New York: Macmillan.

(1996). Sudden infant death syndrome in cross-cultural perspective: Is infant-parent cosleeping protective? *Annual Review of Anthropology* 25:201–216.

Mead M, Macgregor FC (1951). *Growth and Culture: A Photographic Study of Balinese Childhood.* New York: G. P. Putnam's Sons.

Meddis R (1983). The evolution of sleep. In A. Mayes, ed., *Sleep Mechanisms and Functions*, pp. 57–106. London: Van Nostrand Reinhold.

Mitler MM, Carskadon MA, Czeisler CA, Dement WC, Dinges DF, Graeber RC (1988). Catastrophes, sleep and public policy: Consensus report. *Sleep* 11:100–109.

Morelli G, Oppenheim D, Rogoff B, Goldsmith D (1992). Cultural variations in infant's sleeping arrangements: Questions of independence. *Developmental Psychology* 28: 604–613.

Mosko S, McKenna J, Dickel M, Hunt L (1993). Parent-infant cosleeping: The appropriate context for the study of infant sleep and implications for sudden infant death syndrome (SIDS) research. *Journal of Behavioral Medicine* 16:589–610.

Mosko S, Richard C, McKenna J (1997). Infant arousals during mother-infant bed sharing: Implications for infant sleep and sudden infant death syndrome research. *Pediatrics* 100:841–849.

Mosko S, Richard C, McKenna J, Drummond S (1996). Infant sleep architecture during bedsharing and possible implications for SIDS. *Sleep* 19:677–684.

Nakazawa M, Obtsuka R, Kawabe T, Hongo T, Suzuki T, Inaoka T, Akimichi T, Kano S, Suzuki M (1994). Differential malaria prevalence among villages of the Gidra in lowland Papua New Guinea. *Tropical and Geographical Medicine* 46:350–354.

Paige KE, Paige JM (1981). *The Politics of Reproductive Ritual*. Berkeley: University of California Press.

Pankhurst F, Horne J (1994). The influence of bed partners on movement during sleep. *Sleep* 17:308–315.

Potts R (1996a). *Humanity's Descent: The Consequences of Ecological Instability*. New York: Morrow.

(1996b). Evolution and climate variability. *Science* 273:922–923.

Prussin L (1995). *African Nomadic Architecture: Space, Place and Gender*. Washington, DC: Smithsonian Institution Press.

Reyner L, Horne J, Reyer L (1995). Gender- and age-related differences in sleep determined by home-recorded sleep logs and actimetry from 400 adults. *Sleep* 18:127–134.

Sadeh A, Hauri P, Kripke D, Lavie P (1995). The role of actigraphy in the evaluation of sleep disorders. *Sleep* 18:288–302.

Salzarulo P, Fagioli I (1995). Sleep for development or development for waking? Some speculations from a human perspective. *Behav Brain Res* 69:23–27.

Sawczenko A, Fleming PJ (1996). Thermal stress, sleeping position, and the sudden infant death syndrome. *Sleep* 19:S267–270.

Schachter FF, Fuches ML, Bijur P, Stone RK (1989). Cosleeping and sleep problems in Hispanic-American urban young children. *Pediatrics* 84:522–530.

Schieffelin E (1976). *The Sorrow of the Lonely and the Burning of the Dancers*. New York: St. Martin's Press.

Schlegel A, Barry H (1991). *Adolescence: An Anthropological Inquiry*. New York: Free Press.

Schweder RA, Jensen LA, Goldstein WM (1995). Who sleeps by whom revisited. In J. J. Goodnow, P. J. Miller, & F. Kessel, eds., *Cultural Practices as Contexts for Development*, vol. 67, *New Directions for Child Development*, pp. 21–39. San Francisco: Jossey-Bass.

Shostak M (1981). *Nisa: The Life and Works of a !Kung Woman*. Cambridge, MA: Harvard University Press.

Siegel J (1995). Phylogeny and the function of REM sleep. *Behav Brain Res* 69:29–34.

Simons RC, Hughes CC, eds. (1985). *The Culture-Bound Syndromes*. Dordrecht: D. Reidl Publishing.

Stickgold R, Page-Schott E, Hobson J (1994). A new paradigm for dream research: Mentation reports following spontaneous arousal from REM and NREM sleep recorded in a home setting. *Consciousness Cognition* 3:16–29.

Super C, Harkness S (1994). The cultural regulation of temperament-environment interactions. *Researching Early Childhood* 2:59–84.

Super C, Harkness S, van Tijen N, van der Vlugt E, Fintelman M, Kijkstra J (1996). The three R's of Dutch childrearing and the socialization of infant arousal. In S. Harkness & C. Super, eds., *Parents' Cultural Belief Systems*, pp. 447–465. New York: Guilford Press.

Tanchaiswad W (1995). Is sudden unexplained nocturnal death a breathing disorder? *Psychiatry Clinical Neuroscience* 49(2):111–114.

Tobler I (1995). Is sleep fundamentally different between mammalian species? *Behav Brain Res* 69:35–41.

Trevathan WR, McKenna JJ (1994). Evolutionary environments of human birth and infancy: Insights to apply to contemporary life. *Children's Environments* 11:88–104.

Turner KJ, Stewart GA, Woolcock AJ, Green W, Alpers MP (1988). Relationship between mite densities and the prevalence of asthma: Comparative studies in two populations in the Eastern Highlands of Papua New Guinea. *Clinical Allergy* 18:331–340.

Walsh J, Shweitzer P, Anch A, Muehlbach M, Jenkins N, Dickins Q (1994). Sleepiness/alertness on a simulated night shift following sleep at home with triazolam. *Sleep* 14:140–146.

Whiting JWM (1981). Environmental constraints on infant care practices. In R. H. Munroe, R. L. Munroe, & B. B. Whiting, eds., *Handbook of Cross-Cultural Human Development*, pp. 155–179. New York: Garland.

Whiting JWM, Burbank V, Ratner M (1986). The duration of maidenhood across cultures. In J. Lancaster & B. Hamburg, eds., *School-Age Pregnancy and Parenthood*, pp. 273–302. New York: Aldine de Gruyter.

Whiting JWM, Landauer T, Jones T (1968). Infantile immunization and adult stature. *Child Development* 39:58–67.

Whiting JWM, Whiting BB (1975). Aloofness and intimacy of husbands and wives. *Ethos* 3:183–207.

Wikan U (1990). *Managing Turbulent Hearts: A Balinese Formula for Living.* Chicago: University of Chicago Press.

Wolf A, Lozoff B, Latz S, Paludetto R (1996). Parental theories in the management of young children's sleep in Japan, Italy, and the United States. In S. Harkness & C. Super, eds., *Parents' Cultural Belief Systems*, pp. 364–384. New York: Guilford Press.

Worthman CM (1999). Emotion: you can feel the difference. In A. Hinton, ed., *Beyond "Nature or Nurture": Biocultural Approaches to the Emotions*, pp. 41–74. Cambridge: Cambridge University Press.

7. Sleep Patterns of High School Students Living in São Paulo, Brazil

MIRIAM ANDRADE AND L. MENNA-BARRETO

Several authors have verified that adolescents' sleep patterns exhibit some special features that distinguish them from other age cohorts. In summary, they show a sleep phase delay compared with patterns in younger children, a more irregular sleep schedule across the week, and a shorter sleep length on weekdays (Anders, Carskadon, & Dement, 1980; Rugg-Gunn, Hackett, Appleton, & Eastoe, 1984; Strauch & Meier, 1988). Despite the reduced amount of sleep on weekdays, the need for sleep does not decrease and adolescents tend to extend sleep on weekends and holidays (Levy, Gray-Donald, Leech, Zvagulis, & Pless, 1986; Strauch & Meier, 1988; Andrade, Benedito-Silva, Domenice, Arnhold, & Menna-Barreto, 1993; Szymczak, Jasinska, Pawlak, & Zwierzkowska, 1993). They show a high incidence of daytime sleepiness complaints, trouble in falling asleep at night, and difficulty in waking up in the morning (Bearpark, 1986; Andrade, Benedito-Silva, Domenice, Arnhold, & Menna-Barreto, 1993; Saarenpää-Heikkilä, Rintahaka, Laippala, & Koivikko, 1995).

Various factors may relate to adolescents' sleep patterns, probably many of them interacting with one another. Factors include an increase of school and social commitments (Allen, 1992; Manber et al., 1995); psychological variables such as depression, anxiety, and worry (Price, Coates, Thoresen, & Grinstead 1978; Bearpark, 1986; Carskadon, Seifer, Davis, & Acebo, 1991); and ontogenetic changes in the mechanisms of the biological clock. In a previous study, we followed a group of

We are grateful for the collaboration of the students, teachers, and school staff of Centro Específico de Formação e Aperfeiçoamento do Magistério–Butantã, São Paulo, SP, Brazil. Conselho Nacional de desenvolvimento Científico e Tecnológico (CNPq) and Coordenadoria de Aperfeiçoamento de Pessoal de Nível Superior (CAPES) supported this work.

118

12- to 13-year-old Brazilian adolescents for a period of one and a half years and observed significant sleep phase delays on weekends only in the group of adolescents that changed their pubertal stage (Andrade, Menna-Barreto, Benedito-Silva, Domenice, & Arnhold, 1993). The maturational change in the phase of circadian rhythm has also been investigated by means of morningness-eveningness inventories. Carskadon, Vieira, and Acebo (1993) compared the scores of a morningness-eveningness inventory to the bedtime and wake-up time of adolescents of different maturational status. They found that bedtime was significantly associated with pubertal stages, with the more mature adolescents showing later bedtimes. Other surveys with Australian adolescents (Bearpark, 1986) and Japanese adolescents (Ishihara, Honma, & Miyake, 1990) also showed an increase of eveningness character with age. Recently, Carskadon and colleagues (1997) provided additional support to the hypothesis of circadian phase delay during puberty, showing positive correlations of age and Tanner maturational stages with melatonin offset phase.

Despite the evidence of the effect of many factors on the expression of adolescents' sleep-wake cycle, the relative contribution of each one is not well established. Sleep-wake cycle patterns observed in adolescents reflect underlying endogenous and exogenous components of biological rhythmicity. While the endogenous component is a species' feature, the exogenous one may differ according to geophysical conditions and social organization. Since one of the strongest synchronizers of human rhythms is the temporal organization of social activities, sleep-wake cycle patterns are closely related to adolescents' life-styles. Comparisons among different populations provide a general understanding of the characteristics of this age group as well as adolescents' sleep strategies in distinct situations, the sleep-wake cycle's flexibility, and the consequences of modifying sleep patterns. The present work surveys high school students who live in São Paulo City, Brazil, an urban area of approximately 9,810,000 inhabitants, at a latitude of 23 degrees south. The aim of the study is to investigate the temporal patterns of sleep-wake cycle in high school students as well as sleep complaints that may be associated with them.

Method

Ninety-nine female high school students, mean age 16.7 years ± 1.8 years (67% aged 14 to 16 years), participated in this study. They were from middle- to lower-class families and attended the same public school from 7:15 A.M. to 5:05 P.M., Monday to Friday. The general goals of the study were explained to the students, and written consents from their parents were obtained. The adolescents answered a morningness-eveningness inventory and a sleep questionnaire in the classroom in May 1994. The name of the student was identified in the questionnaires. No payment was awarded for participation in the survey.

A Portuguese version of Horne and Östberg's morningness-eveningness inventory was used in the present study (Horne & Östberg, 1976). The result of this inventory is a score ranging from 16 to 86 points: the lower the score the more evening type the person is.

The sleep inventory contained 47 questions that covered the following aspects: health status, sleep complaints, home conditions, and sleep schedules and habits. Sleep complaint answers were provided in a four-choice format: (a) more than once per week, (b) once or more per month, (c) once or more per year, (d) less than once per year. Habitual parasomnia occurrence was assessed by a single question with a multiple-choice answer showing eight types of parasomnia: bruxism, restless sleep ("moving a lot"), sleeptalking, snoring, somnambulism, head bumping, leg movements, and screaming. Sleep quality and wake-up readiness in the morning were evaluated by means of a 10-centimeter visual/analog scale, with the expressions "very good" on the left and "very bad" on the right for the sleep quality scale, and "not difficult" on the left and "very difficult" on the right for the wake-up readiness scale.

Sleep schedules, sleep quality, and wake-up readiness on school days and nonschool days were compared (paired T-Student test). The incidence of spontaneous morning awakening on weekdays and on weekends was analyzed by means of McNemar test. Students were divided into two groups according to their sleep length on weekdays ($<$ 8 hours, n = 55, and $\geq$ 8 hours, n = 44), and daytime sleepiness reports ("more than once per week" plus "once or more per month" n = 49; and rare or no complaint, n = 50). Contingency tables were prepared for sleep-length groups and daytime-sleepiness report groups versus prevalence of sleep complaints. Differences between group means were investigated using unpaired T-Student test. We also investigated the association between daytime sleepiness reports and health status, home conditions, and eveningness scores.

Results

Sleep Complaints

Of the 99 adolescents, 38% had no frequent sleep complaint, 31% reported one sleep problem, 18% reported two sleep problems, and 13% reported three or four types of problems occurring "more than once per week" plus "once or more per month." No adolescent reported taking medicine due to sleep problems. The prevalence of a "more than once per week" complaint of daytime sleepiness was 45%, trouble in falling asleep 14%, night wake-ups 6%, nightmares 4%, and sleep breathing problems 2% (Figure 7.1). The majority of the adolescents (84%) reported at least one type of habitual parasomnia: 70% restless sleep ("moving a lot"), 32% sleeptalking, 10% leg movements, 8% somnambulism, 8% bruxism, 5% snoring, 5% head bumping, and 3% screaming. Sleep problems in at least one person of the family were reported by 42% of the students and, according to adolescents' descriptions, the most common ones were insomnia (n = 13) and night wake-ups (n = 10). No participant reported a history of narcolepsy.

Adolescents who reported frequent daytime sleepiness showed a higher prevalence of sleep problems in general (32% versus 12%, $\chi^2 = 5.7$; p = 0.02) and a tendency for a higher incidence of difficulty in falling asleep at night (35% versus 18%, $\chi^2 = 3.6$; p = 0.06) and restless sleep (79% versus 63%, $\chi^2 = 3.2$; p = 0.07) when compared with the students who did not report frequent daytime sleepiness. We did not

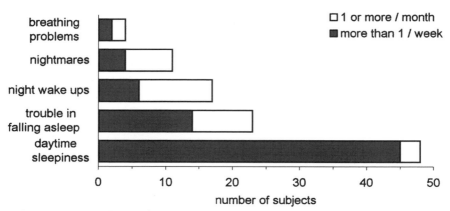

Figure 7.1. Prevalence of sleep complaints reported: more than once per week, once or more per month (n = 99).

find any relation between daytime sleepiness and other types of sleep complaints and parasomnias.

Health Status and Home Conditions

Health problems were reported by 29% of the adolescents surveyed, chiefly sinusitis and rhinitis (n = 10), orthopedic problems (n = 7), different kinds of allergy (n = 7), bronchitis (n = 5), and digestive problems (n = 4). There was no difference in the prevalence of health problems in general between the adolescents who reported frequent daytime sleepiness and the ones who did not report daytime sleepiness (35% versus 25%, $\chi^2 = 1.1$; p = 0.28). The two groups also showed similar incidence of breathing problems (25% versus 16%, $\chi^2 = 1.3$; p = 0.25). The prevalence of habitual alcohol consumption among the adolescents was the same (18%) between the adolescents who reported frequent daytime sleepiness and the ones who did not report daytime sleepiness. Half of the sample reported drinking coffee, 37% of whom reported difficulty in falling asleep, while 16% of the adolescents who did not drink coffee reported the same problem ($\chi^2 = 5.5$; p < 0.05).

The number of people living at the adolescent's house ranged from 2 to 11; in 89% of the cases, 2 to 6 people lived at the same house. About 18% of the adolescents slept alone in the bedroom, 69% shared their bedroom with one or two people, and 13% shared with three to seven people. Just 1% of the adolescents complained of a very noisy bedroom and 2% of a very quiet bedroom. Home conditions were similar between adolescents who reported frequent daytime sleepiness and the ones who did not report daytime sleepiness. The mean number of people living at an adolescent's house (4.0 ± 1.7 versus 3.9 ± 1.5, t = 0.26; p = 0.80) and the number of people sleeping in the same bedroom (1.3 ± 1.1 versus 1.5 ± 1.1, t = −0.57; p = 0.57) were similar for both groups. The majority of the students who reported frequent daytime sleepiness as well as those who did not report daytime sleepiness considered their bedrooms dark (88% versus 86%, $\chi^2 = 0.1$; p = 0.80) and silent (90% but versus 98%, but not enough "noisy" cases to apply chi-square test).

Bedtime, Wake-up Time, and Sleep Length on Weekdays and Weekends

There were significant changes in sleep patterns from weekends to weekdays. Students went to sleep almost 2 hours earlier on weekdays

Table 7.1. Occurrence of Phase Shifts of the Sleep-Wake Cycle from Weekdays to Weekends (n = 99)

Phase Shift	Bedtime, %	Wake Time, %
Advance	10.2	0.0
No modification	7.1	2.0
Delay up to 2.8 hours	59.2	32.3
Delay from 3 to 9 hours	23.5	65.7
TOTAL	100.0	100.0

than on weekends (10:04 P.M. ± 60 minutes versus 11:54 P.M. ± 114 minutes, t = 9.0, p < 0.00001), woke up 3.5 hours earlier (5:48 A.M. ± 32 minutes versus 9:19 A.M. ± 95 minutes, t = 23.5, p < 0.00001), and reduced their sleep length by 1.7 hours (7.7 hours ± 70 minutes versus 9.4 hours ± 108 minutes t = −8.0, p < 0.00001). They reported worse sleep quality (7.7 ± 2.7 versus 8.6 ± 2.3, t = −3.5, p < 0.001) and more difficulty in waking up (6.4 ± 3.3 versus 7.7 ± 3, t = −3.8, p < 0.001) on schooldays than weekends. More students woke up spontaneously on weekends (86%) than on weekdays (18%) (McNemar test χ^2 = 60.7; p < 0.0001). About 22% reported habitual napping, 11% napping more than once per week. There were different weekdays to weekends patterns: some students advanced their sleep onset (10%), others showed no change (7%), some delayed it as long as 2.8 hours (59%), and others reported a 3- to 9-hour delay (23%). No student advanced sleep offset; 2% maintained their wake-up hour, 32% delayed it up to 2.8 hours, and 66% showed a 3- to 9-hour delay (Table 7.1). A sleep-length decrease on weekends was reported by 17% of the students, 3% reported the same amount of sleep as on weekdays, 49% increased sleep length up to 2.8 hours, and 31% had an extra sleep amount of 3 to 8 hours (Table 7.2).

Table 7.2. Occurence of Nocturnal Sleep Length Modification from Weekdays to Weekends (n = 99)

Modification	Sleep Length, %
Decrease	17.4
No modification	3.0
Increase up to 2.8 hours	49.0
Increase from 3 to 8 hours	30.6
TOTAL	100.0

Table 7.3. Comparison between Sleep Characteristics of Longer Sleepers on Weekdays (8 hours) and Shorter Sleepers (<8 hours) by Means of t-Student Test

Characteristic	Shorter Sleepers (mean ± SD)	Longer Sleepers (mean ± SD)	p^a
Weekdays			
Bedtime (hh:mm)	22:47 ± 41 min	21:11 ± 33 min	<.00001
Wake time (hh:mm)	5:43 ± 31 min	5:45 ± 34 min	<.10
Sleep length	6.9 h ± 49 min	8.7 h ± 2.0	<.005
Sleep quality^b	7.0 ± 2.9	6.5 ± 3.5	ns
Wake up readiness^c	6.3 ± 3.2	6.5 ± 3.5	ns
Weekends			
Bedtime (hh:mm)	24:01 ± 114 min	23:45 ± 117 min	ns
Wake time (hh:mm)	9:14 ± 103 min	9:26 ± 85 min	ns
Sleep length	9.2 h ± 100 min	9.7 h ± 116 min	ns
Sleep quality^b	8.3 ± 2.4	9.0 ± 2.1	ns
Wake up readiness^c	7.4 ± 3.3	8.1 ± 2.6	ns

^{a} ns = probability > .10.
^{b} Very good = 10, very bad = 0.
^{c} Not difficult = 10, very difficult = 0.

Relationships between Sleep Patterns and Sleep Complaints

Longer sleepers on weekdays (≥ 8 hours) fell asleep earlier ($t = -12.4$; $p < 0.00001$), reported better sleep quality ($t = 3.17$; $p < 0.005$), and had a tendency to wake slightly later ($t = 1.8$, $p = 0.08$) than shorter sleepers (< 8 hours) on weekdays (Table 7.3). The prevalence of general sleep complaints was higher for shorter sleepers (30% versus 11%, $\chi^2 = 5.0$; $p < 0.05$), as were the incidence of trouble in falling asleep (36% versus 14%, $\chi^2 = 6.5$; $p < 0.05$) and daytime sleepiness (60% versus 41%, $\chi^2 = 3.6$; $p = 0.06$).

As compared with those who were not sleepy, adolescents who reported daytime sleepiness reported a greater increase of sleep length on weekends (132 versus 73 minutes; $t = -2.4$; $p = 0.02$) and showed a tendency to delay bedtime to a lesser degree on weekends compared with weekdays (87 versus 130 minutes, $t = 1.8$; $p = 0.07$). They reported more difficulty in waking up in the morning both on weekdays (5.4 ± 3.3 versus 7.4 ± 3.0, $t = 3.1$; $p < 0.005$) and on weekends (6.6 ± 3.9 versus 8.7 ± 2.1, $t = 3.7$; $p < 0.0005$), and worst sleep quality on weekdays (6.9 ± 3.0 versus 8.5 ± 2.1, $t = 2.9$; $p < 0.005$). The morningness-eveningness score was lower in adolescents who reported frequent daytime sleepiness (53 ± 8 versus 57 ± 8, $t = 2.6$; $p = 0.02$).

Discussion

We analyzed habitual sleep features of a group of high school students who started classes early in the morning (7:15 A.M.) and did not work. Because they studied full-time and received a scholarship, school activities were their main daily occupation, and just 11% practiced sports or attended classes after school. Most of the adolescents did not have health problems or take medication. We believe that the general sleep patterns described are typical of healthy female adolescents of this age group.

Daytime sleepiness was the most prevalent (45%) and most frequent complaint observed in this study. A high incidence of daytime sleepiness complaints has also been reported in studies with different adolescent samples. For instance, Lugaresi, Cirignotta, Zucconi, Mondini, Lenzi, and Coccagna (1983) observed that whereas daytime sleepiness was reported by 9% of a sample of an Italian population, the prevalence was much higher (34%) in the 15- and 16-year-old cohort of the same sample. Saarenpää-Heikkilä et al. (1995) found that daytime sleepiness ("always" plus "frequently") was reported by 18% of 9- to 13-year-old Finnish students and the incidence increased to 24% in the 13- to 16-year-old bracket.

A problem falling asleep was the second most prevalent sleep complaint: 14% of the students reported this problem more than once per week. Tynjälä, Kannas, and Välimaa (1993) found a prevalence of 11% to 27% (at least twice per week) in European students aged 15 to 16 years. Bearpark (1986) observed that 29% of 16- to 17-year-old adolescents reported a problem falling asleep, and she found a relation between this complaint and morningness-eveningnesss character. The incidence of experiencing a problem in falling asleep as well as the prevalence of evening types increased when comparing younger (10- to 11-year-old age bracket) to older (16 to 17 years of age) Australian students.

In the present survey, the students reported no family history of narcolepsy and did not report medicine consumption related to sleep problems. The group of adolescents who reported frequent daytime sleepiness and the group with rare or no sleepiness complaint showed no differences in health status and home conditions. On the other hand, frequent daytime sleepiness was related to a greater prevalence of sleep complaints in general, tendencies toward higher incidence of a problem falling asleep and restless sleep, and lower scores (greater eveningness) on the morningness-eveningness inventory. The eveningness trend of the students with frequent daytime sleepiness may be associated with their higher incidence of having a problem falling asleep, because their spontaneous sleep onset phase might be later than their actual retiring schedule. A problem falling asleep was also associated with higher consumption of coffee, which in turn could reflect a strategy to avoid daytime sleepiness. Previous studies have shown the influence of coffee consumption on sleep onset phase delay, sleep length decrease, and worse sleep quality (Karacan, Thornby, Anch, Boot, Williams, & Salis, 1976; Hicks, Hicks, Reyes, & Cheers, 1983). A schematic representation of the relations between sleep patterns and complaints of high school students observed in our survey is shown in Figure 7.2.

Sleep patterns of Brazilian students were similar (though not identical) to those obtained by means of questionnaires with European (Tynjälä et al., 1993) and American students (Manber et al., 1995) of same age group. Bedtime of Brazilian students was within the range observed in European adolescents aged 15 to 16 years: from 9:48 P.M. to 10:36 P.M. depending on the country. Compared with data in the study of Manber et al. (1995), mean bedtime and wake-up time on weekdays of Brazilian students were half an hour earlier. Weekend sleep schedules of the Brazilian group, on the other hand, were very similar to those of American high school students. Brazilian adolescents' sleep lengths were also very similar to those reported by Manber et al. (1995) on weekends (9.4 versus 9.3 hours), but about 20 minutes shorter on weekdays. Although comparisons between studies must be done with caution because of different methodologies and sample compositions, weekend sleep patterns suggest a similar sleep-wake cycle phase and need for sleep, whereas weekday data probably point out different temporal organization of daily activities, such as school schedules.

Some age tendencies can be revealed when we compare the present study with two other surveys about sleep patterns of Brazilian students (Table 7.4). High school students went to bed at the same time but woke up about 0.5 hour earlier and slept 0.5 hour less on weekdays compared with a younger cohort of female students (12 to 13 years of age) who also lived in São Paulo City and started classes at 7:20 A.M. (Andrade, 1991). On the other hand, bedtime of high school students was 0.8 hour earlier compared with that of college female students (17 to 21 years of age) who studied in the morning (Machado, Varella, & Andrade, 1998). Delays of bedtime and wake-up time on weekends were found in all age groups, but older students showed greater delays. Mean sleep length on weekends was very similar comparing middle school students (9.5 hours) and high school students (9.4), and about 1 hour longer than the sleep length of college students (8.6). The finding that high school students slept less

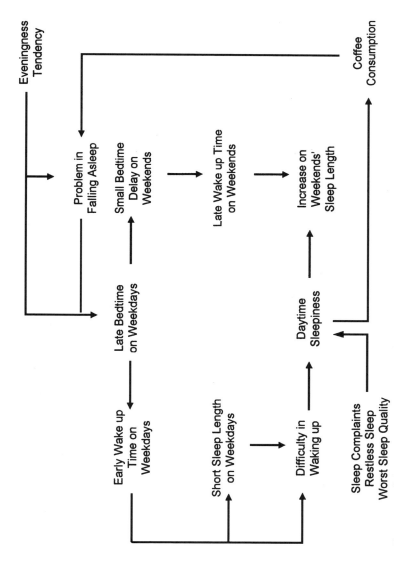

Figure 7.2. Schematic representation of the relations between sleep patterns and sleep complaints.

Table 7.4. Sleep Schedules on Weekdays and Weekends in Three Age
Brackets of Brazilian Female Students Who Began Classes Early
Morning and Did Not Work after School

Characterstic	Middle School 12–13 years (n = 32)	High School 14–16 years (n = 99)	College 17–21 years (n = 47)
Weekdays			
Bedtime (hh:mm)	22:05 ± 50 min	22:04 ± 60 min	22:52 ± 69 min
Wake time (hh:mm)	6:16 ± 16 min	5:48 ± 32 min	6:16 ± 20 min
Sleep length	8.2 h ± 55 min	7.7 h ± 70 min	7.4 h ± 72 min
Weekends			
Bedtime (hh:mm)	23:15 ± 61 min	23:54 ± 114 min	1:20 ± 109 min
Wake time (hh:mm)	8:45 ± 77 min	9:19 ± 95 min	9:55 ± 89 min
Sleep length	9.5 h ± 64 min	9.4 h ± 108 min	8.6 h ± 95 min

Note: Values are means ± SD.

than middle school students on weekdays but slept the same amount
on weekends agrees with previous work done with American students
(Manber et al., 1995). It corroborates the suggestion of other authors
(Strauch and Meier, 1988; Carskadon et al., 1993) that as adolescents
grow older, partial sleep deprivation becomes a chronic situation.

The greater prevalence of sleep complaints found in the shorter sleepers evinces the schoolday sleep restriction consequences. Sleep length on
weekdays was related to the incidence of sleep problems in general and
to sleep quality. The shorter the sleep length, the higher the incidence of
the sleep problems, including difficulty falling asleep, daytime sleepiness, and worse sleep quality. Sleep extension on weekends occurred
even for the group of adolescents who managed to sleep longer than
8 hours on weekdays, suggesting that the amount of sleep on weekdays
was still insufficient.

Bedtime, wake-up time, and sleep length on weekends were very similar between the adolescents who reported frequent daytime sleepiness
and the group with rare or no complaints. The fact that the adolescents
who reported frequent daytime sleepiness increased sleep length more
and showed a smaller bedtime delay on weekends suggests that they
were more sleep-deprived during weekdays than the group with rare or
no complaints. Sleep deprivation could be partially caused by sleep onset phase position, because 35% of the adolescents with frequent daytime
sleepiness reported difficulty in falling asleep. Probably they have more

difficulty in advancing their schedules on weekdays. In our question-naire, we did not discriminate sleep onset problems according to the day of the week, and it would be interesting to verify if there is a lower incidence of difficulty in falling asleep when adolescents are more free to chose their schedules. Moreover, the lower scores of morningness-eveningness inventory of the adolescents with frequent daytime sleepiness supports distinct sleep phase allocation even in a group with very few extreme types (83% were classified as intermediate types).

It is striking that just one student had the habit of maintaining bedtime and wake-up time from weekdays to weekends. About 91% of the adolescents showed sleep onset and offset phase shifts, and there were considerable delays mainly in wake-up time: 66% of the students woke up 3 or more hours later on weekends. The consequences of irregular sleep schedules were recently studied by Manber, Bootzin, Acebo, and Carskadon (1996) in a sample of college students. According to their findings, daytime sleepiness was reduced when students kept a regular sleep-wake schedule. The majority of the adolescents studied in our survey showed both sleep reduction on weekdays and irregular sleep-wake schedules. The role of school schedules seems to be important due to the greater displacement of wake-up time compared with bedtime. Even the 10% of students who reported earlier bedtime on weekends did not wake up earlier.

The delayed sleep phase, irregular sleep time, and daytime sleepiness pattern described by other authors was also observed in the present survey. Additionally, although it represents a general trend for this age group, its expression was more pronounced in a part of the sample. The sleep-wake cycle characteristics were different among adolescents even though they were submitted to the same school schedules. In fact, adolescents exhibited different phase shift types (advance or delay) and magnitude, sleep onset and/or sleep offset displacements and amounts of sleep, yielding distinct individual patterns. We assume that each pattern brings on different consequences that are still not well understood. Even though not all students showed the same pattern, some general risk factors have been identified and should be explored in order to avoid impairment of alertness, performance, and general well-being. Concurrently, an investigation of the interindividual differences that might contribute to the capacity of adolescents to manipulate their sleep schedules should provide a better knowledge of adolescents' sleep needs and complaints.

130   MIRIAM ANDRADE AND L. MENNA-BARRETO

REFERENCES

Allen RP (1992). Social factors associated with the amount of school week sleep lag for seniors in an early starting suburban high school. *Sleep Res* 21:114.

Anders TF, Carskadon MF, Dement WC (1980). Sleep and sleepiness in children and adolescents. *Pediatr Clin N Am* 27:29–43.

Andrade MMM (1991). Ciclo vigília-sono de adolescentes: um estudo longitudinal [Sleep-wake cycle in adolescents: A longitudinal study]. Master's thesis, University of São Paulo.

Andrade MMM, Benedito-Silva AA, Domenice S, Arnhold IPJ, Menna-Barreto L (1993). Sleep characteristics of adolescents: A longitudinal study. *J Adolesc Health* 14:401–406.

Andrade MMM, Menna-Barreto L, Benedito-Silva AA, Domenice S, Arnhold IPJ (1993). Sleep characteristics following change in adolescent maturity status. *Sleep Res* 22:521.

Bearpark HM (1986). Sleep/wake disturbances in Sydney adolescents: A survey of prevalence and correlates. Master's thesis, Macquarie University, Sydney.

Carskadon MA, Acebo C, Richardson GS, Tate BA, Seifer R (1997). An approach to studying circadian rhythms of adolescent humans. *J Biol Rhythms* 12:278–279.

Carskadon MA, Seifer R, Davi, SS, Acebo C (1991). Sleep, sleepiness, and mood in college-bound high school seniors. *Sleep Research* 20:175.

Carskadon MA, Vieira C, Acebo C (1993). Association between puberty and delayed phase preference. *Sleep* 16:258–262.

Hicks AR, Hicks CJ, Reyes JR, Cheers Y (1983). Daily caffeine use and the sleep of college students. *Bull Psychon Soc* 21:24–25.

Horne J, Österberg O (1976). A self-assessment questionnaire to determine morningness-eveningness in human circadian rhythms. *Int J Chronobiol* 4:97–110.

Ishihara K, Honma Y, Miyake S (1990). Investigation of the children's version of morningness-eveningness questionnaire with primary and junior high school pupils in Japan. *Percept Moth Skills* 71, pt. 2:1353–1354.

Karacan I, Thornby JI, Anch M, Boot GH, Williams RL, Salis PJ (1976). Dose-related sleep disturbances induced by coffee and caffeine. *Clin Pharmacol Ther* 20:682–689.

Levy D, Gray-Donald, K, Leech J, Zvagulis I, Pless B (1986). Sleep patterns and problems in adolescents. *J Adolesc Health Care* 7:386–389.

Lugaresi E, Cirignotta F, Zucconi M, Mondini S, Lenzi PL, Coccagna G (1983). Good and poor sleepers: An epidemiological survey of the San Marino population. In C. Guilleminault & E. Lugaresi, eds., *Sleep/wake Disorders: Natural History, Epidemiology, and Long-Term Evolution*, pp. 1–12. New York, Raven Press.

Machado ERS, Varella VBR, Andrade MMM (1998). The influence of study's schedules and work on the sleep-wake cycle of college students. *Biol Rhythm Res* 29:578–584.

Manber R, Bootzin RR, Acebo C, Carskadon MA (1996). The effects of regularizing sleep-wake schedules on daytime sleepiness. *Sleep* 19:432–441.

Manber R, Pardee RE, Bootzin RR, Kuo T, Rider AM, Rider SP, Bergstrom L (1995). Changing sleep patterns in adolescence. *Sleep Res* 24:106.

Price VA, Coates TJ, Thoresen CE, Grinstead OA (1978). Prevalence and correlates of poor sleep among adolescents. *Am J Dis Child* 132:583–586.

Rugg-Gunn AJ, Hackett AF, Appleton DR, Eastoe JE (1984). Bedtimes of 11- to 14-year-old children in north-east England. *J Biosoc Sci* 16(2):291–297.

Saarenpää-Heikkilä OA, Rintahaka PJ, Laippala PJ, Koivikko MJ (1995). Sleep habits and disorders in Finnish schoolchildren. *J Sleep Res* 4:173–182.

Strauch I, Meier B (1988). Sleep need in adolescents: A longitudinal approach. *Sleep* 11:378–386.

Szymczak JT, Jasinska M, Pawlak E, Zwierzykowska M (1993). Annual and weekly changes in the sleep-wake rhythm of school children. *Sleep* 16: 433–435.

Tynjälä J, Kannas L, Välimaa R (1993). How young Europeans sleep. *Health Education Res* 8:69–80.

8. Sleep Patterns and Daytime Function in Adolescence: An Epidemiological Survey of an Italian High School Student Sample

FLAVIA GIANNOTTI AND FLAVIA CORTESI

The developmental changes occurring during adolescence include psychological as well as organic factors and their nature and rapidity are striking. Modifications in sleeping patterns with chronologic age have been well documented and have been related to greater social pressures, as well as normal ontogenetic trends. Several studies have suggested that adolescents, despite an increasing physiological need for sleep, tend to sleep less with age (Simonds & Parrega, 1982; Carskadon, 1990a; Andrade, Benedito-Silva, Domenice, Amhold, & Menna-Barreto, 1993). The sleep-wake cycle tends to become delayed, and many adolescents may experience sleep phase delay syndrome with insufficient sleep (Carskadon, Vieira, & Acebo, 1993). The consequences of chronic insufficient sleep are numerous: daytime sleepiness, mood and behavioral problems, negative effects on daytime functions such as poor school achievement, greater risk of severe accidents, and increased vulnerability to psychoactive substance abuse. Furthermore, in adolescent years expanding social opportunities, including academic demands, changing parent-child relationship, and changing life habits, may also affect the development of adolescent sleep patterns.

Despite the fact that very few epidemiological studies comparing sleep habits in different countries have been conducted, it has been hypothesized that ethnic and sociocultural factors may influence sleep patterns and habits, too (Strauch & Meier, 1988). Although the importance of healthy sleeping habits in this age group has been pointed out in other countries, this topic has not received adequate interest in

This study was conducted under the aegis of the Statistical Division of the Ministry of Italian Public Education. We gratefully thank Fabrizio Cascio for his active help and technical assistance in this research, as well as the students who completed the survey.

132

Italy. Few studies exist of teenagers' sleeping habits and difficulties in our country, and the entire adolescent age range has not previously been studied with the same survey instrument (Lugaresi, Cirignotta, Zucconi, Mondini, Lenzi, & Cuccagna, 1983; Manber, Bootzin, Acebo, & Carskadon, 1996). Therefore, we carried out a questionnaire survey of sleep habits and problems on a sample of adolescents ages 14 to 20 years representative of the Italian high school student population.

Methods

Research data were collected from a sample representative of public high school population in Italy in the academic year 1995–1996. The sample was drawn from 349 schools across the state, according to a two-stage sample procedure involving the selection of a stratified sample of high schools according to geographical regions, and a sample of students stratified to represent the different grades within a high school. Each grade was equally represented. The questionnaires were mailed to schools in March–May 1996. The response rate was 87%. All students suffering from chronic illness and reporting stressful experiences, such as accidents or death among the subject's family or friends, serious illnesses, and family changes in the last year were excluded. The final sample population consisted of 6,632 students (3,987 females and 2,645 males).

A widespread slight prevalence of females among students attending the secondary schools in Italy has already been reported. Data were collected through a modified version of the Sleep Questionnaire for Adolescents by Carskadon (Carskadon, Seifer, & Acebo, 1991). The questionnaire is a comprehensive instrument including items about sleep-wake behaviors during the previous two weeks and the following scales: sleepiness (SS), sleep disturbances (SD), anxiety (ANX), depression (DEP), morningness/eveningness (M/E), and substance use (SUBS). To evaluate the reliability of this questionnaire for an Italian student population, the Italian translation of the integral version of it was given to 1,000 high school students. After this pilot testing we decided to omit items involving unusual life habits for Italian students, such as part-time jobs, and to include some items regarding the use of substances to promote sleep, questions including background, and sociodemographic information such as household composition, living environment (large cities, urban area = cities and towns; rural area = village or country-side), geographical regions (northern, central, and southern Italy) and parents' occupation. This latter information was used as an indicator of socioeconomic status. Students responded anonymously during a class period with a teacher overseeing them.

For the purpose of establishing a developmental picture, we analyzed the data by dividing the entire sample into five age groups as follows: 14–15; 15–16; 16–17; 17–18; > 18 years. Most of the results are based on cross-tabulations by sex and age group. Statistical significances were calculated by means of chi-square (Yates correction), t-test, and analysis of variance (ANOVA). To identify variables related to a perceived poor sleep quality, we examined the relationship among subjective evaluation of poor sleep quality, reported sleep habits, and disturbances. The "Do you consider yourself to be a good or a poor sleeper?" question was used to define sleep quality. Furthermore, to identify predictors of poor sleep quality self-perception and use of substances to promote sleep, multiple logistic regression analyses were performed. In view of significant sex differences, in both cases separate logistic regression analyses were conducted for boys and girls.

Results

In general all girls were postmenarchal, and all boys showed evidence of marked pubertal changes. All of them were free of sleep complaints, but, with age, irregular sleeping habits, as well as sleep difficulties, emerged. Age, and in some cases sex, were important explanatory factors of sleeping habits and sleep difficulties. Therefore results are presented by age group and sex.

Sleeping Habits

As expected, our results confirmed significant changes in sleep patterns with chronological age (see Table 8.1). A reduction of sleep time either during school ($F_{(4,66)} = 59.1$; $p < .0001$) or weekend nights ($F_{(4.66)} = 138.53$; $p < .001$) was found. Between 14 and 19 years the mean sleep time on school nights passed from 8 hours and 30 minutes to 7 hours and 30 minutes. The mean sleep time on school days was about 8 hours for both sexes, whereas on weekends it was less for boys than for girls (sex effect $F_{(1,66)} = 102.63$ $p < .0001$). A tendency to go to bed later ($F_{(4,66)} = 110.7$; $p < .0001$) and less regularly with age was found ($F_{(4,66)} = 179.2$; $p < .0001$) in boys more often than in girls ($F_{(1,66)} = 31.72$; $p < .0001$). Moreover, girls had an earlier bedtime and rise time

Table 8.1. Sleep Patterns among Age Groups

	Age	Girls			Boys		
		Bedtime	Rise Time	Sleep Time	Bedtime	Rise Time	Sleep Time
School nights	14–15	10:15 P.M.	6:45 A.M.	8 h 15 min	10:30 P.M.	7:00 A.M.	8 h 30 min
	15–16	10:30 P.M.	6:45 A.M.	8 h 15 min	10:40 P.M.	7:00 A.M.	8 h 20 min
	16–17	10:45 P.M.	6:45 A.M.	8 h 00 min	11:05 P.M.	7:05 A.M.	8 h 00 min
	17–18	11:05 P.M.	6:50 A.M.	7 h 45 min	11:20 P.M.	7:10 A.M.	7 h 30 min
	>18	11:15 P.M.	6:50 A.M.	7 h 35 min	11:50 P.M.	7:10 A.M.	7 h 20 min
Weekend nights	14–15	11:50 P.M.	9:40 A.M.	9 h 30 min	11:50 P.M.	9:30 A.M.	9 h 40 min
	15–16	11:55 P.M.	9:45 A.M.	9 h 25 min	12:30 A.M.	9:30 A.M.	9 h 00 min
	16–17	12:30 A.M.	9:55 A.M.	9 h 15 min	12:45 A.M.	9:50 A.M.	8 h 55 min
	17–18	12:45 A.M.	10:00 A.M.	9 h 00 min	1:20 A.M.	10:10 A.M.	8 h 50 min
	>18	1:30 A.M.	10:10 A.M.	8 h 40 min	2:00 A.M.	10:20 A.M.	8 h 20 min

(about 20 minutes) on school days. With age, taking naps also became more prevalent during school days (27% at 14 years to 50% at 18 years on weekdays; Pearson chi-square = 259.57; df = 8; p < .001), and napping was more frequent among older adolescent boys (58% vs. 48%; p < .001). Across all age groups, a small percentage of boys and girls (about 8%) used to nap on weekends. The main reason students gave for going to bed on weeknights was being sleepy (about 50%) and on weekends the completion of socializing (about 60%). The latter tended to increase with age. The second reason was watching television, which involved about 30% of students, more on school nights than on weekend nights, and tending to decrease with age. The third reason they gave was doing homework, more reported by girls on weekdays (about 8%). Parental involvement, both at bedtime and rise time, decreased as adolescents got older (bedtime from 3% at 15 years to 0.9% at 18 years, p < .001; risetime from 43% at 15 years to 32% at 18 years, p < .001) on weeknights. On weekends, parental influence at bedtime tended to increase with age but only for girls. We found that most students who went to bed later on school nights than on weekends (about 3% of the whole sample) across all age groups (57% at 14 years to 37% at 18 years) stayed up later to do homework in the evening. This was more common in girls than in boys (p < .01).

As a measure of sleep schedule regularity, we computed the difference between weekend and school-night bedtime and rise time. An irregular sleep schedule (bedtime and rise time higher than 3 hours) was found in 19% of students, in boys more often than in girls (21% vs. 17%; p < .01). With age, irregular sleeping habits increased and, by the age of 16, this gender difference became more evident. Students with irregular sleeping schedules took naps more frequently, got less sleep both on weekdays and weekend nights, complained of daytime sleepiness with a tendency to fall asleep during lessons, and reported more accidents. Furthermore, they used sleeping pills more frequently (see Table 8.2). With regard to circadian patterns, the M/E scale confirmed that in both sexes tendency toward a phase delay preference increased with age (group effect F (4,66) = 18.87; p < .001).

Sleep Difficulties

Current difficulties in falling asleep, defined as sleep latency higher than 30 minutes, were reported in about 21% of students, with a slight but not significant prevalence in girls. Girls suffered from multiple

Table 8.2. Characteristics of Irregular Sleepers School and Weekend Nights Bedtime and Rise Time Difference Greater Than 3 Hours

	Irregular	Regular	p
Week-night sleep duration	7 h 30 min	7 h 55 min	<.01
Weekend sleep	8 h 10 min	9 h 15 min	<.01
Nap	57.0%	37.0%	<.001
Poor school performance	9.7%	6.0%	<.001
Tendency to fall asleep at school	13.4%	6.3%	<.001
Sleeping pills	5.9%	3.6%	<.01
Daytime sleepiness scale	16.5%	13.0%	<.01

nighttime wakings (2–3 times per night) more frequently than boys, and 2.2% of them reported to wake up more than 3 times per night. Long night wakings, lasting more than 30 minutes, were found in about 6% of students with a marked sex difference. Early morning awakenings were found in 23% of students and, also in this case, they were significantly more frequent in girls (see Table 8.3). Long night wakings tended to increase with age for both sexes, whereas difficulties in falling asleep and multiple night wakings remained stable across in all age groups.

Of the whole sample 19.6% considered themselves as poor sleepers. Significantly more girls than boys (21% vs. 17%, p. < 01) reported poor sleep quality. Self-perception of poor sleep tended to increase significantly with age in both sexes (age groups: 14–15 years = 15%; 15–16 years = 18%; 16–17 years = 19%; 17–18 years = 20%; > 18 years = 22.3%; Pearson chi-square = 25.55; df = 4; p < .001). Logistic regression analysis showed that several independent variables – sleep length, sleep onset insomnia, night wakings (either brief, multiple, or prolonged), early morning awakenings, depression, anxiety and evening phase preference – were associated with self-perception of poor sleep. There were no sex differences. Partial arousal disorders and erratic sleep schedules,

Table 8.3. Sleep Difficulties

	% Boys	% Girls	p
Sleep onset insomnia	20.2	22.2	ns
Multiple night wakings	8.1	11.5	<.01
Long night wakings	4.3	6.9	<.01
Early awakening	21.0	25.0	<.01

Table 8.4. Poor Sleep Quality Self-Perception: Logistic Regression Results

	Girls		Boys	
	Odds Ratio (CI 95%)	p	Odds Ratio (CI 95%)	p
Sleep length	.61 (.55–69)	<.0001	.74 (.64–.86)	<.0001
Sleep onset insomnia	1.66 (1.44–1.9)	<.0001	1.24 (1.06–1.36)	<.0001
Night wakings (2–3 per night)	2.51 (1.97–3.2)	<.0001	2.26 (1.59–3.21)	<.001
Night wakings (> 3 per night)	5 (3–8.32)	<.0001	3.42 (1.37–8.51)	<.01
Prolonged night wakings	1.5 (1.1–2)	<.01	1.9 (1.23–2.9)	<.01
Mid-night wakings	1.6 (1.3–2)	<.0001	1.17 (.88–1.56)	ns
Late-night awakenings	1.2 (.93–1.5)	ns	1.54 (1.15–2.07)	<.01
Anxiety scale	1.07 (1.05–1.1)	<.0001	1.02 (1–1.09)	<.001
Depression scale	1.1 (1.09–1.14)	<.0001	1.14 (1.1–1.17)	<.0001
M/E scale	.96 (.94–.98)	<.01	.93 (.91–.96)	<.001
Early awakening	1.50 (1.24–1.81)	<.0001	1.52 (1.18–1.94)	<.0001

although more frequent in poor sleepers, were not statistically significant in relation to self-reported poor sleep quality (see Table 8.4).

Use of Substances to Promote Sleep

We also investigated the use of sleeping pills in Italian adolescents to determine the prevalence and to identify associated factors. Results showed that 4% of students used medication to help themselves to sleep at least once during the past 6 months, but only 1.3% had regularly taken sleeping pills. Female adolescents were more prevalent users of sleeping pills than males (5.3% females vs. 2% males, p < .001). Consumption tended to increase with age (Pearson chi-square df = 4; p < 001). In general, the increase was considerably larger for girls than boys, and sex differences were found in all age groups. Although these differences were minor at age 14–15 (2.8% girls vs. 1% boys; p < .01), female overuse was clear by age 18 (6.7% vs. 2.4%; p < .001) (see Table 8.5).

Anxiolytic benzodiazepines were taken by 44.2% of students, 10% had used aspirin or nonsteroidal antiinflammatory drugs (NSAIDs),

**Table 8.5. Percentage of Boys and Girls Who
Report Using Substances to Promote Sleep**

Age	Boys	Girls	p
14	1.1	2.8	<.01
15	1.6	4.0	<.001
16	1.9	5.8	<.001
17	2.3	6.1	<.001
18	2.4	6.7	<.001

33% had taken herbal teas, and homeopathic remedies were used by 2.6% of students to improve sleep; 6.5% did not specify the type of substance. Some sex differences emerged: girls were prevalent users of anxiolitic benzodiazepines (47.4% vs. 26%; p < .001), whereas in boys the use of over-the-counter remedies (39% vs. 30%; p < .01) and NSAIDs (14.8% vs. 8.3%; p < .01) were more common. Professional help for sleeping problems had been sought by 2.5% of all the sample. Half of the subjects who reported having taken sleeping pills had them prescribed by a general practitioner (51%), whereas in 25% the use was suggested by parents, and 10.3% of these students reported a self-prescription. Anxiolytic benzodiazepines were prescribed by general practitioners in 58.6% of cases, while NSAIDs were suggested by parents in 17% or self-prescribed in 25% of students.

To analyze the data further and determine which independent variables were significantly associated with the condition of using substances to promote sleep, separate logistic regression analyses for boys and girls were performed. Marked sex differences in predicting substance use were found. In females five independent variables (living in urban areas, multiple midnight awakenings, irregular sleep patterns, depressive mood, anxiety and consumption of psychoactive substances) were significantly associated with the use of sleeping pills. By contrast, in boys only depressive mood was associated with the use of sleeping pills. Sleep onset insomnia, sleep length, as well as partial arousal disorders, were not significantly related to the use of sleeping pills (see Table 8.6).

Sociodemographic Factors

Although the socioeconomic level of parents was not correlated with sleep problems, we found that adolescents from single-family homes

Table 8.6. Predictors of Sleeping Pill Use

	Odds Ratio	CI 95%	p
Girls			
Irregular sleep	1.39	0.99–1.19	<.001
Mid-night multiple night wakings	1.9	0.98–3.94	<.05
Depression	1.1	1.0–1.13	<.001
Anxiety	1.06	1.02–1.11	<.0001
Substance use	1.09	1.05–1.14	<.01
Urban area	1.5	1.1–2	<.01
Boys			
Depression	1.13	1.06–1.21	<.001

(8.6%) had more sleep irregularity (11% vs. 8%; p < .001). Moreover, small differences in some sleep habits were found among geographical regions. Students living in southern Italy went to bed significantly later (on average 20 minutes), but their sleep schedules were more regular compared with those living in northern and central Italy. Students living in urban areas tended to sleep less both on weekdays and on weekend nights (on average 30 minutes; p. < 001).

Impact of Sleep on Daytime Function

Sleep problems scale was positively correlated with daytime sleepiness (r = .27; p < .001); increased use of psychoactive substances (r = .32; p < .001); depressive mood (r = .26; p < .01); and anxiety (r = .31; p < .001) while showing a negative correlation with M/E scale (r = .−30; p < .001). Daytime sleepiness increased with age (group effect $F(4,66) = 4.99$; p < .001) and was more common in older adolescents girls (sex effect $F(1,66) = 31.73$; p < .001). By contrast, falling asleep during lessons, which also increased with age (Pearson chi-square = 34.79; df = 4; p < .001), was more frequent in boys (14% of boys vs. 7.8% of girls; p < .001). Regarding academic performance, ANOVA results showed an association between poor self-reported school achievement and increased complaints of daytime sleepiness ($F(4,66 = 21.54$; p < .001), greater use of caffeine, alcohol, and tobacco ($F(4,66) = 54.00$; p < .001), sleep problems ($F(4,66) = 54.11$; p < .001), evening phase delay preference ($F(4,66) = 30.55$; p < .001), anxiety ($F(4,66) = 20.17$; p < .001), and depressive mood ($F(4,66) = 17.21$; p < .01). Furthermore, students who reported attention problems at school (26% of boys, 21% of girls) slept slightly less both on school nights (7 hours 40 minutes vs. 8 hours; p < .001) and on weekend nights (8 hours and 40 minutes vs. 9 hours and 5 minutes; p < .001), had more irregular bedtime (140 vs. 109 minutes; p < .001), and significantly higher scores on all scales, except the M/E scale where they obtained lower scores.

To investigate other factors that can affect the amount and timing of adolescents' sleep, we examined the influence of school starting time, and compared students' sleep patterns attending schools with earlier start times with those enrolled in schools that started later. Despite the small difference in school start time in Italy, ranging from 7:45 A.M. to 8:45 A.M. across all age groups, we found that, in general, students who attended the schools with the earliest start time (before 8:00 A.M.) had more irregular sleep schedules (p < .001), complained of daytime sleepiness (p < .01), tended to fall asleep at school (p < .01), and reported more frequently poor academic performance (p < .05) than those with late school start times (after 8:30 A.M.). Analyzing the differences among age groups, however, we found that students ages 14–15 who started school earlier did not show any problems but reported an earlier bedtime (by almost 30 minutes); by the age of sixteen, school and weekend bedtimes shifted to later times, school-night sleep time progressively decreased, and daytime sleepiness increased with age.

Of the whole sample, 88% reported having had some accidents (at home, at school, driving) There were no age or gender differences. The increased vulnerability to accidents was positively correlated with sleep problems (r = .28; p < .001), daytime sleepiness (r = .20; p < .001), and increased use of stimulants and tobacco (r = .19; p < .001), and less marked but significantly correlated with anxiety (r = .16; p < .01) and depressive mood (r = .11; p < .01).

Discussion

Our data confirm a developmental trend of sleep patterns in adolescence. Similar to other studies (Price, Coates, Thoreson, & Grinstead, 1978; Simonds, 1982; Strauch & Meier, 1988; Carskadon, 1990a; Andrade et al., 1993; Tynjala, Kannas, & Välimaa, 1993; Ledoux, Choquet, & Manfredi, 1994; Gau & Soong, 1995) there is a tendency for sleep duration to get shorter, on either weekdays or weekend nights, as age increased (Table 8.1). Moreover, in all age groups the night sleep duration was longer during weekends than during weekdays, and this difference increased with age. Sleeping habits varied considerably between weekdays and weekends. During weekends bedtimes and rise times were later. Furthermore, a sleep schedule irregularity becomes more evident with age, especially in boys. Of our sample, about 19% of students reported bedtime and rise time differences between school and weekend nights greater than 3 hours. The average shift in bedtime was considerably greater in the older group, supporting the hypothesis that bedtime may get progressively later on weekends due to social pressures as adolescents get older. Moreover, the longer sleep duration during weekends may be a response to insufficient sleep during weekdays. In recent years we have witnessed a controversy over whether the population at large is chronically sleep-deprived. The change in sleep time over the past century has been most dramatic for adolescents. Social pressure, television, and late-night movies compete with sleep, resulting in a rather drastic change in sleep habits and sleep time in adolescents, who now tend to get insufficient sleep. In fact, laboratory data suggested that the need for sleep does not decrease during adolescence (Carskadon, 1990a). Adolescents expand their social lives and tend to spend leisure time with friends more often and later in the evening than before. Parental control at bedtimes decreased with age and among older adolescents, peer group influences over bedtime and sleeping habits, in general, assume greater importance than before. In our sample, parental involvement, both at bedtime and rise time, decreased as adolescents got older. This is different from the report by Carskadon (1990a) concerning the U.S. teens, where parental influence diminishes at bedtime but becomes more important on waking in the morning, but is similar to that reported by Gau for Taipei adolescents (Gau & Soong, 1995). In our study slight gender differences were found regarding parental influence at bedtime, being more common for girls on weekends. This, in our opinion, may be due to the differences in sociocultural contexts, which involves a trend for parents to control girls more than boys. A recent epidemiological study carried out in some European countries on students ages 11–16 years (Strauch & Meier, 1988) found great differences between countries in duration of sleep time with Israeli and Finnish students sleeping the shortest (about 8 hours and 30 minutes) and Swiss children sleeping the longest (over 9 hours). Sleep time among Italian students of the same age group was similar to Israeli adolescents. On the other hand the comparison with the U.S. population (Carskadon, 1990a) showed that American adolescents sleep about 15–20 minutes less than Italians on weekdays, while sleep length on weekends was quite similar. In younger groups bedtime and rise time were quite similar in different countries, whereas a great difference was found in late adolescence both in bedtime and in rise time with U.S. teenagers going to bed more than an hour later than Italians. This difference, in our opinion, may be due to different educational systems; in fact, in Italy 18-year-olds are still attending high school and living with their families, while in the United States they may already be attending college. This implies more parental control for the Italian population in late adolescence, resulting, probably, in more regular sleep habits.

Compatible with the results of Carskadon (1990a) and Gau and Soong (1995), we observed in this study that girls went to sleep and woke up earlier (about 20 minutes) on weekdays. The earlier rise time in girls may be due, as already pointed out, to the habit of spending more time in preparing for school (Price et al., 1978; Carskadon, 1990b; Carskadon, Seifer, Davis, & Acebo, 1991). Similar to other studies, daytime sleepiness increased with age, and there was a tendency for increased napping among older adolescent boys, who reported also more sleep schedule irregularity. Rather than maintaining healthy sleep habits, many Italian adolescents resort to stimulants, brief naps, or sleeping late on weekends to improve their level of daytime alertness. In fact, the teens in this study reported a shorter sleep duration, associated with irregular sleep schedules, resulting in teens' getting insufficient sleep. Likewise, decreased sleep and irregular sleep schedules were negatively related to daytime functions such as mood, tendency of increased use of psychoactive substances and sleeping pills, poor school performance, and increased vulnerability to accidents. In particular, as already documented by Carskadon, Wolfson, Tzischinsky, and Acebo (1995), we found a strong association between self-reported school difficulties, attention problems, daytime sleepiness complaints, shorter sleep time duration, and more irregular sleep schedules.

Regarding the effect of school start time on sleep, we found that by age 16 adolescents starting school earlier reported shorter sleep length, sleepiness complaints, falling asleep at school, and attention problems more frequently than their peers enrolled in schools with later start times. Again, results regarding older adolescents are similar to those reported by Carskadon et al. (1995) and Tynjala (1993); however, young adolescents with early school starting times in our sample did not show any of these problems except a tendency to have later bedtimes. Therefore, the sleep loss in older adolescents may be due to increasingly later bedtimes. We hypothesize that these age group differences in our sample of Italian adolescents may be due to reduced parental control at bedtime, and increasing social pressure at around the age of 16.

Living environment and geographical regions, although less important than other factors such as age and sex, seemed to influence sleeping habits of Italian teenagers. Adolescents living in southern Italy, although reporting a later bedtime, seemed to have a more regular sleep schedule than their peers living in the northern and central regions. Moreover students living in the urban areas tended to sleep less at night than those living in rural areas. These slight differences seem, in our opinion, related to different sociocultural contexts, which determine different styles of living. In fact, it seems that social pressures and facility to expand social lives, such as socializing with friends more often and later in the evening, is easier for adolescents living in big towns and in central and northern regions. Although the socioeconomic level of parents was not related to sleep problems, adolescents from single-family homes showed more sleep irregularity, probably due to different life-styles such as reduced parental control over bedtime.

The rates of students reporting inability to fall asleep (21%) are quite similar to those reported by other studies (United States 24%, Taiwan 27.2%, Australia 22.85%) (Bearpark & Michie, 1987; Carskadon, 1990a; Gau & Soong, 1995) but less than that reported to Choquet and colleagues (1988) for the French population (40%). In contrast to other studies (Price et al., 1978; Bearpark & Michie, 1987; Gau & Soong, 1995), we found only a slight, but not significant, increased prevalence in girls. In one epidemiological study carried out in some European countries (Strauch & Meier, 1988), the rates of inability to fall asleep varied from 10% for Austrian adolescents to about 30% for Finnish students, with a trend to decrease with age. In contrast, Bearpark reported an increased prevalence of difficulty falling asleep with age in the Australian population, significant in girls but not in boys (Bearpark & Michie, 1987). By contrast, in our sample we did not find significant differences among age groups. As already reported, girls had multiple night wakings more frequently than boys. The rates for wakenings found in our sample (12%) are similar to those reported for the Australian population (11.4% girls, 10.8% boys), but lower than that reported by Choquet and colleagues (1988) for the French population (16% boys, 25% girls), and by Price et al. (1978) for the U.S. adolescents (20%). We found also a high incidence (23%) of early morning awakenings without gender differences; this figure is similar to that reported by Choquet et al. (1988) for French adolescents (24%). In contrast to other studies (Bearpark & Michie, 1987; Choquet et al., 1988) that reported an increase of night wakings with age particularly for girls, we found that in girls the prevalence of night wakings is stable across all age groups, and in boys the rates decreased with age. Moreover, poor sleep self-perception occurred with sufficient frequency in healthy Italian adolescents (19%), with marked significant prevalence in girls (21%). Our results, similar to other studies (Simonds & Parraga, 1982; Patois, Valatx, & Alperovitch, 1993), suggest that adolescents who describe themselves as poor sleepers showed significant differences in daytime feelings and mood, feeling more depressed, anxious, and less alert and reporting more evening phase preference. In our sample, difficulties in falling asleep as well as multiple and prolonged night wakings, early morning awakenings, and shorter sleep length played an important role in predicting poor sleep quality self-perception. On the contrary, sleep schedule irregularity was not related to poor sleep quality.

Despite the relative incidence of sleep problems, professional help was sought by only 2% of the whole sample. A small percentage of Italian adolescents (4%) had occasionally used substances to help themselves to sleep, and only 1.3% had regularly taken sleeping pills. Although sex differences were found in all age groups, the increase in the use among girls between the age of 14 and 18 years led to a very marked difference by late adolescence, which may persist, as shown by other studies, throughout adulthood. Our results are similar to those reported for other adolescent populations (Kirmil-Gray, Eagleston, Gibson, & Thoresen, 1984; Manni et al., 1996). About half of the adolescents who reported using medication took benzodiazepines; the others took over-the-counter medications, including aspirin or homeopathic remedies. About one-third of students have taken medications suggested by relatives or parents or that were self-prescribed. One explanation is that cultural differences in family networks and parenting might lead some students to be more predisposed to use substances to promote sleep as a way of coping with sleep problems. Contrary to the report of Patois et al. (1993), who found difficulties with falling asleep related to the use of sleep medication in both sexes, we found striking sex differences. In our study, the girls' multiple nightwakings and sleep schedule irregularity were strongly associated with the use of sleeping pills as well as depressive mood, anxiety, living in an urban area, and an increased use of psychoactive substances. In contrast, in males only depressive mood played an important role in predicting the use of sleeping pills.

Although the use of medications to enhance sleep was not very common in Italian adolescents, the trend, which increases with age, to use a chemical solution may persist in adult life and become a risk factor for habitual use. As a general conclusion, sleep patterns of Italian adolescents seem to be similar to those of previous studies carried out in other countries. The slight differences found may be due to different sociocultural contexts, as well as data collection methods, or age groupings, or differences in formulation of questions related to sleeping habits and sleep difficulties. Our results also point out that Italian adolescents experience more unhealthy sleeping habits and difficulties in late adolescence. Age and, in some cases, sex are important explanatory factors.

In this sample of Italian teenagers, we observed a marked prevalence of sleep irregularity and unhealthy sleep habits, shorter sleep duration, daytime sleepiness, more attention problems, poor school performance, and a tendency to use stimulant substances in males; however, sleep problems were more common among the girls. This difference became stronger as age increased; in the older age group there was a marked prevalence of sleep problems in girls.

This study confirms that the roots of sleep problems may lie in the adolescent period and that a complexity of contributing factors (cultural, biological, and developmental) may influence sleeping habits and problems. Therefore multiple points of intervention for prevention and change should start as early in the life course as possible to alert adolescents, parents, educators, and health officials to the dangers of unhealthy and irregular sleeping habits in adolescence.

REFERENCES

Andrade MMM, Benedito-Silva AA, Domenice A, Arnhold IPJ, Menna-Barreto
    L (1993). Sleep characteristics of adolescents: A longitudinal study. *J Adolesc
    Health* 14:401–406.
Bearpark HM, Michie PT (1987). Prevalence of sleep/wake disturbances in
    Sidney adolescents. *Sleep Res* 16:304.
Carskadon MA (1990a). Patterns of sleep and sleepiness in adolescents. *Pediatrician* 17(1):5–12.
    (1990b). Adolescent sleepiness: Increased risk in a high-risk population. *Alcohol Drugs–Driving* 5–6:317–328.
Carskadon MA, Seifer R, Acebo C (1991). Reliability of six scales in a sleep
    questionnaire for adolescents. *Sleep Res* 20:421.
Carskadon MA, Seifer R, Davis SS, Acebo C (1991). Sleep, sleepiness, and mood
    in college-bound high school seniors. *Sleep Res* 20:175.

Carskadon MA, Vieira C, Acebo C (1993). Association between puberty and delayed phase preference. *Sleep* 16(3):258–262.

Carskadon MA, Wolfson A, Tzischinsky O, Acebo C (1995). Early school schedules modify adolescent sleepiness. *Sleep Res* 24:92.

Choquet M, Tesson F, Stevenot A, et al. (1988). Les adolescents et leur sommeil: Approche epidemiologique. *Neuropsychiatrie de l'enfance* 36(10):399–410.

Dahl RE, Matty MK, Nelson B, Al-Shabbout M, Ryan ND (1992). The effects of sleep restriction in normal adolescents. *Sleep Res* 21:117.

Gau SF, Soong WT (1995). Sleep problems of junior high school students in Taipei. *Sleep* 18(8):667–673.

Kirmil-Gray K, Eagleston JR., Gibson E, Thoresen CE (1984). Sleep disturbance in adolescents: Sleep quality, sleep habits, beliefs about sleep, and daytime functioning. *J Youth Adolesc* 13:375–384.

Ledoux S, Choquet M, Manfredi R. (1994). Self-reported use of drugs for sleep or distress among French adolescents. *J Adolesc Health* 15(6):495–502.

Lugaresi E, Cirignotta F, Zucconi M, Mondini S, Lenzi PL, Coccagna G (1983). Good and poor sleepers: An epidemiological survey of the San Marino population. In C. Guilleminault & E. Lugaresi, eds., *Sleep/Wake Disorders: Natural History, Epidemiology, and Long-Term Evolution*, pp. 1–12. New York: Raven Press.

Manber R, Bootzin RR, Acebo C, Carskadon MA (1996). The effects of regularizing sleep-wake schedules on daytime sleepiness. *Sleep* 19(5):432–441.

Manni R, Ratti MT, Marchioni E, Castelnovo G, Murelli R, Sartori I, Galimberti CA, Tartara A (1997). Poor sleep in adolescents: A study of 869 17-year-old Italian secondary school students. *J Sleep Res* 6(1):44–49.

Patois E, Valatx JL, Alperovitch A (1993). [Prevalence of sleep and wakefulness disorders in high school students at the Academy of Lyon.] *Rev Epidemiol Sante Publique* 41(5):383–388.

Price VA, Coates TJ, Thoresen CE, Grinstead OA (1978). Prevalence and correlates of poor sleep among adolescents. *Am J Dis Child* 132:583–586.

Simonds JF, Parraga H (1982). Prevalence of sleep disorders and sleep behaviors in children and adolescents. *J Am Acad Child Psychiatry* 21(4):383–388.

Strauch I, Meier B (1988). Sleep need in adolescents: A longitudinal approach. *Sleep* 11:378–386.

Tynjälä J, Kannas L (1993). Sleeping habits of Finnish school children by sociodemographic background. *Health Prom Int* 8:281–289.

Tynjala J, Kannas L, Välimaa R (1993). How young Europeans sleep. *Health Educ Res* 7:69–80.

9. Risks of Driving While Sleepy in Adolescents and Young Adults

MARY A. CARSKADON

In 1989 motor vehicle accidents were the second largest single cause of death in persons aged 15 to 24 years in the United States (U.S. Department of Commerce 1992). Sleepiness is increasingly recognized as a causal factor in crashes and may be a particular risk in chronically sleep-deprived young people (Carskadon, 1990, 1993). For example, data from a series of 4,333 automobile crashes attributed to the driver's falling asleep (but not being intoxicated) in North Carolina from 1990 through 1992 demonstrated that the peak age of the driver in such crashes was 20 years (Pack, Pack, Rodgman, Cucchiara, Dinges, & Schwab, 1995). Furthermore, 55% of the sleep-related crashes involved a driver younger than 25 years old. This disproportionate age distribution of fall-asleep crashes singles out young people as a singularly high-risk group.

We have learned much about the sleep processes and sleep pattern development of adolescents over the past 20 years, enough to be confident in saying that many high school and college-aged young people do not obtain adequate sleep to maintain full alertness. High school students, in particular, go to bed late, wake up early, and sleep on average about 7 hours and 15 minutes a night (Wolfson & Carskadon, 1998). On the other hand, we have good evidence that adolescents probably

I dedicate this paper to the memory of a valued colleague and cherished friend, Helen M. Bearpark, Ph.D., who was struck by a motor vehicle and killed on December 19, 1996. Helen was committed to research in the area of driving and sleepiness, as well as sleep apnea and insomnia, and she provided the impetus for the second survey reported in this paper while training as a postdoctoral fellow in my group (Bearpark, Thacher, & Carskadon, 1996). This research was supported by a grant from the National Institutes of Health, MH45945. I also thank Pamela V. Thacher, Ph.D., who provided valuable assistance to this project, and Christine Acebo, Ph.D., who provided expert assistance with the data analyses and editing.

need at least 9 hours to 9 hours and 15 minutes of sleep a night to maintain optimal alertness (Carskadon, Orav, & Dement, 1983). Even with 9 hours of sleep, however, adolescents are not as alert as when they slept that amount as are preadolescents (Carskadon, 1982). Furthermore, during the course of pubertal development, the pattern of sleep propensity changes in a way that leads to a decrease of midday alertness, and this pattern appears to be maintained as humans age (Carskadon & Dement, 1987). In addition, college students in general obtain even less sleep than adolescents and sleep on quite erratic schedules (Carskadon & Davis, 1989; Manber, Bootzin, Acebo, & Carskadon, 1996). The consequence of these patterns is that young people carry a large sleep debt.

In addition, the driving skills and judgment of this group are not well polished, and the risk of continuing to drive while sleepy is hence exacerbated in younger drivers. We have performed two surveys in an attempt to gauge more clearly the level of risk for driving while sleepy in adolescents and young adults (Carskadon, 1994; Bearpark et al., 1996). In the first study, the questions considered were those bearing on how the risk of sleepy driving is perceived and how this risk perception compares with the perception of driving under the influence of alcohol. The second analysis examined factors that might help identify those young people at greatest risk for automobile crashes due to falling asleep.

Study 1: Risk Perception in Adolescents and Young Adults

Participants

Two groups of students were evaluated. The high school group included 191 students: 78 males (mean age = 16.6 ± 0.8 years) and 113 females (mean age = 16.5 ± 0.8 years) of whom 96% were Caucasian. These students all attended the same suburban Rhode Island public high school. The collegiate group included students enrolled in an introductory neurosciences course at Brown University, a sample of 182 students: 81 males (mean age = 19.4 ± 2.0 years) and 101 females (mean age = 18.9 ± 1.8 years) of whom 58% were Caucasian, 30% were Asian-American, and the remainder were other racial or ethnic groups. The project was approved by the E. P. Bradley Hospital Institutional Review Board (IRB) for the Protection of Human Subjects, and college students signed an abbreviated consent form (which was separated from the data sheets) before completing the anonymous survey during class. The high school group did not sign a consent form but were told to turn in a blank form if they did not wish to complete the survey. No compensation was provided.

Methods

Students were given a one-page anonymous form to complete and turn in at the start of a class period. A copy of the survey items is shown in Figure 9.1. The survey included two sets of questions about driving: one set focused on alcohol, and the second set of identical items focused on sleepiness. The alcohol and sleepiness items were presented in reverse order on half the forms. Analyses included ANOVA for group (high school or collegiate) and sex effects, chi-square with Yates correction for continuity when $df = 1$, and Spearman correlations, all with a p value of .05 required for statistical significance.

Results

As expected, the collegiate group reported more years of driving experience than did the high school students ($F = 160.3$, $df = 1,324$, $p < .001$), and slightly more college students were drivers than high school students. For some of the analyses, only those with driving experience were assessed; for others, we took into account all the students.

When we examined the scores on the risk questions ("indicate your thoughts on the risks of driving while impaired ... by sleepiness or alcohol"), we found that the high school students rated driving while impaired by alcohol as riskier than driving while sleepy ($F = 147.7$, $df = 1,187$, $p < .001$). A similar pattern occurred among the college students ($F = 157.1$, $df = 1,171$, $p < .001$). As illustrated in Figure 9.2, college students rated driving impaired by sleepiness or by alcohol as significantly riskier than did high school students ($F = 9.95$, $df = 1,358$, $p = .002$). Furthermore, females in both groups rated driving while sleepy or while impaired by alcohol as more risky than did males ($F = 10.79$, $df = 2,358$, $p = .001$). In both the high school and collegiate groups, the alcohol and sleepy driving risk scores were correlated at a statistically significant level (high school: $r = .42$, $df = 189$, $p < .001$; collegiate: $r = .45$, $df = 174$, $p < .001$).

We attempted to identify whether personal experience with incidents involving driving while impaired by alcohol or sleepiness might influence risk perception. Table 9.1 summarizes the number of students who drive, who report having experienced impairment while driving, and

Driving Impairment Survey

1. What is your sex?   [1] male [2] female   2. What is your age? _____   3. What is your race? _____
4. Do you drive?   [1] no   [2] yes   5. If yes, for how many years? _____
6. Have you ever driven while impaired by **sleepiness**? no [1]   yes [2] _____
7. If yes, please make 2 lists:
   <u>List 1</u>:   How did you know you were impaired?

_____

_____

   <u>List 2</u>:   What did you do to help reduce your impairment?

_____

_____

8. Have you ever or do you know anyone <u>personally</u> who has had an accident (or been the victim of an accident) due to being impaired by **sleepiness** while driving? [2] no   [2] yes
   (If no, skip to item 9; if yes, answer the items below.)
   * **who was it?**   [1] yourself   [2] a family member   [3] a friend
   * extent of **damage**:   [1] none/slight   [2] car damage was repairable   [3] car was "totaled"
   * extent of **injury**:   [1] none/slight   [2] injury requiring hospitalization   [3] someone died
   * who was **at fault**?   [1] you or the person you know   [2] another driver
9. Check one box below to indicate your thoughts on the risk of driving while impaired by **sleepiness**:

   extremely risky   moderately risky   risk free
   [1]   [2]   [3]   [4]   [5]   [6]   [7]

10. Have you ever driven while impaired by **alcohol**? no [1]   yes [2]
11. If yes, please make 2 lists:
    <u>List 1</u>:   How did you know you were impaired?

_____

_____

<u>List 2</u>:   What did you do to help reduce your impairment?

_____

_____

12. Have you ever or do you know anyone <u>personally</u> who has had an accident (or been the victim of an accident) due to being impaired by **alcohol** while driving? [1] no   [2] yes
    (If no, skip to item 13; if yes, answer the items below.)
    * **who was it?**   [1] yourself   [2] a family member   [3] a friend
    * extent of **damage**:   [1] none/slight   [2] car damage was repairable   [3] car was "totaled"
    * extent of **injury**:   [1] none/slight   [2] injury requiring hospitalization   [3] someone died
    * who was **at fault**?   [1] you or the person you know   [2] another driver
13.   Check one box below to indicate your thoughts on the risk of driving while impaired by **alcohol**:

    extremely risky   moderately risky   risk free
    [1]   [2]   [3]   [4]   [5]   [6]   [7]

Figure 9.1. This figure shows Form A (sleepiness questions first) of the Driving Impairment Survey used in study 1.

who report *personal* knowledge of automobile accidents attributed to either cause. Significantly more students reported having driven while impaired by sleepiness than by alcohol (chi-square = 31.79, df = 1, p < .001). If students reported having experienced driving while impaired by alcohol, then they tended to minimize risks of driving while impaired by alcohol compared with students who never experienced

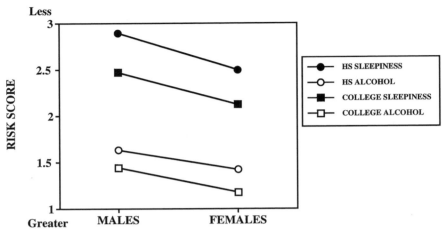

Figure 9.2. The mean risk scores reported by students for sleepiness- (filled symbols) and alcohol-related (open symbols) driving impairment are summarized in this figure. Note that the larger values indicate *decreasing* risk scores, that is toward "risk free." The high school group is indicated by the circles and the collegiate group by the squares. Females rated both behaviors as riskier than did males; college students rated both behaviors as riskier than did high school students.

such impairment ($F = 23.70$, $df = 1,318$, $p < .001$). Similarly, students having experienced sleepiness while driving gave scores indicating less risk of sleepy driving than those who denied having driven while sleepy ($F = 9.83$, $df = 1,319$, $p = .002$).

Table 9.1. Reported Experience with Alcohol- and Sleepiness-Related Driving

	High School Group		Collegiate Group	
	Males (n = 83)	Females (n = 113)	Males (n = 81)	Females (n = 101)
Number who drive	69	93	79	89
Mean years driving	1	1	3.2	2.9
Number who drive while impaired by alcohol	19	20	19	14
Number who drive while impaired by sleepiness	47	57	56	62
Number aware of alcohol-related accident	47	76	42	62
Number aware of sleepiness-related accident	35	11	40	44

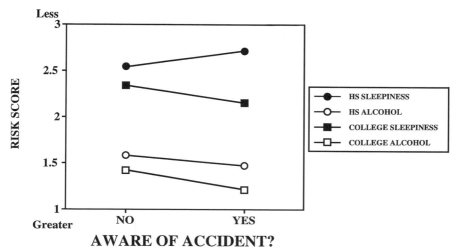

Figure 9.3. The mean risk scores shown in this figure are segregated depending on whether students reported personal knowledge of an accident. Symbols are as in Figure 9.2. These data showed no significant effect of accident knowledge on risk scores; however, the high school students show a trend for *reduced* risk attribution if they have personal knowledge of a sleep-related accident.

More students overall reported personal experience of an alcohol-related accident than a sleepiness-related accident (chi-square = 4.09, df = 1, p = .04); no group or sex differences were found for these variables. Students who reported knowing of accidents caused by alcohol rated the risk of such impairment greater than those who denied such personal knowledge (F(1,249) = 3.84, p = .012). In contrast, knowledge of sleepiness-related accidents had minimal effect on sleepiness risk scores in the college group and even showed a trend for lessened risk attribution associated with personal knowledge of accidents in high school students (Figure 9.3).

Another interesting aspect of this study included the responses students wrote to the open-ended items asking about how they could tell if they were impaired by sleepiness or alcohol and what actions they would take to reduce their impairment. The responses are summarized in Tables 9.2 and 9.3, in which the distribution of answers is presented in categories, such as symptoms that affected the eyes (blurred vision, heavy eyelids, difficulty keeping eyes open, etc.). Summed values will exceed 100% because many students reported multiple answers. Because of the nature of these data and the subjective judgments involved in categorizing the responses, no analyses were performed.

**Table 9.2. Responses to Open-Ended Items Regarding
Knowledge of Impairment (percentage of students)**

How do you know when you are impaired by sleepiness?	
Eyes are blurred, heavy, difficulty keeping open, etc.	74.4
Realize drifting or swerving out of lane	16.7
Decreased concentration	15.5
Feel drowsy, sleepy, or tired	15.5
Notice head bobbing, nodding, rolling, or drooping	14.3
Notice memory gaps, spacing out, zoning out	14.3
Yawning	9.5
Falling asleep, dozing	8.3
How do you know when you are impaired by alcohol?	
Decreased reaction time	23.1
Vision impaired, blurred, double	19.2
Decreased attention or concentration	15.4
Feel dizzy, tipsy, groggy	15.4
Number of drinks consumed	15.4
Decreased coordination, driving skills	11.5

Nevertheless, clear differences in the patterns of "symptoms" and countermeasures for alcohol and sleepiness impairment are apparent.

Study 2: Factors Associated with Increased Risk

Participants

This survey study included students at Brown University enrolled in introductory psychology or neuroscience courses. Only data from participants with driver's licenses were considered for these analyses. Participants included 115 men and 169 women, with a median age of 19 years (mean = 19.5, SD = 1.6). These students reported that they had been driving for a median of 3.0 years (mean = 3.4 ± 1.5).

Methods

As in the previous study, approval was granted from the E. P. Bradley Hospital IRB, and participants completed the brief questionnaire at the beginning of a class period. This survey took place 2 years later than the survey in study 1; thus, the likelihood of overlapping samples is small. In addition to general demographic questions, participants were asked to estimate how much they usually sleep at night as well as the frequency of

Table 9.3. Responses to Open-Ended Items Regarding Countermeasures (percentage of students)

What do you do to reduce impairment by sleepiness?	
Turn up the volume (or increase the tempo of music = 4.8)	72.6
Open the window	48.8
Talk to one's self or a passenger	19.0
Drink caffeine	16.7
Stop the car (to nap = 7.1%, to exercise = 4.8%, just stop = 2.4%)	14.3
Eat or drink (not caffeinated, just in general)	10.7
Move, dance, stretch	9.5
Let someone else drive who is not sleepy	2.4
What do you do to reduce impairment by alcohol?	
Drive slowly	42.3
Increase attention, care, focus, concentration	34.6
Wait, sober up, stop drinking	23.1
Nothing	15.4
Open the window	11.5
Eat something	7.7
Drink caffeine	3.8
Turn up the volume	3.8
Pray	3.8

experiencing sleepiness while driving. They were also asked a number of items related to the frequency of experiencing sleepiness at other times, including falling asleep during class, taking preplanned naps during the daytime, experiencing trouble waking up in the morning, and arriving late for or totally missing morning classes due to sleepiness. Responses to all items were given on a 4-point scale with the following values: (1) never, (2) rarely (less than once per week), (3) occasionally (1 or 2 times per week), (4) frequently (more than twice per week). The scores for responses on these items were summed within subjects to yield an "excessive daytime sleepiness" (EDS) score. Data were analyzed using t-tests and chi-square.

Results

As shown in Table 9.4, men reported having experienced a "near miss" while sleepy or had experienced falling asleep while driving more frequently than did women. On the other hand, the actual number of

Table 9.4. Sex Differences in Responses to Sleep-Related Driving
Items in Study

	Percent of Yes Responses		Men versus Women	
	Men	Women		
Survey Item	(n = 115)	(n = 169)	Chi-square	p
Have you ever had an accident due to sleepiness while driving?	3.5	3.0	.6	ns
Have you ever had a "near miss" due to sleepiness while driving?	37.4	18.3	12.9	< .001
Have you ever fallen asleep while driving?	27.2	15.5	5.8	< .02

accidents attributed to sleepiness did not show a sex difference. In order to evaluate factors that might identify those young adult drivers at greater risk, we classified students into two groups. Those who reported either an accident due to sleepiness or *both* a near miss due to sleepiness or having fallen asleep while driving were classified as the "high-risk" group (n = 36). The "low-risk" group comprised the drivers who reported none of these behaviors (n = 184). The high-risk group included 24.3% of the male sample and only 12% of the female sample, a statistically significant overrepresentation of males (chi-square = 5.6, df = 1, p < .02). In addition, the students in the high-risk group had been driving longer than those in the low-risk group (t = 5.4, p = .02). Reported total sleep time did not distinguish the high- and low-risk groups: mean total sleep time in the high-risk group was 415 (± 71) minutes and in the low-risk group was 421 (± 62) minutes. Drivers with EDS scores greater than 1 standard deviation above the mean (6.2 ± 2.5) were classified as "EDS positive" (n = 58), and these students composed a significantly higher proportion of the high-risk driver group (chi-square = 4.5, df = 1, p = .03).

Discussion

These two small surveys indicate several important factors regarding the risks of driving while sleepy in high school and college students. Both studies, for example, showed that a high number of students reported driving behavior affected by sleepiness. In study 1, 67% of students who drive reported having driven while impaired by sleepiness. Twenty percent of the second sample reported having fallen asleep while driving. As with the study by Horne and Reyner (1995), we found males overrepresented in the high-risk group and a tendency for those with signs of excessive sleepiness during other activities (e.g., falling asleep in classes) to be at greater risk for sleepy driving behavior.

Although these young people constitute a high-risk group, their perceptions of the risks of sleepy driving do not seem adequate to mitigate this high-risk status, The college students reported greater perceived risk associated with both alcohol- and sleepiness-impaired driving than did high school students, with females rating risks of both as greater than did males. In general, however, the students rated alcohol impairment as a greater driving risk than sleepiness impairment. Of interest is that students who reported experience with alcohol-impaired driving or sleepy driving minimized their risk attribution for such behaviors. These students may reason that if they survived the experience, it cannot be extremely risky. Additionally, they may deny that behaviors they are engaged in carry a risk. Furthermore, students with personal knowledge of accidents involving alcohol thought of alcohol and driving as riskier than those without such personal knowledge. On the other hand, personal knowledge of accidents attributed to sleepiness had no significant effect on perceived risk of driving sleepy in either high school or college students. As illustrated in Figure 9.3, the high school students who had personal knowledge of sleep-related accidents tended to report *reduced* risk.

Discrepancies between risk attribution of alcohol-impaired and sleepy driving may indicate that these young people have been socialized to the risks of alcohol and driving through years of exposure to educational programs warning against drinking and driving. Traffic safety programs in general have focused on alcohol risks and seatbelt safety, yet sleepiness while driving has received little attention in traffic safety or driver training programs. Failure of accident exposure to affect risk attribution for sleepy driving may be another indication of a general ignorance about sleepiness and traffic accidents. Educational programs that focus on risks of sleepy driving may improve risk attribution and consequently driving safety. Targeted efforts are currently underway by the National Sleep Foundation and the American Automobile Association Foundation for Traffic Safety; however, routine incorporation of the information in driver training programs may be necessary. The students' assessments of impairment and counter-measures raise additional concerns. Most experts would agree that the most effective sleepiness countermeasures are far down on students' lists, reported by a small percentage of young people.

REFERENCES

Bearpark HM, Thacher PV, Carskadon MA (1996). Sleep-related motor vehicle accidents and sleepy driving in young adults. *Sleep Research* 25:92.
Carskadon MA (1982). The second decade. In C. Guilleminault, ed., *Sleeping and Waking Disorders: Indications and Techniques*, pp. 99–125. Menlo Park, CA: Addison Wesley.
    (1990). Adolescent sleepiness: Increased risk in a high-risk population. *Alcohol, Drugs and Driving* 5–6:317–328.
    (1993). Sleepiness in adolescents and young adults. *Proceedings: Highway Safety Forum on Fatigue, Sleep Disorders, and Traffic Safety*, pp. 28–36. Albany, NY: Institute for Traffic Safety Management and Research.
    (1994). The risk of sleepy driving: A survey of adolescents and young adults. *Sleep Research* 23:115.
Carskadon MA, Davis SS (1989). Sleep-wake patterns in the high-school-to-college transition: Preliminary data. *Sleep Research* 18:113.
Carskadon MA, Dement WC (1987). Daytime sleepiness: Quantification of a behavioral state. *Neuroscience and Biobehavioral Review* 11:307–317.
Carskadon MA, Orav EJ, Dement WC (1983). Evolution of sleep and daytime sleepiness in adolescents. In C. Guilleminault & E. Lugaresi, eds., *Sleep/Wake Disorders: Natural History, Epidemiology, and Long-Term Evolution*, pp. 201–216. New York: Raven Press.
Horne JA, Reyner LA (1995). Sleep related vehicle accidents. *British Medical Journal* 310(6979):565–567.
Manber R, Bootzin RR, Acebo C, Carskadon MA (1996). The effects of regularizing sleep-wake schedules on daytime sleepiness. *Sleep* 19(5):432–441.
Pack AI, Pack AM, Rodgman D, Cucchiara A, Dinges DF, Schwab CW (1995). Characteristics of crashes attributed to the driver having fallen asleep. *Accident Analysis and Prevention* 27:769–775.
U.S. Department of Commerce, Economic & Statistical Administration, Bureau of the Census (1992). *112th Edition Statistical Abstract of the U.S.* Lanham, MD: Bernan Press.
Wolfson AR, Carskadon MA (1998). Sleep schedules and daytime functioning in adolescents. *Child Development* 69(4):875–887.

10. What Can the Study of Work Scheduling Tell Us about Adolescent Sleep?

ROGER H. ROSA

Recent surveys indicate that at least half of adolescents who attend school are also part of the commercial work force, and half of those employed work more than 20 hours per week (Steinberg & Dornbusch, 1991). Such extensive work schedules have led to concerns about possible detrimental effects on the development or well-being of adolescents who work these schedules and also attend school. In one study, for example, increasing hours of employment were associated with poorer school performance, higher psychological stress, more frequent substance abuse, and reduced parental supervision (Steinberg & Dornbusch, 1991). Other studies have reported that students working the most hours tended to obtain the least sleep and were the most sleepy during the day (Carskadon, 1989–1990, 1990). Such studies raise the distinct possibility that increased sleepiness associated with the working hours of adolescents could place those individuals at risk of accident or injury or at a developmental disadvantage. The purpose of the present review is to examine the association between working hours, sleep, and sleepiness to determine whether there are parallels to adolescent sleep that may help focus future sleep research in this age group.

Both laboratory and field studies of work scheduling have demonstrated a reliable association between working hours, sleep quantity and quality, and waking alertness. Both the timing of working hours within a day (circadian timing) and the number of hours worked in a day or week can affect sleep and alertness.

Circadian Timing of Work and Sleep

Sleep and subsequent waking alertness will be affected adversely to the degree that working hours intrude upon the normal nighttime sleeping hours. This tendency is most obvious in night-shift workers who must sleep during the daytime. Both retrospective cross-sectional surveys and prospective sleep-diary types of studies have indicated that night-shift workers consistently obtain less sleep than day or evening shift workers (Knauth, Landau, Droge, Schwitteck, Widynski, & Rutenfranz, 1980). Furthermore, night-shift workers often report their daytime sleep to be lighter, more fragmented, and less restful than sleep at night (Walsh, Tepas, & Moss, 1981; Lavie et al., 1989). Increasing experience with shift work apparently does not result in adaptation of sleep patterns, because older shift workers still show decreased daytime sleep (Tepas, Duchon, & Gersten, 1993). The sleep loss associated with these schedules results in increased sleepiness while awake, which may affect the worker's ability to perform activities safely and efficiently, both on and off the job. Increased sleepiness in shift workers on the job has been demonstrated with subjective reports (Folkard, Monk, & Lobban, 1978), objective performance testing (Wilkinson, Allison, Feeney, & Kaninska, 1989), and electroencephalographic (EEG) recordings showing brief sleep episodes while at work (Torsvall, Åkerstedt, Gillander, & Knutsson, 1989).

Night shift is not the only shift that can reduce the amount of sleep. Questionnaire studies have suggested that very early starts for morning shift can truncate sleep taken before that shift and also increase self-perceived sleepiness and fatigue during subsequent waking hours (Knauth et al., 1980; Kecklund & Åkerstedt, 1995). Work site surveys suggest that reduced sleep prior to an early morning shift probably is a result of difficulty in advancing the evening retiring time to try to obtain an adequate amount of sleep (Folkard & Barton, 1993). This observation is consistent with laboratory studies of circadian sleep propensity, which have demonstrated very long sleep latencies when sleep is attempted in the early evening (Lavie, 1986). Social incentives also could play a role in delaying retiring, as the early evening is a typical time to meet with family and friends. Data from a recent collaboration between the Finnish Institute of Occupational Health (FIOH) and the U.S. National Institute for Occupational Safety and Health (NIOSH) is shown in Figure 10.1 to illustrate the difference between days when sleep is constricted by going to work early and days when no such constriction exists. As shown, total sleep before the first 6:00 A.M. morning shift of the week, and sleep between morning shifts, is approximately two hours less than sleep after the last morning shift of the week. Sleep during

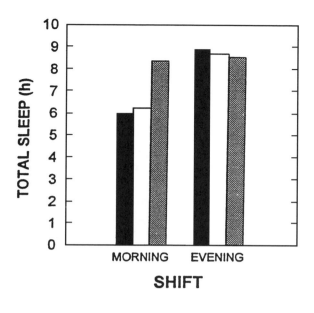

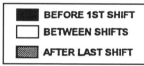

Figure 10.1. Questionnaire reports of steelworkers' habitual sleep before, during, and following a week of morning or evening shifts.

those days is also shorter than sleep at any time while working evening shifts. The apparent "rebound" increase of two hours observed after the last morning shift suggests an accumulated sleep debt across a week of morning shifts.

Such individual factors as age also might influence the ability to adjust to early-morning start times. A frequently observed feature of aging is a tendency toward "morningness" or a preference for earlier retiring and arising times in older compared with younger people (Monk et al., 1991; Ishihara, Miyake, Miyasita, & Miyata, 1992). Our collaborative study with FIOH illustrates some effects of morning start times and age on sleep and alertness (Rosa, Härmä, Pulli, Mulder, & Näsman, 1996). That study evaluated the impact of a one-hour delay of shift start and end times on worker sleep and alertness at a Finnish steel corporation.

Rescheduling Shift Starting Times: Effects on Sleep and Alertness

Two steel mills on rotating three-shift schedules were involved in the study. Both factories were from the same corporation and located in the same geographical area. The new shift schedule was established at site 1, which was a rolling mill where steel billets were processed into wire. Site 2, where no change of schedule occurred, was an ore processing mill that produced steel billets. Most of the work at both sites was automated, requiring workers to monitor processes and operate self-propelled machinery, but there also were operations that required heavy physical labor from some workers.

The change of schedule at site 1 was based partly on a preliminary questionnaire evaluation which indicated that nighttime sleep prior to the 6:00 A.M. morning shift was as brief as daytime sleep following night shift. In addition, questionnaire ratings of fatigue during morning shift at that site were as high as those given for night shift. These results contrasted with responses from the second factory which had shift starting times delayed by 1 hour. Morning shift sleep length at site 2 was considerably longer than night shift sleep and morning fatigue ratings were lower than night ratings. From these results it was hypothesized that a delay in starting times might improve morning shift sleep and fatigue. Therefore, a new schedule was established at site 1 with all start-end times delayed by 1 hour (morning shift start at 7:00 A.M.). The later start-end times were in effect throughout the study at site 2.

The new shift schedule was evaluated with the Standard Shiftwork Index (SSI) questionnaire administered to all factory workers. More extensive measures were made in a smaller group of workers using electronic activity monitors (actigraphs) and daily diaries to quantify home sleep, as well as using onsite computerized tests to quantify alertness at the work site. Base line testing was accomplished 4–6 months prior to the establishment of the new schedule, and follow-up testing occurred at the end of a 4-month trial period under the new schedule. For comparison, the same tests were given twice at the same times of year at site 2 where no change of schedule occurred. Workers participating in the study ranged in age from 18 to 62 years. For some analyses, the workers were divided at age 40 into younger (mean age = 31) and older groups (mean age = 50) to test for age-related differences in sleep or alertness.

Results indicated overall differences associated with age but no interaction of age with the change in schedule. Younger workers scored

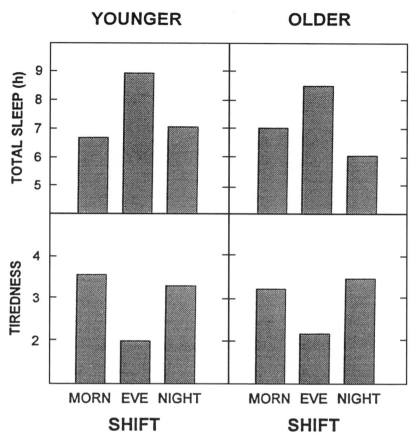

Figure 10.2. Questionnaire reports of total sleep and feelings of fatigue during work for morning, evening, and night shifts in younger and older steelworkers.

lower in "morningness" preference on the SSI, which, as shown in Figure 10.2, was reflected in less sleep than older workers prior to morning shift and more sleep than older workers after evening or night shifts. Similarly, as shown in Figure 10.2, younger workers felt more fatigued than older workers on morning shift and less fatigued on evening and night shifts.

With respect to the schedule change, we were able to demonstrate that as little as a 1-hour delay in morning shift starting times could reliably increase total sleep time prior to morning shift. As shown in Figure 10.3, both the actigraph and daily diary measures of total sleep time increased after the schedule change at site 1, whereas

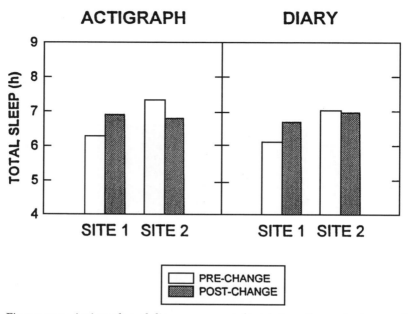

Figure 10.3. Actigraph and diary measures of total sleep time prior to morning shift at two steel mills, before and after a delay of shift starting times at site 1.

corresponding increases in total sleep were not apparent at site 2 where no change of schedule occurred. Self-reports of overall fatigue during morning shift recorded on the SSI and periodic self-ratings of sleepiness recorded by computer during the shift also improved after the change in schedule, as shown in Figure 10.4. Similar changes were not apparent at site 2. Examination of retiring and arising times indicated that increases in sleep could be attributed to later awakening times and not to earlier evening bedtimes. Despite increases in sleep and alertness after the schedule change, however, sleep still was constricted by the morning shift and a rebound in sleep length remained after the last morning shift of the week.

To summarize, the results provide strong evidence that early morning start times in the working world restrict the opportunities for sleep, which in turn contribute to sleepiness and fatigue during work. The most convincing support for this argument is that sleep and sleepiness were responsive to an apparently minor change in the start time of morning shift. The results also indicate that younger adults were affected by early starts more than older adults, as the younger group obtained less sleep and reported more morning sleepiness and fatigue at work.

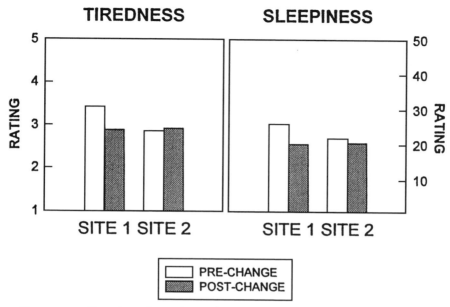

Figure 10.4. Questionnaire ratings of overall fatigue and computer-recorded ratings of periodic sleepiness during morning shift at two steel mills, before and after a delay of shift starting times at site 1.

Extended Work Hours and Sleep

Another factor limiting the opportunity for sleep is the number of hours of work in a day or week. Studies of extended workdays in adults suggest that sleep loss increases in proportion to the number of scheduled work hours per week. An extreme example of extended workdays is a person working double 8-hour shifts in response to chronic understaffing or the occasional absence of co-workers. Such a schedule allows for no personal time unless a portion of the average 8-hour sleep period is sacrificed. Working double shifts, however, is less common than working a regularly scheduled 10- or 12-hour shift. Nonetheless, under the more common extended-workday schedules, sleep still is sacrificed. Studies of extended work shifts conducted by NIOSH have demonstrated both a gradually accumulating sleep debt over a 4-day week of 12-hour shifts, and decreased worker alertness during the 12-hour shifts (Rosa, Colligan, & Lewis, 1989; Rosa & Bonnet, 1993).

The NIOSH studies were conducted on control room operators (ages 25 to 59) at a power plant and on control room and field operators at a natural gas utility. At both work sites, measurements were taken

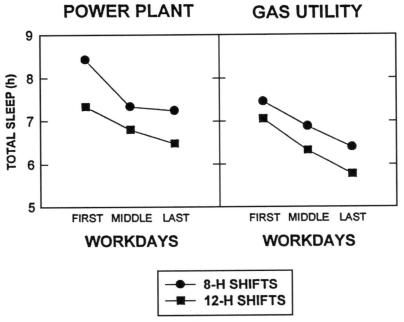

Figure 10.5. Diary measures of total sleep time across the workweek during 8-hour and 12-hour shift schedules at a power plant and a natural gas utility.

during the original 8-hour rotating shift schedule 5 to 7 workdays per week and again several months after a change to a 12-hour rotating shift schedule having 3 or 4 workdays per week. In a method similar to the steel mill study, workers recorded sleep quantity and quality in daily diaries and performed computerized tests of alertness periodically during their work shifts.

Results from both work sites suggested an accumulating sleep debt across the workweek. As shown in Figure 10.5, total sleep decreased across the week during both shift schedules, but the decrease was more acute during the 12-hour shift schedule. Data in Figure 10.6 from diary items recorded at the power plant also are consistent with accumulated sleep loss: frequency of napping decreased, latency to sleep decreased, and subjective depth of sleep increased across a week of 12-hour shifts. At the natural gas utility, we asked the workers specifically whether sleep was sacrificed because of work. As shown in Figure 10.7, increases in such reports were most apparent during the 12-hour shift schedule. This sleep debt was attributed partially to reduced daily personal time

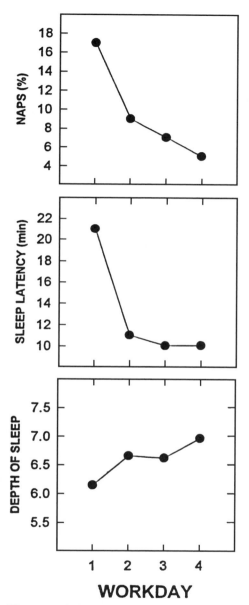

Figure 10.6. Diary measures of nap frequency, latency to sleep, and depth of sleep across a 4-day week of 12-hour shifts at a power plant.

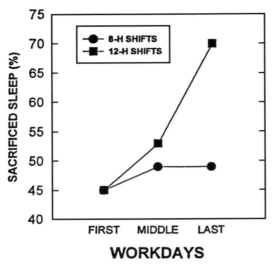

Figure 10.7. Diary reports of sacrificing sleep across the workweek during 8-hour and 12-hour shift schedules at a natural gas utility.

afforded by the extended workdays, which resulted in sleep being sacrificed for the sake of social-domestic obligations.

Discussion

Review of studies of work scheduling in adults points to at least two major factors affecting sleep and sleepiness: the circadian timing of work and the total number of hours of work. These factors interfere with sleep to the degree that they directly or indirectly intrude upon the nighttime hours normally allotted to sleep. An early morning work start reduces sleep length because it is difficult to go to bed early enough on the night before work. Working extended hours either directly overlaps the nighttime sleep period or forces other important waking activities to be accomplished at that time.

The degree to which these work schedule factors are relevant to adolescent sleep depends on the timing of the adolescent's primary "job" (going to school) and how many additional hours are worked in a week. Studies of adult work shift timing probably are relevant to adolescents, because adolescents often are required to begin school very early in the morning. Limited bus transportation has required many municipalities to stagger school starts for different age groups so that all students can take advantage of municipally provided transportation. Consequently, high school students often start school very early in order to accommodate a later start for students in the younger grades. These early starts could increase the likelihood of truncated morning sleep and associated waking drowsiness in a manner similar to that observed in adult morning shift workers. Consistent with this argument, the younger adults in our steel mill study had the most difficulty with early morning shifts. In addition, studies directly measuring adolescent sleep suggest that adolescents have at least as much difficulty with early morning awakening as the young adults in our study (Carskadon, 1989–1990, 1990).

It is also quite likely that the study of extended workdays in adults is applicable to adolescents. Attending school for 35 hours per week combined with 20 hours per week at a part-time job amounts to an extended work schedule for adolescents that is characterized as both demanding and fatiguing by most adult workers. Studies of extended workdays in adults suggest that sleep loss increases in proportion to the number of work hours scheduled in a week. The likelihood of greater sleepiness and fatigue associated with sleep loss and extended workdays could place working adolescents at greater risk of poor school performance or having an accident or injury. Studies of student working hours by Carskadon and colleagues are consistent with this suggestion. Those researchers observed that students working the most hours tended to obtain the least sleep and were the most sleepy during the day based both on EEG assessment (the multiple sleep latency test) and on subjective reports of intrusive sleepiness while driving or frequent loss of attention during class (Carskadon, 1989–1990, 1990).

Research directly examining the degree to which work schedule effects on sleep and fatigue differ in adults and adolescents is rare. There is some suggestion that adolescents have a greater sleep need than adults which could exacerbate the effects of work-related sleep debt (Carskadon, 1990). Young people, however, usually have fewer domestic duties than adults, which could allow greater opportunity for sleep. Examination of the interaction of work scheduling with other work-related fatigue factors is scarce in adults and nonexistent in adolescents. Virtually no work site research has compared different job tasks, workloads, or work pacing under the same work schedules, and social elements have been recognized but not studied systematically in terms of how they might affect fatigue. Environmental exposures on the job can affect fatigue and may be potentiated by sleep loss and increased sleepiness. Chemical solvents, for example, cause drowsiness (Dick, 1988), and noise, vibration, or heat can produce performance decrements (for reviews, see Hockey, 1983). It is unclear, however, whether there are differences in sensitivity to these factors between mature adults and developing adolescents.

In conclusion, the study of work and work schedule effects on adults may provide clues to guide research into the development of sleep and expression of sleepiness in adolescents. Definitive recommendations, however, cannot be given at the present time. It is hoped, however, that studies such as those presented here can contribute to a framework on which future recommendations can be made.

REFERENCES

Carskadon MA (1989–90). Adolescent sleepiness: Increased risk in a high-risk population. *Alcohol, Drugs and Driving* 5/6:317–328.
      (1990). Patterns of sleep and sleepiness in adolescents. *Pediatrician* 17:5–12.
Dick RB (1988). Short duration exposures to organic solvents: The relationship between neurobehavioral test results and other indicators. *Neurotoxicology and Teratology* 10:39–50.
Folkard S, Barton J (1993). Does the "forbidden zone" for sleep onset influence morning shift sleep duration? *Ergonomics* 36:85–91.
Folkard S, Monk TH, Lobban MC (1978). Short and long-term adjustment of circadian rhythms in "permanent" night nurses. *Ergonomics* 21:785–799.
Hockey R (1983). *Stress and Fatigue in Human Performance.* Chichester: John Wiley and Sons.
Ishihara K, Miyake S, Miyasita A, Miyata Y (1992). Morningness-eveningness preference and sleep habits in Japanese office workers of different ages. *Chronobiologia* 19:9–16.
Kecklund G, Åkerstedt T (1995). Effects of timing of shifts on sleepiness and sleep duration. *Journal of Sleep Research* 4 (suppl. 2): 47–50.
Knauth P, Landau K, Droge C, Schwitteck M, Widynski M, Rutenfranz J (1980). Duration of sleep depending on the type of shift work. *International Archives of Occupational and Environmental Health* 46:167–177.
Lavie P (1986). Ultradian rhythms in human sleep: III. Gates and "forbidden zones" for sleep. *Electroencephalography and Clinical Neurophysiology* 63: 414–425.
Lavie P, Chillag N, Epstein R, Tzischinsky O, Givon R, Fuchs S, Shahal B (1989). Sleep disturbances in shift workers: A marker for maladaptation syndrome. *Work and Stress* 3:33–40.
Monk TH, Reynolds CF, Buysse DJ, Hoch CC, Jarrett DB, Jennings JR, Kupfer DJ (1991). Circadian characteristics of healthy 80-year-olds and their relationship to objectively recorded sleep. *Journal of Gerontology* 46:M171–M175.
Rosa RR, Bonnet MH (1993). Performance and alertness on 8-hour and 12-hour rotating shifts at a natural gas utility. *Ergonomics* 36:1177–1193.
Rosa RR, Colligan MJ, Lewis P (1989). Extended workdays: Effects of 8-hour and 12-hour rotating shift schedules on performance, subjective alertness, sleep patterns, and psychosocial variables. *Work and Stress* 32:1–32.

Rosa RR, Härmä M, Pulli K, Mulder M, Näsman O (1996). Rescheduling a three-shift system at a steel rolling mill: Effects of a 1-hour delay of shift starting times on sleep and alertness in younger and older workers. *Occupational and Environmental Medicine* 53:677–685.

Steinberg L, Dornbusch SM (1991). Negative correlates of part-time employment during adolescence: Replication and elaboration. *Developmental Psychology* 27:304–313.

Tepas DI, Duchon JC, Gersten AH (1993). Shift work and the older worker. *Experimental Aging Research* 19:295–320.

Torsvall L, Åkerstedt T, Gillander K, Knutsson A (1989). Sleep on the night shift: 24-hour EEG monitoring of spontaneous sleep-wake behavior. *Psychophysiology* 26:352–358.

Walsh JK, Tepas DI, Moss PD (1981). The EEG sleep of night and rotating shift workers. In L. C. Johnson, D. I. Tepas, W. P. Colquhoun, & M. J. Colligan, eds., *Biological Rhythms, Sleep, and Shift Work*, pp. 371–381. New York: Spectrum.

Wilkinson R, Allison S, Feeney M, Kaninska Z (1989). Alertness of night nurses: Two shift systems compared. *Ergonomics* 32:281–292.

11. Accommodating the Sleep Patterns of Adolescents within Current Educational Structures: An Uncharted Path

KYLA L. WAHLSTROM

The attempt to make significant changes in education systems is often likened to trying to change the course of a supertanker ship – with the inertia for the present course being extraordinarily powerful and with changes often occurring only in small degrees. Such is the case for attempting to change the current start time for high schools. The path toward making that change is replete with real and presumed obstacles in the form of facts and misperceptions.

The School Start Time Study, presented here, was initiated at the request of several school superintendents and was completed with the administrative and financial support of seventeen school superintendents in the Minneapolis–St. Paul area. Information was gathered from participating school districts about the issues and impact of a potential change in the starting time for their high schools. The perspectives of key stakeholder groups, including students, teachers, parents, school administrators, and community members, were sought. They responded to concerns in the areas of transportation, athletics and other school activities, community education, food service, human resources and contractual agreements, elementary school start time, and crime statistics.

In particular, one suburban school district (Edina) in the Minneapolis–St. Paul area shifted its high schools to a later start time for the 1996–1997 school year. Its experiences provide vital information because the residents are living with a school start time change. Included in this report is a brief case study of the Edina school district.

It is important to note that most of the participating districts in this study are in one of two athletic conferences located in the west metropolitan area. The reasoning for this apparent selectivity is that changing the starting time for the secondary schools has an impact on other school districts within the same activities conference, with respect to the start time for games and cocurricular activities that involve students from two or more school districts. Therefore, the superintendents sought to have common information so that the interrelational aspect of the discussion could occur as well.

Review of the Literature: An Overview

The impetus for the development of the study presented here is based on research information from studies of the sleep patterns and sleep needs of the adolescent. For a more comprehensive view of the findings, please refer to works cited at the conclusion of this chapter and to other chapters within this book. For purposes of brevity within this chapter, the following are some of the essential elements being cited by local advocates seeking to change to a later start:

Sleep Research

- All living organisms appear to have rhythmic patterns at the cellular level known as circadian rhythms.
- Circadian rhythms are generated internally and develop without any social or environmental cues.
- Natural circadian patterns are very resistant to change.
- Sleep deprivation is associated with information-processing and memory deficits; increased irritability, anxiety, and depression; hypersexuality; decreased creativity and ability to handle complex tasks.
- As teenagers move through teenage years, they need increasing amounts of sleep.
- Nine hours per night is the necessary amount to avoid behaviors associated with sleep deprivation.
- Risks with teenage sleep deprivation include mood and behavior problems, increased potential for drug and alcohol use, and vulnerability to accidents.
- Twenty percent of all high school students fall asleep in school (Maas, 1995).
- Over 50% of students report being most alert after 3:00 P.M. (Allen & Mirabile, 1989).

- Forced awakening does not appear to reset the circadian rhythm, and school sleep lag is worse for earlier starting schools (Allen, 1991). Additional weekend sleep does not alleviate this negative effect.
- Students who evidence a sleep lag syndrome correspond to those having poorer grades. Causation is not implied here, but the relationship does statistically exist (Allen, 1992; Carskadon, 1993; Wolfson & Carskadon, 1998).

Time of Day for Learning

- The use of Dunn's Learning Styles Inventory assisted one school in changing the time of day that various forms of instruction were employed with the result being an improvement in student achievement and a reduction in behavior problems (Stone, 1992).
- Performance typically peaks in the afternoon (Kraft & Martin, 1995), although others believe this depends on the individual.
- Individuals classified as "morning types" performed better on measures of speed and response in the morning, while "afternoon types" performed better in the afternoon (Anderson, Petros, Beckwith, Mitchell, & Fritz, 1991).
- Afternoon reading instruction produced the greatest increase in reading scores as compared with morning instruction (Barron, Henderson, & Spurgeon, 1994).
- Callan (1995) suggests that administering the SAT only in the morning may discriminate against some students.

Stakeholder Reports

The information from each of the groups that has a stake in the discussion and outcome of changing the starting time for high schools can be usefully examined as separate categories first, before looking at the common themes among them. This is because many of these stakeholder groups believe that they each have the most critical reasons and hold the deciding factors for whether a change is feasible or a wise move. Indeed, each group interviewed has a legitimate reason for being consulted during this discussion; however, the factors and concerns are incredibly interrelated and no single group holds the trump card, even though it may think it does.

Transportation

Costs

The seventeen transportation directors interviewed individually by phone emphasized the need to stagger the high school, middle school, and elementary school start times to cut down the number of drivers and buses needed and thus contain costs. School districts are limited in their transportation funding by the legislature. Three directors mentioned another possible implication of high school starting last: there might be extra transportation costs if the bus drivers would be then working overtime hours because of the later scheduled activities (sports, etc.).

Safety

When asked about safety concerns, most directors (12 of 17) did talk about the possible danger of having elementary students outside in the dark, either in the early morning or coming home late from school – depending on when the elementary start and dismissal times are. However, several directors noted that in their past experiences, once changes were made, people habituated to it fairly quickly and with little extended complaining.

Athletics and Activities

Three people were interviewed by phone in each of the 17 districts (N = 51): the athletic director, a coach, and either the activities director or a fine arts teacher (or sometimes both if the activities director was also the athletic director). In the interviews the faculty responded to questions about the possible impact of a later high school or middle school start time on after-school athletics and activities.

Athletics

Overall, the majority of athletic directors and coaches believed that a 1-hour-later start time would cause some difficulties, ranging from minor to major problems. Nine of them stated clearly that they prefer to keep the school day as it is. However, about one-third of the athletic directors and coaches thought it would be "possible" or "manageable" to start one hour later. Others were undecided as to whether the change would be manageable or not. Four of them said they would prefer a later school start time, primarily for the sake of student academics. Also, five individuals mentioned that a half-hour later school start time would work better than the present school time, but that more than a half-hour change would begin to cause conflicts. A few others said there would be a large impact unless the other schools changed their school time also. Eleven of those interviewed mentioned that practice time could or would be cut back if school started later.

Daylight-Darkness Concern

Another major concern was the limited daylight to finish games, meets, and practices. Twenty of the interviewees brought up this issue, saying that certain sports would be affected by darkness in the late fall, the winter months, and early spring. The major concerns were how to fit events in before darkness, yet not have students miss school. Some interviewees pointed out that to get students to away games and have them warmed up before the event, they have to leave immediately after school even on the current schedule.

Eleven athletic directors or coaches mentioned that the major concern would be the impact on the younger grades' sports teams – the freshman, sophomore, and junior varsity teams. Presently, these games (e.g., football and soccer games) usually start at 4:00 P.M., and the fields they use are not lit. With a later start, the games might not end before dark.

Facility Availability for Community Groups

One concern frequently mentioned regarding a later school day is the effect it would have on community education and youth programs. Twenty-four study participants brought up the concern that community sports for adults and youth start right after the high schools' practices. Generally, the cities or suburbs have agreements with the school districts to have students use facilities (school and city facilities) after school and for games so that the community can take over after school practices are finished.

Many interviewees mentioned that there is a big demand on the limited sports' facilities in their city because of all the adult and youth programs. Gymnasium space at the schools is in particularly high demand. In addition, ice arenas, softball fields, and the football and soccer fields are often shared between the schools and the larger community. Changing to later start times for the community activities "would increase the tensions," as one athletic director explained it, and allow less time for adults, younger children, and families to participate in community sports.

In addition, many student athletes work after practices, so if the school day and practices began later this could impact the student athlete's job in a number of ways: working less, working later, or not working during the week. Indeed, two athletic directors and two fine arts teachers thought that moving the school day back might cause less after-school student participation. Students may choose work over an after-school activity or may participate in fewer school activities. However, at the Edina school where the change has already occurred, the three people interviewed seemed to feel "the positives have outweighed the negatives" concerning the later high school starting time.

Cocurricular Activities and Fine Arts

Seventeen activities directors and five teachers who instruct in one or two of the areas of music, debate, speech, and drama were interviewed. The overall sentiment was that the fine arts and clubs would not be nearly as affected by a later high school start time as would the athletic programs. The interviewees were split evenly between believing the school time should stay as it is and believing it would be manageable to move the time back.

Some of the same concerns were raised by the fine arts directors and teachers as were raised by the athletic directors and coaches. However, two major differences make the fine arts programs much less affected by a later start time than athletics: there are many fewer interdistrict competitions in the fine arts programs, and the use of facilities is not a major issue as in athletics. A concern raised by five individuals was the belief that, with a later school start time, there might be less student participation because of greater time constraints, with students being involved in other things like work and athletics.

Middle School

Of the 51 interviewees, 5 commented specifically about middle school, or junior high, athletics and activities. In general, the middle schools would also be impacted by a later school day, but probably not nearly as much as the high schools. Middle schools have fewer athletic programs and after school fine arts programs than do high schools. Also, the middle school students are employed less than the high school students, and thus would still be involved in sports without a job getting in their way. However, the middle schools would have some of the same problems as the high schools in fitting in their practices and games before it gets dark and before the community wants to use the facilities.

Community Education

The community education departments in the districts involved in the study all have similar programs that service preschool age children through adults, and some of the districts also offer senior citizen programs. Of the 17 districts, 16 responded to telephone calls about their community education programs. In general, the directors spoke positively about their flexibility; they said they would change as necessary to provide services for all community members.

Facilities

The majority of community education directors reported that facilities would be impacted the most by a change in school start times. Currently, in most districts the demand for gymnasium space far exceeds supply; gyms are used every weekday and Saturdays. A change in school start and end times would influence practice times and space for middle, junior, and senior high school athletic programs. Scheduling pools was also a problem in some districts, as was available ice time in others. This varied considerably from district to district.

School-Age Child Care

All districts offered school-age child care, although some programs were contracted out to the local YMCA. Hours generally run from 6:00 A.M. to 6:30 P.M., with some slight variation. Most directors said that a change in the school start and end times might affect the number of children enrolled in the before and after school programs. If elementary schools started earlier, the number of children enrolled before school may drop, while the numbers might increase in the afternoon. That would impact the staffing of those programs.

Adult Enrichment

Community education directors reported that most of the adult enrichment programs do not begin until after 6:00 P.M. in the evenings and there likely wouldn't be an impact if the schools started and ended later.

Moreover, a similar concern expressed by a number of community education directors was the importance of a common start and end time for all levels of schools, to make sure there is consistency – that is, all elementary, all middle or junior high schools, and all senior high schools should begin and end at the same time in the district or metro area. It may be beneficial for the middle school to end earlier because it would leave more time for students to be involved in extracurricular activities.

Related to the community education study, four park and recreation directors were contacted to see if there would be any impact on their programs if the high schools' start and dismissal times were later. The directors said there would not be an impact, with the exception of use of ice arenas after school (in the late afternoon). The high school hockey teams would have to practice in the morning and/or have their afternoon practices cut back, which both of the Edina High School's hockey teams have done because of their later school day.

Food Service

Food service directors were contacted in four school districts. If wide differences had emerged among those four, additional food service directors would have been contacted. As it was, the information provided revealed great similarities from one district to another, and it appears to be representative of the broad issues associated with a potential change in the starting times of the local schools.

Lunch times would have to change if the schools started later or earlier in most districts. For several districts, changing the start time may create difficulties because some kitchens only have a serving site with no preparation facilities. One food service director said a later start time may result in establishing a breakfast program.

Many district food programs also prepare meals for senior citizens, including Meals on Wheels, and for district child care services. The coordination and timing of providing those meals would likely be affected by shifting the start times of certain schools.

Some districts' workers are unionized and others are not. Thus, changing the employees' schedules may or may not be a problem. The food service workers in one district often are semiretired and work as needed; changing their start time would not be an issue.

Contractual Agreements

Part of the study was to determine if there would be any implications for school or employee contract agreements with changing the start time for schools. Interviewed were six human resource directors who are in charge of their districts' employee contract agreements with the teachers, secretaries, custodians, food service workers, and others. The response given by all six interviewees was that the employee contracts refer to the employees of the school working a certain amount of hours each day, but the contracts do not mention specific start and end times. The starting-ending time for work may become part of the negotiations discussion, even though it would not become part of the written contract language.

Elementary Directors

Thirteen curriculum directors, elementary directors, and elementary principals whose districts are participating in this study were contacted. Current elementary school start times in the 17 districts range from 8:25 to 9:40 A.M.

Nearly all of the respondents volunteered the belief that morning is the best time of day to learn, and thus having a longer morning with an earlier start for teaching would be an advantage. One elementary principal said teachers prefer mornings for the most intensive study because children are more alert and ready to learn then. Several respondents noted that a longer morning would be better educationally, but children might need a break of some sort.

One elementary principal particularly noted that a start time of later than 9:00 A.M. is too late: teachers perceive a loss of good learning time. Also, there is difficulty scheduling elementary field trips in the afternoon because buses are usually transporting secondary students and are therefore not available.

One principal said that the parental response to starting elementary schools earlier in the morning will be "situational." Some families have older siblings who would leave for school later and could make sure the younger children get off to school first. Or a parent could get the child off to school in the morning before leaving for work. Several respondents believed that an earlier elementary start would likely mean that someone would at least be home in the early morning to supervise young children, as opposed to leaving them alone to get themselves off to school, which is often the case now. An elementary director thought that parents would adjust, and overall it may be easier in terms of family schedules. After-school child care is generally easier to arrange than early-morning care.

Several respondents referred to the fact that darkness is a concern at this time of year for little ones. Currently, some elementary students are dropped off at 4:15 in the afternoon when it is nearly dark in the winter. Several principals were not sure whether dark mornings are worse than dark late afternoons. An assistant superintendent noted that, in geographically small districts, darkness and safety were not problems because they have short bus runs.

Employers Report

The School Start Time Study sought to determine if later high school start and dismissal times would impact local employers of the students. Names of employers were furnished by the school districts. In addition to speaking to fifteen employers, interviewed were three Chamber of Commerce directors and a teacher who works with the 9th grade Work Experience Career Exploration Program (WECEP), which helps 9th grade students fulfill work study during the second half of the school day. The 15 businesses contacted included 6 fast food restaurants, 3 supermarkets, 3 department stores, 2 mall retail stores, and 1 manufacturing company.

The overall impression that the employers, managers, and human resource workers gave was that there would be little or no impact from a later school dismissal time. Four employers stated there would be an impact in the after-school work shifts, but when asked if a 1 hour later start time would have an impact, three said that 1 hour would not make much of an impact, that they "could deal with it" or that they are "flexible." Most of the employers said that their high school employees either do not start right after school or that they could "adjust the day workers'" shifts to accommodate a later arrival of the students.

Impact on 14- and 15-year-old students who work centered on the fact that, by law, they can only work 3 hours a day during the school week and not after 7:00 P.M. However, one of the employers pointed out that it would not be a problem as long as the students could start by 4:00 P.M.

The three Chamber of Commerce directors thought there would be no or little impact. One director thought the employers might benefit from a later school time because their student workers would be better rested for work.

Crime Statistics Report

Juvenile crime in the state of Minnesota has been increasing at a high rate. According to the Minnesota Department of Safety's Bureau of Criminal Apprehension, the number of juvenile arrests rose by 52.5% between 1990 and 1995, placing the 1995 total at 68,212. This number represents 29.5% of all apprehensions made in the state during that year. In addition, 13- to 18-year-olds were apprehended more often than any other age group of a similar 5-year age span. Juveniles tend to perpetrate crimes and be arrested in groups of two or more, in contrast with adult arrests which occur in single incidents. Therefore, the number of arrest incidents versus the number of juvenile persons arrested will be two different statistics and needs to be considered in understanding this data. Finally, juvenile "nuisance behaviors" are not reported because they are not arrests per se and therefore may be underrepresented in the statistics.

For the purposes of this study, it would be desirable to know when these crimes are occurring. Unfortunately, most state crime bureaus, including the Minnesota Bureau of Criminal Apprehension, do not separate juveniles from adults when compiling crime data based on the time of day crimes were committed. There is national data available from the FBI, however, that suggest that on school days, juvenile crime peaks between 2:00 P.M. and 4:00 P.M. and decreases throughout the evening hours. In contrast, the number of crimes committed by adults increases during the day and evening hours, with the peak occurring around midnight. Finally, these data reveal that the frequency of juvenile crime is about four times greater in the hours after school than during curfew hours.

School Start Times outside the Metropolitan Area

Eight smaller and larger towns and cities outside of the seven-county metropolitan area were contacted to get an idea of when their schools begin. Seven of the school districts contacted have a high school start time between 8:05 and 8:30 A.M. Generally, the junior high and elementary schools start at approximately the same time as the high schools. In smaller districts all grade levels ride together on one bus run. The buses begin picking up the students living farthest away from one hour to one and a half hours before school starts. As a result, some adolescent students living farthest from school may still suffer from a lack of adequate sleep because of the need to arise early to catch the bus.

Teacher Survey

All secondary teachers and a random sample of elementary teachers from all districts participating in the study were surveyed (N = 3,460). The survey questions centered around times of the day for school start and end times in terms of optimal student learning and optimal instruction times. Elementary teachers were also asked about perceived issues for student safety if youngsters are coming to school while it is still dark outside. Open-ended comments were solicited after each question to amplify the response. Tables 11.1 and 11.2 contain the teacher responses to the question of best starting time to enable optimal learning.

Table 11.1. Secondary Teacher Survey:
Optimal Start Time of First Class for
Majority of Students

Time	Number	Percentage
6:00	5	0.2
6:30	3	0.1
7:00	20	0.7
7:15	32	1.1
7:30	318	10.7
7:45	157	5.3
8:00	1037	35.0
8:15	291	9.8
8:30	696	23.5
8:45	77	2.6
9:00	250	8.4
9:30	19	0.6
9:45	1	0.0
10:00	12	0.4
Other	9	0.3
No opinion	37	1.2
TOTAL	2,964	100.0

Table 11.2. Elementary Teacher Survey:
Optimal Start Time of First Class for
Majority of Students

Time	Number	Percentage
6:00	1	0.1
7:15	1	0.1
7:30	14	2.0
7:45	14	2.0
8:00	159	23.0
8:15	97	14.0
8:30	287	41.5
8:45	57	8.2
9:00	52	7.5
9:30	7	1.0
10:00	2	0.3
Other	1	0.1
TOTAL	692	100.0

Student Survey

A stratified random sample of students in the secondary schools of the participating districts was asked to complete the "Sleep Habits Survey," a 62-item questionnaire developed and normed by E. P. Bradley Hospital at Brown University in Providence, Rhode Island (Wolfson & Carskadon, 1998). A total of 280 classrooms were sampled, with a return rate of 98.57%. Overall, approximately 10.8% of the total population of 66,394 students was sampled (N = 7,168).

Summary of Findings

All six grade levels (7–12) show the same general increase in reported academic grades associated with later start times; however, for all six grade levels the pattern is different. The increase in academic grades associated with later start times is greater at the early start time for students in grades 7 and 8, with the most rapid increase between 7:30 and 8:00 A.M. The patterns in grades 11 and 12 are very similar and contrast with those found in grades 7 and 8. For 11th and 12th graders, they have a gradual increase in academic grades, which accelerates rapidly from the 8:00 to 8:30 A.M. start time and beyond.

It is important to note that these findings do not indicate causality (i.e., that later start times will necessarily cause academic grades to

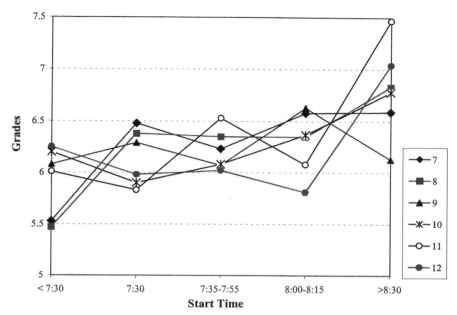

Figure 11.1. Mean Grades by Start Time and Grade Level

improve), but there is clearly a statistical relationship between these two variables that may be explained by other variables (e.g., less depression, less struggle to stay awake in class) that change when the start time of school is changed (see Figure 11.1).

Other findings from the student survey are consistent with the findings noted in the literature reviewed in the beginning of this chapter. The "picture" of our students is very similar to that of the students studied in other locations in the United States. Finally, there were no gender differences. The relationship between start time and reported academic grades is basically the same for boys and girls, with the girls consistently reporting a higher level of academic grades. This finding is visible in the essentially parallel lines seen in Figure 11.2.

Parent Survey

A random sample of parents was contacted by telephone in each of the 17 school districts (N = 765). Roughly 15 parents in each of the three age levels (elementary, middle or junior high, and high school; n = 45 parent respondents per district) were asked questions about the time their child leaves home in the morning, as well as what time they thought would

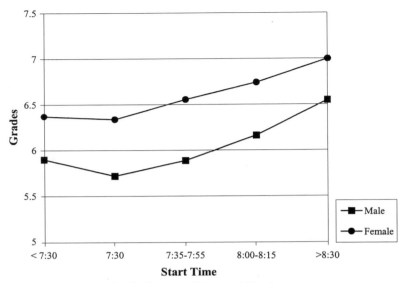

Figure 11.2. Mean Grades by Start Time and Gender

be the preferred leaving time, given the age of their child. A follow-up
question was then asked about why that time was preferred. Parents
of elementary age children were also asked to name the earliest leaving
time from home that would be safe for the child (see Tables 11.3 and 11.4.)

Table 11.3. What Would Be the Best Leaving Time for Your
Child? (percentage of respondents)

Time	Elementary	Middle/Junior High	Senior High
Before 7:15	0	3	9
7:15	1	11	11
7:30	4	16	15
7:45	2	13	7
8:00	23	28	31
8:15	10	5	7
8:30	28	13	9
8:45	9	1	0
9:00	14	4	2
9:15	1	0	0
9:30	1	0	0
9:45	1	1	0
No preference	4	5	5
Unsure	1	1	1

Table 11.4. Could You Tell Me Why You Selected That Time?
(percentage of respondents)

	Elementary	Middle/Junior High	Senior High
Allows sleep	24	39	45
Able to get ready	33	25	18
Current time works	165	95	7
Better schedule	11	7	6
Light outside	3	8	10
Time to go to work	9	5	6
Will learn more	1	1	5
Leave with siblings	1	3	1
Avoid traffic	0	0	1
Unsure	3	2	1

Edina Case Study

As noted at the beginning of this chapter, Edina is the only local district to have purposefully made the move to a later start time for its high school. Edina, a suburb of Minneapolis, changed its high school's starting time from 7:25 to 8:30 A.M. with corresponding changes in closing times from 2:05 to 3:10 P.M. To reach that decision in the spring of 1996, there was a small amount of fact-finding and discussion before a vote at a school board meeting confirmed this as an administrative decision. The district quietly made the change with little public notice, until the fall of 1996 when the studies of adolescent sleep needs became widely discussed, and Edina became the district to watch. The case of Edina is important because the respondents are speaking from personal experience and not from speculation about what "might" happen if the district were to change, as is the case in the other 16 districts involved in this study.

Edina Teachers Focus Group Summary

In the fall of 1996, eight Edina high school teachers participated in a discussion after school about their experiences and perceptions during the first term under the 65 minute later start time. They discussed their impressions and observations regarding the impact on students and learning, changes in teaching behavior, and other pertinent issues.

There was general agreement among all eight who said that, during the first hour, they do not have "people with their heads down on the desk; they seem to be more engaged in what they're doing and to be more focused." Flexibility for both students and staff was also mentioned by a number of the teachers. There is flexibility for students to come in early and take tests, get academic help, study, and so on. The teachers did wonder if students will continue to come in early in a couple years when the later start time is the "norm."

Staff meetings in the morning are now possible instead of always after school. Guest speakers are more likely to come to a first hour class with the later start time. Many teachers commented that there's now time in the mornings to conduct meetings with parents, which was not the case in previous years.

In general, teachers come at the same time in the morning as they did in previous years, but this year they have time to process and prepare new and timely information to incorporate into teaching: "I teach a lot of business courses and I use daily news, so I have time to go over some newspapers, jump on the Internet, and find out what some of the top stories are for the day," one teacher commented; "I think our day has gotten longer." This notion was reiterated by a number of faculty who said most of them come to school at the same time but stay longer in the afternoon. A few of them mentioned that they miss the late afternoon break between school and dinner to wind down, exercise, or run errands.

Generally, parents seem to be in favor of the later start time. One teacher called the parents of all 160 students in her classes and asked if they saw a difference in the behavior of their children. She reported "it was just an overwhelming 'yes'; there was a difference within what was happening at home and in the family, particularly the behaviors and attitudes."

A drawback to the later start time was noted by one teacher. "What we're losing at the moment is some of the students involved in these athletics and sports who leave early from their 6th hour to get to the activities." Another stated, "I don't think [students missing part of their 6th hour for activities] is anything that can't be worked out once people are aware of the facts."

In support of the later start time, a teacher commented, "I've heard a steady stream of positives from parents, and especially from students. I polled the senior class and it was 8 to 1 in favor of the change. The overwhelming response is positive; the only issue that ever comes up that's kind of negative is the impact that it does have on sports and school activities, because of the time pressure. But I think a number of those concerns might be addressed by taking a look at how long we run practices. . . . How much time do we *really* need for practices, and how can we be more effective with our use of time for extracurricular activities?"

When asked if the students have changed their bedtimes, one teacher commented that she asked her classes this question and said there has not been a big change. She went on to say, "[The students] say they may stay up a little bit later to do their homework, because they have a little bit more time knowing they can sleep in, which is the positive side to this. But they're not just staying up for the sake of staying up."

One teacher added that she went to the school's health service "to inquire if there was a difference this year in terms of students not feeling well." She was told that there has been a "tremendous difference" this year over last year. Last year, 39 students had been sent home for illness compared to 25 this year during the same time period. They added that there could be any number of factors for this change, but part of it could be the later start time, and that kids are eating breakfast more often now.

Edina Student Focus Group Summary

Eight students from Edina High School were interviewed regarding the later school start time. The students were asked to speak not only from their own perspectives, but also to share what they have heard from their classmates about the later school start time.

The students were first asked what the biggest difference or change was as a result of the later school start time. A couple of the students immediately answered, "I get more sleep." One student replied, "I feel more awake in the first hour – I'm less likely to fall asleep." They have observed that fewer students are sleeping during school. One student said that after-school activities are now shorter, so they have less time to practice these various activities.

Most students said that they go to bed around the same time as they did last year and get up later, getting extra sleep. One student commented that he naturally is not sleepy until later at night. Last year he tried to go to sleep at 9:30, but it did not work, and he "couldn't fall asleep until 11:30." Now he goes to bed at 11:30, and the later school start time allows him to get a good night's sleep. Another student said that his body doesn't "shut down" until midnight, so that is when he goes to bed. Not all students are getting more sleep, however. A few said they go to bed later this year, so they end up getting about the same amount of sleep as last year. One student commented that she would like to go to bed at the same time as she did last year, but has to stay up an hour later because she has more homework.

The students talked about some of the drawbacks to the later start time as well. For instance, one student said that the only thing that her classmates do not like about the change is that "they get home late after sports." Another student agreed. Still another added that some of his friends who work have complained about the change. He said, "last year they could work from 3:00 to 5:00 P.M. Now they are forced to work at a later time." One student mentioned that she knew somebody who had to quit her job because, with the new school schedule, she doesn't have enough time to work. However, she added that if a student really wants to work, he or she can if they manage their time well.

Originally, there was some concern that, with the later school time, students would begin to fade by the end of the school day. Although one student commented that "kids are more excited to leave school by the end of the day than a year before," other students agreed that the last hour of the day, 6th hour, has not been negatively impacted.

A few students said they are doing better academically because they are more awake. One student shared, "I have only fallen asleep once in school this whole year, and last year I fell asleep about three times a week." Another student added that she's "more alert" and doesn't "zone out as much." On a similar note, a student said, "I feel I pay better attention because my sleep schedule is closer to my normal sleep pattern." Two students added that it feels a lot better now that they leave for school when it is light out, whereas last year during the winter it was dark when they left for school.

Another positive aspect of the later school start is that there is time before school for students to make up tests, attend review sessions for important tests, and join activities that meet before school. Also, the students mentioned that they have eaten breakfast more often this year as compared to last.

Edina Counselors Focus Group Summary

Four Edina high school counselors participated in a focus group meeting to discuss the impact of their district's later school day. They were asked what was most striking or interesting to them regarding the school start time moving back 65 minutes.

One counselor said she had asked 50 to 60 students about how they are doing with the later start time. She said she "can't think of one student who did not like the change and most students are really appreciative" of the later start. She added that the students are booked solid all day with extracurricular activities and work, and that they like having the extra hour in the morning. Sometimes they use that time to meet before school for their extracurricular activities.

One respondent mentioned she has spoken with a few students who are morning-oriented and would prefer an earlier start, but "the overwhelming response is favorable to starting at 8:30." She added, "I think the kids are more alert . . . and they are 'with you' at 8:30." Last year was not always like that. She thinks the students are now getting more sleep.

When asked about any changes in student behavior, one counselor noted that stress referrals for students who feel a lot of academic pressure are "significantly down." She thinks students feel they have more personal time with the later start time. However, another counselor added that the later start time is hard on the teachers who coach extracurricular activities after school, because they do not get home from school until the early evening.

One issue brought up and echoed by all respondents was that the new schedule makes conferences between counselors and parents easier to schedule. Parents appreciate the convenience of later meetings, and they feel more free to ask the counselor for a 4:00 P.M. or even later meeting.

The counselors stated that the school climate is better this year. It appears to be more "calm" and "positive." The attitude and behavior of the students appears to be significantly better than past years. However, again, the counselors were not sure if this change is related to the new start time or not.

Edina Administration Focus Group Summary

Several Edina High School administrators participated in a focus group regarding the later high school start time. They were asked about any differences they see this year at Edina High School because of the schedule change.

One administrator started by stating, "there is an alertness in the students coming into school that I haven't seen in many, many years. I have also heard fewer complaints from the students about not getting enough sleep." Another administrator added, "the school as a whole seems more calm – there are fewer students loitering in the halls at the start of first hour."

The school attendance rate for first period is better. Also, parents whose children have had trouble in previous years getting to school on time are supportive of the change, and these parents are more likely to be supportive of school policies when their children are late now.

One administrator asked some of the student athletes and coaches about their impressions of the later school day. He said, "the change has been well received, by and large. If I had to put a percentage on the positives versus the negatives, I would have to say 85% have been in favor of the later start." "However," he added, "we need to run through the whole year to get a fair assessment of the impact on athletics. There will be more of an impact in the winter and spring with student athletes getting out of their last period class early for 'away' competitions." This fall some students have been dismissed about 20 minutes early for away games.

The administrators have also noticed that the teachers are less rushed in the morning and are more available to assist students. The later start time is of benefit to students who couldn't get academic help after school because of extracurricular activities and who can now come in before school. One administrator added that it is also easier for group activities, such as marching band, to practice in the morning.

Concerning discipline issues, one administrator commented that he was not sure he has seen much change. However, he reiterated the point that was made earlier, that attendance for the first hour is presently not a problem. In past years the lack of attendance first hour "had been a big deal."

The administrators noted that the halls seem to be calmer. Also, one administrator said that the students are better behaved in the lunch-room. The administrators were not sure where best to place attribution for these changes, but they seemed to believe the later start time has had a positive impact on the overall climate of the school.

Parent Written Survey Report from Edina School District

Parents who attended parent-teacher conferences on November 25 and 26, 1996, at Edina High School were asked to complete a written survey concerning their impressions of the change in the starting time of the high school. The total number of surveys returned represented

18.8% of the families with children at the school. Related to the total enrollment at the school, 11.8% of parents of seniors, 20% of parents of juniors, and 22.7% of parents of sophomores responded. Although this group of parents is self-selected because of their participation in school conferences, the significantly positive rate of response to the later start time should not be dismissed or undervalued.

When asked: "Are you pleased with the later start time for high school students?" responses of "Yes," "No," and "Not sure" were as follows: sophomores: 96, 6, and 4; juniors: 84, 4, and 1; seniors: 48, 2, and 0. Total responses for "Yes" were 228 (93%); for "No," 12 (5%); and for "Not sure," 5 (2%). Fifteen surveys included families with multiple students at the high school, and these data are included within the individual class figures.

Parents also included lengthy written comments as a part of the survey. Parents of seniors described several advantages: "takes time to eat breakfast"; "more rested, healthier, awakens more easily, has not overslept this year"; "more rested and less hurried"; "long overdue – would be nice for middle school too"; "student is a backup at home as a responsible person to get grade schooler off"; "more alone time with each child"; "he is better rested and more alert all day"; "time to meet teacher or make up test in the A.M."; "better grades, better focus"; and "I have had students at Edina High School for the past six years, and this is THE best change." They pointed out a few disadvantages as well: "she starts doing her homework later"; "we don't see our son in the morning"; "phone calls later into the P.M."; and "needs to leave 6th hour for sports too often."

Sophomore and junior students' parents also shared their views. Parents of juniors pointed out the following advantages: "Both of us get more sleep. Now can you change middle school?"; "She is able to adjust and use her time better, especially with all the early evening activities this age group has – it allows her more time for homework"; "Stick with it, it's much better overall"; "I get to talk with her at breakfast"; "He is rested and is doing much better academically this year"; "Parents are raving about the late start for EHS. Should have done this years before, BRAVO!"; "psychological benefits even if she doesn't get any more sleep"; "has time to review in A.M. on day of test"; "everyone is not so rushed"; and "traffic patterns have eased up." They noted few disadvantages: "dinner hour later"; "jobs start at 3:30 P.M."; "prefer to get a jump start on the day; conflicts with after school sports practices and early dismissals for meets."

Parents of sophomores reported the following pros: "I am so relieved that Edina had the wisdom to follow the advice of the Minnesota Medical Association . . . definitely keep it"; "less stressful mornings"; "breakfast is never missed"; "fix the middle schools too!"; "not as much time to kill in the afternoons – very pleased"; "The later start time is very beneficial both relative to grades and to energy level"; "We have family time before school"; "Keep it . . . would like to see middle school start later. Buy more buses if needed"; "my child can meet with teachers before school for help if necessary." And, some of their drawbacks were: "Only problem is regarding sports – athletes need to miss classes in order to get to meets"; "Our child does not come home from extracurricular activities until 6:30 P.M. and is up early for weights – we don't get the benefit of a late start"; "They stay up later and the amount of sleep is the same"; "calls from friends late at night; won't go to bed"; "eating dinner later because of school sports, no time for a job."

Discussion

The bottom line finding of the study is that any decision to change the starting time of schools, from elementary to high school, is highly politically charged and extraordinarily complex. The interrelatedness of the stakeholder groups must always be taken into account, even when one of the factors or groups becomes the dominant feature in the decision-making process. Failure to acknowledge the needs and concerns of each group may lead to charges of reaching an incomplete decision and may well cause a change to be reversed. When this happens, public trust in the school district's capability to reach a sound and wisely considered decision may be tarnished or eroded for many years to come.

This chapter was subtitled "an uncharted path" for good reason. The experiences of the Edina school system are viewed skeptically by many. This is because Edina is a geographically small district with high socioeconomic status. Many districts that are considering making the change to a later start find if difficult to assure skeptics and naysayers that Edina's experiences are, indeed, relevant because the findings are largely unconnected to money or size – that is, sleepy adolescents are sleepy adolescents no matter how much money a district has.

Other factors impeding a potential change have arisen during many meetings among superintendents. These include the fear that public discussion about a later start time may negatively impact the outcome of an upcoming bond levy referendum to raise school taxes. Also, several superintendents are concerned that a public, unhappy about discussions about a later start time for school may not support the renewal of their contract. In all of these cases, the superintendents are purposely remaining quiet about the topic. They intend to wait until someone or some group other than themselves initiates a community dialogue about the merits of altering the starting times of the schools.

The current debate in the schools and in the newspapers centers around a small subgroup of articulate students who are active in many sports and cocurricular activities who fear that they will have to cut back on all that they do. These students speak of a later start time having a negative impact upon being selected for the "best" colleges when they will have fewer activities to list on their résumés. Comments such as those hit home with their parents as well, thus causing a ground swell of opposition to making the change – an opposition that, one is reminded, is based upon supposition and speculation.

Educational debate has always been laden with local values and tends to be deeply political in nature. For this study to be accepted and the findings trusted by those reading this report, the study had to be conducted in a manner to avoid bias, with the results and implications provided to the reader in neutral language as findings of fact only. Thus, as intended, there are no specific recommendations as to "the best" starting time for any grade level.

Most likely, those persons engaged in the dialogue about changing the starting time of schools will find the issues and arguments of one stakeholder group more compelling than others, thus forming an opinion around that information. It is therefore incumbent upon the group that hopes to prevail to argue a most convincing case for its point of view, taking into full account the values of the community and the community's history with other change initiatives. If the researchers on adolescent sleep needs believe that their findings are crucial to the well-being of young people today, then they need to get their message out in clear language, while at the same time being publicly cognizant of the dynamics of school politics and administrative decision making. Without a strategic approach, the forces to maintain the status quo in the schools will prevail. At least adding the sleep research into the equation will round out the discussion. If all sides contribute, a well-informed decision about whether a change in school start time is feasible and wise will be the result.

196   KYLA L. WAHLSTROM

Appendix: Overview of Findings from Metropolitan Minneapolis: 1995–1996 to 1999–2000

In 1997 the schools in Metropolitan Minneapolis instituted a new high school schedule. The class schedule of 7:15 A.M. to 1:45 P.M. was changed to run from 8:40 A.M. to 3:20 P.M. We have followed outcomes of over 18,000 students in these schools in the 2 years prior to and the 3 years after the change and have recently begun to summarize this longitudinal data set. At present, however, we are only able to provide a brief excerpt from the mountains of data.

Our analyses of the longitudinal data found statistically significant improvements for graduation rates, rates of continuous enrollment, tardiness, and attendance. We provide here examples of our findings for a few outcome variables. (In each example, the first number indicates the finding before the schedule change and the second number provides the rate after the late start was implemented.) Average daily attendance increased from a mean of 70% for 9th graders in 1995–1996 to a mean of 77% for 9th graders in 1999–2000. The mean attendance rate for that same group of 9th graders rose from 70% in 1995–1996 to 83% as 12th graders in 1999–2000. The dropout rate decreased by 2% per year for all students (39% in 1995–1996 to 33% in 1999–2000), and the number of students continuously enrolled in the same high school for 2 or more years increased on average about 10% each year since the later start time was instituted.

Overall, the group most positively affected by the later start time comprised the African American students, whose rates in every outcome indicator showed statistically significant positive gain. African American students constituted nearly 40% of the total student population in Minneapolis. Also, students of all ethnic groups who were chronically tardy are now getting to school for their first hour of class, and thus have shown a reduced likelihood of dropping out of school due to attendance problems. We also analyzed the letter grades earned by all students in grades 9–12 during the 3 years prior to the change versus the grades earned in the 3 years after the change. These data indicate a slight improvement in grades earned overall, but the differences were not statistically significant.

These findings are certainly encouraging outcomes for those who favor delaying the starting time for high school students. Our efforts make clear, however, that identifying the specific gains of such a schedule change is an enormous challenge. One of the most compelling findings from our time-consuming and intensive data analysis is that using the letter grades earned as the single or primary indicator of the success of such a change is likely to be a problem for *any* district. Furthermore, if a district fails to take into account other gains such as changes in attendance, tardiness, graduation, and continuous enrollment, letter grades alone paint an incomplete picture.

The complete findings of our longitudinal study can be found on our web site as they become available: <http://education.umn.edu/carei/Programs/start_time/default.html>.

REFERENCES

Allen RP (1991). School-week sleep lag: Sleep problems with earlier starting of senior high schools. *Sleep Research* 20:198.
  (1992). Social factors associated with the amount of school week sleep lag for seniors in an early starting suburban high school. *Sleep Research* 21:114.
Allen RP, Mirabile J (1989). Self-reported sleep-wake patterns for students during the school year from two different senior high schools. *Sleep Research* 18:132.
Anderson M, Petros TV, Beckwith BE, Mitchell WW, Fritz S (1991). Individual differences in the effect of time of day on long-term memory access. *American Journal of Psychology* 104(2):241–255.
Barron BG, Henderson MV, Spurgeon R (1994). Effects of time of day instruction on reading achievement of below grade readers. *Reading Improvement* 31(1):59–60.
Callan RJ (1995). Early morning challenge: The potential effects of chronobiology on taking the scholastic aptitude test. *Clearing House* 68(3):174–176.
Carskadon MA (1993). Sleepiness in adolescents and young adults. In *Proceedings: Highway Safety Forum on Fatigue, Sleep Disorders, and Traffic Safety*, pp. 28–36. Albany, NY: Institute for Traffic Safety Management and Research.
Kraft M, Martin RJ (1995). Chronobiology and chronotherapy in medicine. *Disease-a-Month* 41(8):501–575.
Maas J (1995). Asleep in the fast lane: Everything you should know about sleep but are too tired to ask. Paper presented at the Master's Forum.
Stone P (1992). How we turned around a problem school. *Principal* 72(2):34–36.
Wolfson AR, Carskadon MA (1998). Sleep schedules and daytime functioning in adolescents. *Child Development* 69(4):875–887.

12. Bridging the Gap between Research and Practice: What Will Adolescents' Sleep-Wake Patterns Look Like in the 21st Century?

AMY R. WOLFSON

According to psychologists, sociologists, and educators, as well as anec-
dotal reports and stories from parents and teachers, adolescents growing up in the United States are portrayed as stormy, moody, persistent,
entitled, self-centered, independent, and emotional. Sleep researchers,
parents, and teachers have added that adolescents are frequently sleepy
and exhausted. This intense developmental stage is marked by physiological, cognitive, emotional, and psychosocial changes. Among the host
of changes that accompany adolescence are alterations in sleeping and
waking patterns. During adolescence, quality, quantity, and timing of
sleep are influenced by changing academic demands, new social pressures, altered parent-child relationships, and increased time spent in
part-time jobs, extracurricular activities, and sports. Likewise, the way
adolescents sleep critically influences their ability to think, behave, and
feel throughout adolescence. Researchers have documented that adolescents growing up in the late 1990s and early part of this decade are
not getting enough sleep; however, countermeasures have not been
developed to reverse this trend.

Although sleep consumes approximately one-third of our lives (50%
at early school age), it is often ignored by developmental psychologists,

Research presented in this chapter was supported by funds from the National Institutes
of Health (NIH), MH 45945. My work on this chapter would not have been possible
without the guidance and support from my mentor, colleague, and friend, the director of
the E. P. Bradley Hospital and Brown University Sleep Laboratory, Mary A. Carskadon,
Ph.D. I also thank Christine Acebo, Ph.D., who provided expert advice on data analysis
for the 1994 survey of 3,000 high school students. Many others assisted with this timely
research, including Orna Tzischinsky, Catherine Darley, Jennifer Wicks, Elizabeth Yoder,
Liza Kelly, Jeffrey Cerone, Camille Brown, François Garand, Eric Kravitz, and Christopher
Monti.

pediatricians, educators, and others who devote their lives to working with children and adolescents. For example, sleep is rarely mentioned in textbooks on adolescent development, child-adolescent sleep topics are infrequently presented at the Society for Research on Child Development meetings (.3% of presentations at the 1995 biennial SRCD meeting), and pediatricians get very little training in sleep medicine. This chapter examines current knowledge of the factors that influence adolescents' sleep-wake patterns and discusses how adolescent sleep researchers, school administrators, health care providers, and policy makers must bridge the research-practice gap so that adolescents can be alert (not sleep-deprived) and successful in school.

Philosophers, psychologists, and other theorists throughout history, such as Aristotle, John Locke, G. Stanley Hall, and Carol Gilligan (Brown & Gilligan, 1992), have viewed the transition or crossroads from childhood to adulthood as a time of vulnerability as well as an opportunity for developing a life-style that promotes health, physical and psychological well-being, and empathy. They argued that special attention should be given to helping and supporting adolescents through this period so that they can become healthy and successful adults. Unfortunately, over the past several decades adolescents have been viewed with disrespect, disregard, and antagonism. More than 30 years ago, U.S. teenagers were seen as idealistic. In contrast, currently they are viewed as one of the main roots of our nation's social ills (e.g., drug abuse, juvenile crime, teen pregnancy, gangs, violence). This chapter argues that one explanation for adolescents' academic difficulties, behavior problems, and disengagement from school relates to society's reinforcement of irregular and short sleep-wake schedules through early morning school start times and pressure to work long hours after school. Data suggest that adolescents are starting school at increasingly earlier times, working increasingly longer hours after school, and sleeping fewer hours than in the past. If this trend continues, teenagers will have difficulty successfully negotiating the transition into adulthood. We must focus on how to make things more manageable for adolescents as opposed to setting up systems that are likely to promote failure.

Throughout this chapter I refer to a large-scale survey study that my colleagues and I (Acebo, Wolfson, & Carskadon, 1997; Wolfson & Carskadon, 1998) conducted in the fall of 1994. Some of the findings have been reported in other papers (Acebo et al., 1997; Wolfson et al., 1998), whereas some of the data discussed here has not been presented previously. Specifically, an eight-page sleep habits survey was administered to 9th–12th grade students in four public high schools from three districts in the Providence metropolitan area with a response rate of 88%. The four schools had start times between 7:10 and 7:20 A.M. The survey was completed anonymously by 3,120 (48% boys, 52% girls). The students' ages ranged from 13 to 19. More than 91% of the students from schools A, C, and D noted that they were Caucasian, whereas school B was more diverse (75% Caucasian, 25% multiracial). Students from all four schools reported that 81% to 85% of their mothers *and* fathers were employed. The survey items queried students about usual sleeping and waking behaviors over the past two weeks (e.g., total sleep, bedtimes and rise times, work, sports and study hours, depressed mood, daytime sleepiness, academic performance, and substance use).

Developmental Changes in Adolescents' Sleep

As described earlier in this book (Carskadon, Chapter 2 in this volume), there are striking changes in sleep-wake schedules, sleep quality, and total sleep times during adolescence. In the United States, parents, school administrators, and teenagers themselves have assumed that adolescents do not really need as much sleep as preadolescents. A myriad of surveys and field studies have shown that teenagers usually obtain much less sleep than school-age children, from 10 hours during middle childhood to less than 7 hours by age 17 (Williams, Karacan, & Hursch, 1974; Carskadon, 1982; Carskadon, 1990a; Allen, 1992; Wolfson & Carskadon, 1998). Furthermore, numerous studies have observed that adolescents tend to stay up increasingly later over the high school years, get up extremely early for school, and, as a result, get increasingly less sleep over the course of adolescence. For example, the 3,120 high school students surveyed in Rhode Island were getting only 7 hours, 20 minutes total sleep on school nights, and school-night and weekend total sleep decreased linearly across ages 13 to 19 by 40 to 50 minutes (Wolfson & Carskadon, 1998).

Although surveys document that teenagers are getting increasingly less sleep over the high school years, laboratory studies show that adolescents do not have a decreased need for sleep across puberty (Carskadon, Harvey, Duke, Anders, & Dement, 1980; Carskadon, Orav, & Dement, 1983; Carskadon, 1990a). In fact, Carskadon et al. (1980) clearly demonstrated that sleep quantity remained constant at approximately 9.2 hours across all pubertal stages.

In addition, adolescents tend to delay their phase of sleep by staying up later at night and sleeping in later in the morning than preadolescents (Carskadon, Vieira, & Acebo, 1993; Dahl & Carskadon, 1995). One manifestation of this process is that adolescents' sleep patterns on weekends show a considerable delay (as well as lengthening) versus weekdays, with sleep onset and offset both occurring significantly later. This sleep phase shift is attributed to psychosocial factors and to biological changes that take place during puberty. For example, in the longitudinal study described earlier, as children reached puberty, they were less likely to wake up on their own and lab staff needed to wake them up (Carskadon et al., 1980). Carskadon et al. (1980) noted that they probably would have slept more than 9 hours if undisturbed.

Carskadon and her colleagues have shown that this adolescent tendency to phase delay may be augmented by a biological process accompanying puberty. Their group examined self-reported puberty scores (Carskadon & Acebo, 1993) and phase preference (morningness-eveningness) scores of over 400 pre- and early pubertal 6th graders (Carskadon, Vieira, & Acebo, 1993). These data documented that morning types reported going to bed earlier, rising earlier, and waking up spontaneously more often than evening types. In contrast, evening types were more likely to report staying up past 3:00 A.M. and sleeping past noon. Furthermore, pubertal 6th grade girls were more evening type than prepubertal 6th graders (Carskadon et al., 1993). Andrade, Benedito-Silva, and Domenice (1993) and Ishihara, Honma, and Miyake (1990) also reported an adolescent delay of sleep phase in Brazilian and Japanese teenagers, respectively. A recent study examined the circadian timing system more directly in early adolescents by measuring the timing of melatonin secretion. Findings from this study led to the hypothesis that a developmental delay of circadian phase may occur in young humans (Carskadon, Richardson, Tate, & Acebo, 1997).

The changes from childhood to adolescence in sleep need, sleep-wake schedules, and circadian timing of sleep have several ramifications for the teenagers themselves, and for the context in which they live, attend school, work, and interact with their families. Although research suggests that the circadian phase delay and sleep needs of adolescents are similar across cultures, environmental constraints, such as school schedules, leisure time activities, and employment demands are highly culturally determined. In the next few sections, the relationship between sleep-wake patterns, school start times, and work schedule demands for U.S. teenagers are explored.

Environmental Constraints That Affect Sleep-Wake Patterns

School Start Times

Researchers of adolescent development have focused mainly on the ways in which adolescents' backgrounds and personal characteristics help or hinder them as they progress through the junior and senior high school years. In contrast, the social ecology approach emphasizes how social demography (e.g., single-sex schools, minority enrollment) and organizational characteristics (e.g., schedules, tracking, number of grades in the school) of the school influence adolescent behavior and development. Historically, schools have started early in the morning throughout the United States. Additionally, many U.S. school districts use a three- or four-bell schedule where high schools open first, followed by middle or junior high schools, and then elementary schools with one or two starting times (Nudel, 1993). In a preliminary survey of 40 high school schedules posted on the Internet from throughout the United States, 48% started at 7:30 A.M. or earlier, whereas only 12% started between 8:15 and 8:55 A.M. School districts claim that they have developed these schedules for a variety of reasons, such as bus schedules, parent work schedules, ideal learning times, and pressure from high school student employers. This early high school start time is a significant, externally imposed constraint on teenagers' sleep-wake schedules; for most teens waking up to go to school is neither spontaneous nor negotiable. In combination with factors such as late night activities or jobs, early morning school demands often significantly constrict the hours available for sleep. Szymczak, Jasinska, Pawlak, and Zwierzykowska (1993) followed Polish students ages 10 and 14 years for over a year and found that all slept longer on weekends and during vacations as a result of waking up later. These investigators concluded that the school duty schedule was the predominant determinant of waking times for these students. Similarly, several surveys of high school students found that students who start school at 7:30 A.M. or earlier obtain less total sleep on school nights due to earlier rise times (Carskadon & Mancuso, 1987; Allen & Mirabile, 1989; Allen, 1991; Wolfson & Carskadon, 1998).

In a laboratory and field study, Carskadon and her colleagues evaluated the impact of a 65-minute advance in school start time on 25 9th graders across the transition to 10th grade (Carskadon, Wolfson, Tzischinsky, & Acebo, 1995; Wolfson, Tzischinsky, Brown, Darley, Acebo, & Carskedon, 1995). Specifically, junior high school started at 8:25 A.M. and high school started at 7:20 A.M. in this large urban school district. The initial findings demonstrated that students slept an average of 40 minutes less in 10th grade compared with 9th grade due to earlier rise times, and they displayed an increase in the multiple sleep latency test (MSLT)-measured daytime sleepiness (laboratory measure of sleepiness described in Chapter 2; Carskadon, Dement, Mitler, Roth, Westbrook, & Keenan, 1986). In addition, evening-type students had more difficulty adjusting to the earlier start time than did morning types, and higher scores on an externalizing behavior problems scale (Youth Self-Report, Achenbach, 1991) were associated with less total sleep and later bedtimes (Brown et al., 1995; Wolfson et al., 1995).

Work Hours and Other After-School Activities

Adolescents spend a significant portion of their time engaged in leisure activities and an even more substantial amount of time in the part-time labor force. In studying adolescence, social scientists have given primary attention to the family, school, and peer group as central contexts for development. Today, however, high school education and employment are simultaneous activities. In fact, the tendency for teenagers to work in the paid labor force has increased substantially in the past 20 years. According to the U.S. Department of Labor (1996), nearly 43% of 16- to 19-year-olds who are enrolled in school are also employed throughout the year. Although some high school students work only in the summer, nearly 90% of 11th and 12th graders in the National Survey of Families and Households who worked for pay worked for at least part of the academic year (Manning, 1990). Greenberger and Steinberg (1986) and Steinberg, Brown, and Dornbusch (1996) argued that high school students' employment is distinctly an American phenomenon. Moreover, middle-class high school students are more likely to work than students from economically disadvantaged homes (Greenberger & Steinberg, 1986).

Researchers looked at the short-term and long-term effects of working part-time while attending high school. A number of studies concluded that increased hours of work are correlated with lowered grade point averages (GPA), lowered sense of well-being and self-image, increased absenteeism, lateness, cutting classes, cheating, and the use of cigarettes, marijuana, and alcohol (Greenberger & Steinberg, 1986; Yamoor & Mortimer, 1990). Specifically, researchers demonstrated that students with lower GPAs are more likely to work and, therefore, have less time available for schoolwork (Wirtz, Rohrbeck, Charner, & Fraser, 1988). In contrast, Greenberger and Steinberg's (1986) survey of workers in four California high schools pointed out that employment was associated with punctuality, dependability, and personal responsibility. Their study suggested that employed students maintain grades, even while working long hours, by manipulating their schedules to avoid courses that require a heavy time investment (e.g., math, science, foreign language). Similarly, D'Amico (1984) reported that students who work less than 20 hours per week are less likely to drop out of high school, and that long work hours depress grades for 10th and 11th graders but not 12th graders. Unfortunately, these studies did not assess the relationship between high school work hours and sleep-wake schedules. Teenagers who work more than 20 hours per week may avoid academically demanding courses, obtain poor grades, miss school, and exhibit other negative behaviors because they are exhausted from not getting enough sleep.

Adolescents are also not getting enough sleep because of after-school commitments to athletic teams and other activities. School schedules demand increasingly earlier rise times. At the same time, academic pressures, extracurricular activities, and work hours require later and later bedtimes. In an analysis of the 3,120 high school students from the Wolfson and Carskadon study (1998), it is clear that adolescents spend a large percentage of their time working for pay as opposed to studying, playing sports, participating in other extracurricular activities, or sleeping. Over the high school years, total work hours increased linearly across ages 13 to 19 from 11 hours to 22 hours, whereas participation in sports, extracurricular activities, and study hours changed minimally (see Figure 12.1). Steinberg et al. (1996) would argue that high school students are increasingly more disengaged from school and school-related activities.

Especially in 11th and 12th grade, work hours occupy a significant amount of the adolescent's time. Fifty-two percent of the 1,712 Rhode Island students in 11th and 12th grades reported that they hold part-time jobs, and 56% of those who work do so for 20 hours or more per week (M = 21.1, SD = 10.0). On average, males reported that they work 2 more hours than their female peers (21 vs. 19 hours). In comparison to this intense involvement in after school work hours, only 29% reported participating in sports (M = 9.2, SD = 6.8) and 28% were involved in extracurricular activities (M = 5.9, SD = 5.8). While 66% of the 11th and 12th graders reported that they spend time on homework and studying, the mean number of hours spent studying was only 7 hours, 8 minutes per week. In addition, 37% of these 11th and 12th graders are working 2 to 5 weekdays after school in the afternoon and/or evening hours.

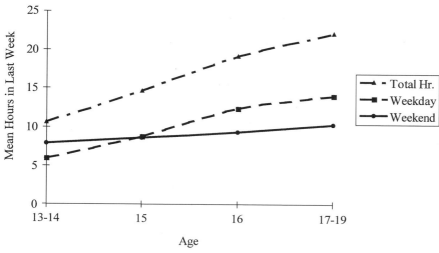

Figure 12.1. Hours spent working.

Obviously, outside of school hours, these juniors and seniors are spending their time in the work force. Hours working after school compete with time for doing homework and time for sleeping. Based on data from several studies (Carskadon, 1990b; Steinberg et al., 1996; Wolfson & Carskadon, 1998), an average 11th or 12th grader's weekday schedule would be similar to the schedule displayed here:

11:00 P.M. Bedtime
6:10 A.M. Rise time
7:00 A.M. Leaving home for school
7:30 A.M. School start time
2:30 P.M. School closing time
3:00 P.M. After school sports
5:00 P.M. Part-time job
9:30 P.M. Homework, socializing, television
11:00 P.M. Bedtime.

Carskadon (1990b) previously documented a relationship between hours spent at jobs, sleep patterns, and daytime sleepiness. These new data demonstrate that the 11th and 12th grade students who work 20 hours or more have more problematic sleep-wake habits than students who work less than 20 hours or who do not work at all. Specifically, the high-work group reported significantly less total sleep and later bedtimes on school nights (e.g., total median sleep time 6 hours, 57 minutes vs. 7 hours, 17 minutes). In addition, students working more than one evening per week reported less school-night total sleep than students working during the day or not at all. The high-work group in the more recent sample as well as from the survey conducted in the late 1980s (Carskadon, 1990b) reported more symptoms of daytime sleepiness, such as more difficulty staying awake in classes or while studying; increased sleep-wake behaviors (e.g., arriving late to class due to oversleeping or feeling tired, dragged out, or sleepy during the day); and reported greater use of caffeine, alcohol or drugs, and tobacco. Figure 12.2 depicts the significant relationship between work status and scores on the sleep-wake behaviors scale (Carskadon, Seifer, & Acebo, 1991).

In both surveys, the high school students also reported being sleepy while driving a car (Carskadon, 1990b). In the 1994 data, 10% of the 11th and 12th graders who were spending 20+ hours per week versus 8% of those working less than 20 hours per week admitted to struggling to stay awake and/or having fallen asleep at the wheel. Adolescents who work more than 20 hours a week and/or have other time-consuming demands on their schedule are likely to develop a sleep-wake pattern of minimal sleep, excessive sleepiness, decreased alertness, and increased risk-taking behaviors (e.g., substance abuse, driving while tired).

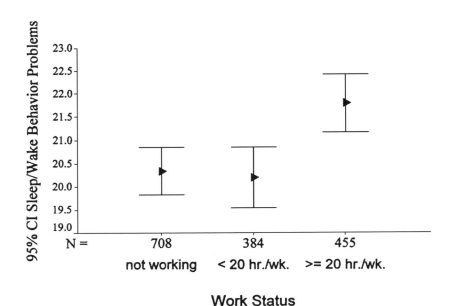

Figure 12.2. Sleep-wake behavior problems according to work status.

Impact of Sleep-Wake Patterns on Adolescents' Quality of Life

Academic Performance

When the United States is contrasted with other industrial nations, it has the lowest economic support for education, the lowest rate of parental involvement in schools, the poorest performance on high school achievement tests, and the lowest number of hours spent in school (Ravitch, 1995). Furthermore, sleepy adolescents – that is, those with inadequate sleep – seem to encounter increased academic difficulties. Wolfson and Carskadon's study of over 3,000 high school students (1998) found that high schoolers who described themselves as struggling or failing in school (i.e., obtaining Cs, Ds, and Fs) reported that they obtain less sleep, have later bedtimes, and more irregular weekday-weekend sleep schedules than students who report better grades (i.e., As, Bs). Other surveys of high school students reported that more total sleep, earlier bedtimes, and later weekday rise times were associated with better grades in school (Allen, 1992; Link & Ancoli-Israel, 1995; Manber et al., 1995). Epstein, Chillag, and Lavie (1995) surveyed Israeli elementary, junior high, and senior high school students and reported that less total sleep time was associated with daytime fatigue, inability to concentrate in school, and a tendency to doze off in class. Persistent sleep problems have also been associated with learning difficulties throughout the school years (elementary through high school grades) (Quine, 1992). Studies of excessive sleepiness in children and adolescents due to delay phase sleep disorder, narcolepsy, or sleep apnea have also reported negative effects on learning, school performance, and behavior (Guilleminault, Winkle, & Korobkin, 1982; Dahl, Holttum, & Trubnick, 1994; Dahl & Carskadon, 1995). One explanation for these results is that students who get more sleep and maintain more consistent school and weekend sleep schedules obtain better grades because of their ability to be more alert and to pay greater attention in class and on homework.

Emotional and Behavioral Well-Being

Research is in the early stages of investigating the complex relationship between adolescents' sleep patterns and their daytime behaviors. Although studies have concluded that associations between sleep-wake patterns and daytime functioning exist, the direction of this relationship is not clear. In addition, several of the studies have looked at younger children as opposed to adolescents. Inferences and conclusions about sleep and daytime functioning in younger children may or may not apply to adolescents. Clinical experience shows that adolescents who have trouble adapting to new school schedules and other changes (e.g., new bed and rise times, increased activities during the day, increased academic demands) may develop problematic sleeping behaviors leading to chronic sleepiness. Several studies indicate an association between sleep, stress and emotional well-being. For example, studies have found that sleep-disturbed elementary school–age children experience a greater number of stresses (e.g., maternal absence due to work or school; family illness or accident; maternal depressed mood) than non-sleep-disturbed children (Kataria, Swanson, & Trevathan, 1987). Likewise, sleepy school-age children may have poorer coping behaviors (e.g., more difficulty recognizing, appraising, and adapting to stressful situations) and display more behavior problems at home and in school (Fisher & Rinehart, 1990; Wolfson et al., 1995).

In the Rhode Island survey of over 3,000 high school students, many of the teenagers complained about feeling depressed, fatigued, and falling asleep in classes and noted that they used a variety of mood-altering substances. Specifically, 51% of the 9th through 12th graders reported that they feel tired or dragged out nearly every day, 30% rarely had a good night's sleep in recent weeks, 27% admitted that they fell asleep and/or struggled to stay awake while in class, and 34% reported that they use 2–4 substances (e.g., caffeine, alcohol, cigarettes) at least once a day.

Wolfson and Carskadon (1998) examined a priori defined groups of high school students based on their sleep times and schedules. The extreme groups of students were defined as follows: long (≥ 8 hours 15 minutes) versus short (≤ 6 hours 45 minutes) school-night total sleep time; large (≥ 120 minutes) versus small (≤ 60 minutes) weekend delay; and high (≥ 120 minutes) versus low (≤ 60 minutes) weekend oversleep. High school students who had longer total sleep times, small weekend delays, and low weekend oversleeps were defined as having adopted adequate sleep habits, whereas students with shorter sleep times, large weekend delays, and high weekend oversleeps were defined as having adopted less than adequate sleep habits. Students with short school-night sleep reported increased levels of depressed mood, daytime sleepness, and problematic sleep behaviors in comparison with longer sleepers. Likewise, students with more irregular sleep schedules had more behavior problems and increased substance abuse (e.g., cigarettes and marijuana).

Analogous findings were reported by researchers in New Zealand, France, and Canada. Morrison, McGee, and Stanton (1992) compared four groups of 13- and 15-year-olds in New Zealand: those with no sleep problems, those indicating they needed more sleep only, those reporting difficulties falling asleep or maintaining sleep, and those with multiple sleep problems. They concluded that adolescents in the sleep-problem groups were more anxious, had higher levels of depression, and lower social competence than those in the no-sleep-problem group. Similarly, in a sample of over 500 French and French-Canadian high school students, suicidal ideation and self-reported depression were associated with tiredness, less total sleep, and more sleep disturbances (Choquet, Kovess, & Poutignat, 1993). These studies all strongly suggest that adolescents with inadequate total sleep, irregular school-night to weekend sleep-wake schedules, and/or sleep disturbances struggle with behavior problems, academic difficulties, and substance abuse.

Implications of the Factors Imposing on Adolescents' Sleep-Wake Patterns

The interplay among sleep-wake schedules, circadian rhythms, environmental constraints, and behavior during adolescence results in an increasing pressure on the nocturnal sleep period, producing insufficient sleep in many teenagers and ultimately changes in daytime functioning (Carskadon, 1995). For children and preadolescents, society structures time for nighttime sleep, parents are more likely to set bedtimes, and school begins later in the morning. Prepubescent children are thus more likely to have earlier bedtimes and to wake up before the school day begins (Petta, Carskadon, & Dement, 1984). In contrast, due to behavioral factors (social, academic, and work-related, as well as environmental constraints such as school schedule and job hours), and circadian variables (pubertal phase delay), teenagers have later bedtimes, earlier rise times, and therefore, decreased time available to sleep (Carskadon et al., 1995). As a result, adolescents get to bed late, have difficulty waking up in the morning, and struggle to stay alert and to function successfully during the daytime.

The Next Generation of Students

Clearly, a number of variables impact the American high school student. High school students are influenced by society's values toward education. Educators and social scientists have pointed out that two trends reveal educational values: the devaluing or trivializing of education; and the competing interests of media, consumerism, and employment upon studying (Prather, 1996). The studies presented in this chapter demonstrate a third trend – the devaluing of emotional and physical health, particularly sleep. With increasingly earlier high school start times, increasingly more time spent in after school employment, increasing consumerism, diminished time for sleep, and possibly increased illness and injury rates (Acebo et al., 1997), what will high school students' sleep-wake patterns will look like in the 21st century?

In light of the growing number of hours students are spending in the work force relative to all of their other activities (which do not appear to change over these years), I examined the impact of increasing work hours on total sleep in high school students. Among the nearly 40% of high school students who work an average of 19.5 hours/week (SD = 10.7 hours), for every 10 hours that they work, 14 minutes of sleep is lost per night (see Figure 12.3). On a weekly basis, the typical student who works approximately 20 hours per

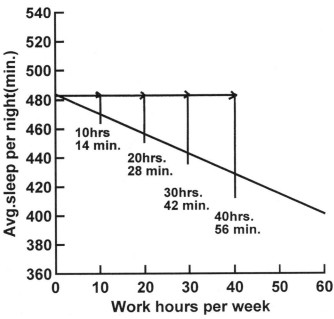

Figure 12.3. Work and lost sleep. For every 10 hours of work, 14 minutes of sleep is lost per night.

Table 12.1. Characteristics of the 21st-Century High School Student's Sleep-Wake Habits

School-night total sleep time less than 7 hours
School-night bedtime later than 11:00 P.M.
School-morning rise time prior to 6:00 A.M.
School start times earlier than 7:00 A.M.
More than 25 after-school work hours
Increased disengagement from school
Weekend sleep-wake schedule delayed by 2 or more hours
Decreased academic performance and less than 45 minutes per night study time
Increased emotional and behavioral difficulties
Increased sleepy-driver automobile accidents and other injuries

week will lose 3 hours, 20 minutes of sleep per week. At the extreme, the 5% of students who are working full-time and attending school are losing approximately 1 hour of sleep per night or 7 hours of sleep per week. If these data hold true, we are faced with an increasing sleep debt for adolescents in the United States with academic, emotional, and health consequences. Table 12.1 illustrates the typical adolescent's sleep-wake patterns in the next century if the trends of the 1990s continue.

Countermeasures: Bridging the Gap between Research and Practice

At this juncture, how can sleep and adolescent development researchers work with school administrators, parents, and teachers to guarantee that adolescents obtain more sleep and engage more in school in the next decade? In recent years sleep researchers have suggested that public schools delay high school start times from, for example, 7:30 to 9:00 A.M. to increase the likelihood that teenagers will sleep more. School principals and superintendents, however, have been reluctant to start high schools at later morning times. For example, last spring, in a suburban school district in Connecticut, more than 620 students and parents signed a petition urging the district to reject a plan to start high school at 7:30 A.M., 10 minutes earlier than the previous year (Stansbury, 1996; Dunne, 1996). One of the student leaders presented the petition along with relevant information from research studies conducted by Carskadon, Wolfson, and others to the board of education. However, the school superintendent, high school principals, and other board members and administrators stuck with their plan to move the start time to

7:30 A.M. to lengthen the school day. Dunne (1996) reported that the administrators emphasized that the regulation of school hours are the responsibility of the administration; however, the board has plans to evaluate the consequences of the earlier start time. Although this is a case example and not a large-scale study of researcher–school administrator relations, many school districts are reluctant to rethink the timing of the school day, which may result in large-scale systemic changes. Wahlstrom describes the Minneapolis–St. Paul experience of delaying start times in Chapter 11 of this volume.

A number of barriers interfere with establishing working relationships between sleep researchers and educators. Sleep researchers are reluctant to collaborate with school administrators because they fear that they will have to compromise on experimental design; likewise, school administrators argue that the researchers do not understand the economic constraints of running a public school system (e.g., bus schedules, time for after-school sports before dark, parent work schedules). Researchers, educators, and parents must be able to speak each other's languages and to understand and respect each other's expertise to combine their talents to improve adolescents' sleep-wake patterns and their engagement with school.

Three requirements for productive connections are interdisciplinary communication skills, experiences that develop mutual respect, and enthusiastic support from the field of sleep research and sleep medicine. First of all, sleep researchers who want to work actively with school systems must publish, present, and discuss their findings at conferences and in journals and other publications that are subscribed to by educators and child development specialists. Second, educators are much more likely to consider sleep clinicians and researchers' recommendations when they come out of a collaborative process. For example, school districts may be more likely to change school start times as a part of a pilot project that involves students' input, parents' concerns, school transportation departments' goals, and teachers' pedagogical questions. Finally, the sleep field needs to increase professional training in child and adolescent sleep development at the undergraduate level in medical and nursing schools, and in masters and doctoral programs in education and psychology. These components should strengthen the discipline and increase the likelihood that schools will take adolescents' sleep needs seriously in designing curriculums, schedules and school reforms.

Over the past decade, sleep and circadian rhythm researchers have worked with industry, highway safety organizations, the National

Aeronautics and Space Administration, hospitals, and other organizations that rely on 24-hour operations. Increasingly more programs have been developed and implemented on the individual and systemic level to promote performance, productivity, and safety in 24-hour operations (Rosekind et al., 1995; Monk, 2000). However, few interventions, countermeasures, and/or systemic changes have been implemented for the high school setting to promote academic performance, motivation, engagement, and health and safety for adolescents. Systemic and individual countermeasures may potentially stop the increasing adolescent sleep debt and improve adolescents' sleep hygiene and daytime functioning in school. Similar strategies have been developed for pilots, truck drivers, and shift workers (Rosekind et al., 1995).

School and Community Countermeasures and Systemic Changes

School systems and sleep researchers should continue to evaluate the benefits of later school start times for junior and senior high school students. Although research has not definitively proved an ideal school start time, the data strongly indicate that many current school start times are too early. For example, students with later school start times report the same average bedtimes as students with earlier school start times, but they have later rise times (Carskadon et al., 1995). One argument for increasingly earlier school start times has been to lengthen the school day; however, school reform studies have concluded that extending the quantity of time in school does not necessarily improve academic performance (Adelman, 1996). In addition to changing school start times, it is also important to evaluate school schedules. Are there certain times of day that adolescents perform better, feel more motivated, and are more likely to engage in their education? Data suggest that junior and senior high school students are more owl-like than elementary school–age children (Carskadon & Acebo, 1993). Therefore, high school students may be more involved and obtain better grades in late morning and afternoon classes in comparison to elementary school children.

The goal of countermeasures is to improve school performance and alertness. Because it may be difficult to change class schedules and school start times to an hour that meets everyone's needs (e.g., students, administrators, teachers), active learning that involves more social interaction may be a useful strategy for fighting sleepiness in junior and senior high schools. Although the usefulness of napping for high school students is not well researched, napping is one of the countermeasures that has been tested for adults and college students (Gorin, Kelly, Wolfson, 1994; Rosekind et al., 1995). Rosekind et al.'s study demonstrated that a planned 40-minute nap improved reaction time and vigilance performance and alertness for long-haul crew members. Similarly, first-year college students who took planned, early afternoon naps reported more effective coping strategies than students who took no naps or erratic, spontaneous naps (Gorin et al., 1994). Future studies should evaluate the effectiveness of scheduled naps (e.g., nap rooms) as a way to improve alertness and performance for high school students.

The studies reviewed in this chapter also indicate that high school students are employed in after-school jobs for far too many hours and that work hours further decrease time for sleep. Ideally, if high schools started later and, therefore, ended later, teenagers would have less time to work. Over the past 2 decades schools have started increasingly earlier, and during the same period high school students have increased their hours in the paid labor force. For working adolescents, child labor laws should be adequate not only to protect them from occupational risks but also to insure that they have time to sleep and that their ability to learn in school is not adversely affected. Communities must begin to limit high school students' time in after-school jobs. Presently, 29 states have no limits at all on the numbers of hours that students may work each week during the academic year and 13 states allow 40 or more hours of employment per week. Eight states have some restrictions on weekly hours of employment during the school year; however, only 2 states actually limit employment to 20 hours per week or less (Steinberg et al., 1996). In addition to limiting teenagers' time in after-school jobs, employers should pay more attention to their adolescent employees' school performance and health (e.g., sleep requirements).

Countermeasures for Sleepiness: Student Strategies

Although the large-scale, systemic countermeasures discussed in the previous section are crucial, they take a long time to develop, are difficult to implement, and may be costly. In comparison, individual-focused strategies may be important in the short-run and may be efficacious for many adolescents. The following six preventive strategies or sleep hygiene guidelines are recommended for adolescents:

1. Minimize sleep loss by keeping consistent, regular bedtimes and rise times throughout the week.

2. As emphasized in the previous section, planned 25- to 45-minute naps can improve alertness and performance. Prior studies have shown that *prophylactic napping* is helpful for adults who must work for prolonged hours to prevent sleepiness from increasing to a level that impairs one's ability to function (Dinges & Broughton, 1989).

3. A presleep routine is helpful for adolescents so that they unwind and relax before going to bed. During evening hours, high school students tend to socialize on the phone with friends, watch television, play video games, and/or log on to the Internet or pursue other computer activities. An established sleep routine breaks the connection between the psychological stressors and stimulating activities of the day and the sleep period (Rosekind et al., 1995).

4. Circadian strategies are particularly relevant to adolescents. Because adolescents experience a phase delay and are sleepy later in the evening, it is helpful to reduce the amount of light that teenagers are exposed to in the evening, including the light from television(s) and computer(s), to prevent a further delay of bedtime and augment morning light.

5. Avoid alcohol, caffeine, nicotine, and other drugs as they have well-documented disruptive effects on sleep (see reviews by Rosekind et al., 1995; Zarcone, 2000). Steinberg et al. (1996) reported that students who work long hours use drugs and alcohol about 33 percent more often than students who do not work. Similarly, in the 1994 survey of high school students in the Providence area, the 11th and 12th graders working more than 20 hours per week reported greater substance use than those working fewer hours. Moreover, students with more irregular sleep-wake habits and less total weekly sleep used more substances. Clearly, some adolescents are further aggravating their sleep debt through their use of caffeine, nicotine, and alcohol.

6. Regular exercise may be helpful for adolescents' sleep hygiene. Morning exercise advances the circadian clock, whereas exercise in the late evening may delay the phase of sleep. However, additional research is needed to elucidate the relationship between the different types and quantity of exercise, sleep, and circadian rhythms, especially for adolescents. These adolescent-focused countermeasures combined with more systematic changes may help to improve the quantity and quality of adolescents' sleep and, as a result, school engagement and daytime functioning.

Conclusions

Although a tremendous amount of well-researched information is available on adolescents' sleep-wake patterns, sleepiness, school and job schedules, and daytime functioning, research in these areas is still in its youth. This is particularly true in the application of this research knowledge to creating programs and new policies that will increase the time available for adolescents to sleep and reengage in school. Outcome studies need to evaluate and compare the effects of school schedule changes, revisions in adolescent labor regulations, and sleep hygiene education programs. The development of countermeasures, continued research, and ongoing dialogues between sleep researchers, educators, parents, and adolescents themselves will help reverse the early school start time, increased work hours, and increased sleep loss trends that face the teenager at the turn of the 21st century.

REFERENCES

Acebo C, Wolfson A, Carskadon M (1997). Relations among self-reported sleep patterns, health, and injuries in adolescents. *Sleep Research* 26:149.

Achenbach TM (1991). *The Child Behavior Checklist.* University of Vermont, Department of Psychiatry.

Allen RP (1991). School-week sleep lag: Sleep problems with earlier starting of senior high schools. *Sleep Research* 20:198.

(1992). Social factors associated with the amount of school week sleep lag for seniors in an early starting suburban high school. *Sleep Research* 21:114.

Allen RP, Mirabile J (1989). Self-reported sleep-wake patterns for students during the school year from two different senior high schools. *Sleep Research* 18:132.

Andrade MMM, Benedito-Silva EE, Domenice S (1993). Sleep characteristics of adolescents: A longitudinal study. *Journal of Adolescent Health* 14:401–406.

Bearpark HM, Michie PT (1987). Prevalence of sleep/wake disturbances in Sydney adolescents. *Sleep Research* 16:304.

Brown C, Tzischinsky O, Wolfson A, Acebo C, Wicks J, Darley C, Carskadon MA (1995). Circadian phase preference and adjustment to the high school transition. *Sleep Research* 24:90.

Brown LM, Gilligan C (1992). *Meeting at the Crossroads: Women's and Girl's Psychology Development.* Cambridge, MA: Harvard University Press.

Carskadon MA (1982). The second decade. In C. Guilleminault, ed., *Sleeping and Waking Disorders: Indications and Techniques*, pp. 1–16. Menlo Park, CA: Addison-Wesley.

(1990a). Patterns of sleep and sleepiness in adolescents. *Pediatrician* 17:5–12.

(1990b). Adolescent sleepiness: Increased risk in a high-risk population. *Alcohol, Drugs and Driving* 5–6:317–328.

(1995). Sleep's place in teenagers' lives. *Proceedings of the Biennial Meeting of the Society for Research in Child Development*, p. 32 (abstract). Indianapolis, IN, March 31.

Carskadon MA, Acebo C (1993). A self-administered rating scale for pubertal development. *Journal of Adolescent Health Care* 14:190–195.

Carskadon MA, Dement WC, Mitler MM, Roth T, Westbrook PR, Keenan S (1986). Guidelines for Multiple Sleep Latency Test (MSLT): A standard measure of sleepiness. *Sleep* 9:519–524.

Carskadon MA, Harvey K, Duke P, Anders TF, Dement WC (1980). Pubertal changes in daytime sleepiness. *Sleep* 2:453–460.

Carskadon MA, Mancuso J (1987). Sleep habits in high school adolescents: Boarding versus day students. *Sleep Research* 17:74.

Carskadon MA, Orav EJ, Dement WC (1983). Evolution of sleep and daytime sleepiness in adolescents. In C. Guilleminault and E. Lugaresi, eds., *Sleep/Waking Disorders: Natural History, Epidemiology, and Long-Term Evolution*, pp. 201–216. New York: Raven Press.

Carskadon MA, Richardson GS, Tate BA, Acebo C (1997). An approach to studying circadian rhythms of adolescent humans. *Journal of Biological Rhythms* 12(3):278–289.

Carskadon MA, Seifer R, Acebo C (1991). Reliability of six scales in a sleep questionnaire for adolescents. *Sleep Research* 20:421.

Carskadon MA, Vieira C, Acebo C (1993). Association between puberty and delayed phase preference. *Sleep* 16(3):258–262.

Carskadon MA, Wolfson A, Tzischinsky O, Acebo C (1995). Early school schedules modify adolescent sleepiness. *Sleep Research* 24:92.

Choquet M, Kovess V, Poutignat N (1993). Suicidal thoughts among adolescents: An intercultural approach. *Adolescence* 28(111):649–659.

Comstock G (1991). *Television and the American Child*. San Diego, CA: Academic Press.

Dahl RE, Carskadon MA (1995). Sleep and its disorders in adolescence. In R. Ferber & M. Kryger, eds., *Principles and Practice of Sleep Medicine in the Child*, pp. 19–27. Philadelphia: Saunders.

Dahl RE, Holttum J, Trubnick L (1994). A clinical picture of childhood and adolescent narcolepsy. *Journal of the American Academy of Child and Adolescent Psychiatry* 33:834–841.

D'Amico R (1984). Does employment during high school impair academic progress? *Sociology of Education* 57:152–164.

Dinges DF, Broughton RJ, eds. (1989). *Sleep and Alertness: Chronobiological, Behavioral, and Medical Aspects of Napping*. New York: Raven Press.

Dunne DW (1996). School daze: Classes start so early that kids are sleep deprived. *Hartford Courant*, August 26, 1996.

Epstein R, Chillag N, Lavie P (1995). Sleep habits of children and adolescents in Israel: The influence of starting time of school. *Sleep Research* 24A:432.

Fisher BE, Rinehart S (1990). Stress, arousal, psychopathology and temperament: A multidimensional approach to sleep disturbance in children. *Personality and Individual Differences* 11(5):431–438.

Gorin A, Kelly L, Wolfson A (1994). First year college students: Effects of coping intervention on sleep hygiene and cognitive arousal. *Sleep Research* 23:124.

Graham L, Hamden L (1987). *Youth Trends: Capturing the $200 Billion Youth Market*. New York: St. Martin's Press.

Greenberger E, Steinberg L (1986). *When Teenagers Work: The Psychological and Social Costs of Adolescent Employment*. New York: Basic Books.

Guilleminault C, Winkle R, Korobkin R (1982). Children and nocturnal snoring: Evaluation of the effects of sleep related respiratory resistive load and daytime functioning. *European Journal of Pediatrics* 139:165–171.

Ishihara K, Honma Y, Miyake S (1990). Investigation of the children's version of the morningness-eveningness questionnaire with primary and junior high school pupils in Japan. *Perceptual and Motor Skills* 71:1353–1354.

Kataria S, Swanson MS, Trevathan GE (1987). Persistence of sleep disturbances in preschool children. *Pediatrics* 110(4):642–646.

Link SC, Ancoli-Israel S (1995). Sleep and the teenager. *Sleep Research* 24a:184.

Manber R, Pardee RE, Bootzin RR, Kuo T, Rider AM, Rider SP, Bergstrom L (1995). Changing sleep patterns in adolescence. *Sleep Research* 24:106.

Manning W (1990). Parenting employed teenagers. *Youth and Society* 22:184–200.

Monk T (2000). Shift Work. In M. H. Kryger, T. Roth, & W. C. Dement, eds., *Principles and Practice of Sleep Medicine*, pp. 600–605. Philadelphia: Saunders.

Morrison DN, McGee R, Stanton WR (1992). Sleep problems in adolescence. *Journal of the American Academy of Child and Adolescent Psychiatry* 31(1): 94–99.

Nudel M (1993). The schedule dilemma. *American School Board Journal* 180(11): 37–40.

Petta D, Carskadon MA, Dement WC (1984). Sleep habits in children aged 7–13 years. *Sleep Research* 13:86.

Prather JE (1996). What sociologists are learning about the next generation of students: Are we prepared to teach in the 21st Century? *Sociological Perspectives* 39(4):437–446.

Quine L (1992). Severity of sleep problems in children with severe learning difficulties: Description and correlates. *Journal of Community & Applied Social Psychology* 2(4):247–268.

Ravitch D (1995). *National Standards in American Education: A Citizen's Guide*. Washington, DC: Brookings Institution.

Rosekind MR, Gander PH, Gregory KB, Smith RM, Miller DL, Oyung R, Webbon LL, Johnson JM (1995). Managing fatigue in operational settings: An integrated approach. *Behavioral Medicine* 21(4):166–170.

Stansbury R (1996). West Hartford students oppose earlier start time. *Hartford Courant*, July 26, 1996.

Steinberg L, Brown BB, Dornbusch SM (1996). *Beyond the Classroom: Why School Reform Has Failed and What Parents Need to Do*. New York: Simon & Schuster.

Szymczak JT, Jasinska M, Pawlak E, Swierzykowska M (1993). Annual and weekly changes in the sleep-wake rhythm of school children. *Sleep* 16(5):433–435.

U.S. Department of Labor (1996). Annual Statistics.

Williams R, Karacan I, Hursch C (1974). *EEG of Human Sleep*. New York: J. Wiley & Sons.

Wirtz PW, Rohrbeck CA, Charner I, Fraser BS (1988). Employment of adolescents while in high school: Employment intensity, interference with schoolwork, and normative approval. *Journal of Adolescent Research* 3(1):97–105.

Wolfson AR, Carskadon MA (1998). Sleep schedules and daytime functioning in adolescents. *Child Development* 69(4):875–887.

Wolfson, AR, Tzischinsky O, Brown C, Darley C, Acebo C, Carskadon MA (1995). Sleep, behavior, and stress at the transition to senior high school. *Sleep Research* 24:115.

Yamoor CM, Mortimer JT (1990). Age and gender differences in the effects of employment on adolescent achievement and well-being. *Youth and Society*, 22(2):225–240.

Zarcone VP (2000). Sleep hygiene. In M. H. Kryger, T. Roth, & W. C. Dement, eds., *Principles and Practice of Sleep Medicine*, pp. 657–661. Philadelphia: Saunders.

13. Influence of Irregular Sleep Patterns on Waking Behavior

CHRISTINE ACEBO AND MARY A. CARSKADON

Two consistent findings in the literature on adolescent sleep patterns are that time spent sleeping on school nights decreases from childhood through adolescence, and that differences between weekend and school-night sleep schedules are large for many teenagers (Billiard, Alperovitch, Perot, & James, 1987; Strauch & Meier, 1988; Carskadon, 1990; Szymczak, Jasinska, Pawlak, & Swierzykowska, 1993). In general, school-night sleep is restricted because of early school start times, whereas on weekends, bedtimes and rise times are later and total sleep time is longer. In a recent large survey of over 3,000 high school students, Wolfson and Carskadon (1998) found such irregular bedtimes related to self-reported academic difficulty in school, daytime sleepiness, depressed mood, and sleep-wake behavior problems. Lower amounts of self-reported total sleep time were also related to more difficulties with daytime functioning. We suspect that these difficulties in daytime function may result in part from disturbances in both the homeostatic and circadian timing systems regulating sleep-wake behavior.

Evidence from other studies in children and adolescents supports the importance of total sleep time and sleep schedule regularity as predictors of daytime functioning. Several other survey studies have linked total sleep time with grades, daytime fatigue and struggles to

This work was funded by National Institutes of Health (NIH) grant MH45945. We thank Amy Wolfson, Ronald Seifer, Camille Brown, Catherine Darley, François Garand, Liza Kelly, Eric Kravitz, Christopher Monti, Orna Tzischinsky, Beth Yoder, Jennifer Wicks, and Tony Spirito for their assistance with this project. This chapter is based on a paper presented at the UCLA Youth Enhancement Service Conference on Contemporary Perspectives on Adolescent Sleep Patterns, Los Angeles, CA, April 17–20, 1997.

stay awake, and difficulties concentrating in class (Allen, 1992; Epstein, Chillag, & Lavie, 1995). Results from a longitudinal study of teenagers across the 9th to 10th grade transition demonstrated that students decreased sleep by an average of 20 minutes across the transition because of earlier school start times and showed an increase in daytime sleepiness as measured by the Multiple Sleep Latency Test (Carskadon, Wolfson, Acebo, Tzischinsky, & Seifer, 1998). Results from other survey studies have indicated that adolescents with irregular sleep-wake schedules are more likely to report high levels of daytime sleepiness (Billiard et al., 1987) or to express a need for more sleep (Strauch & Meier, 1988). Acebo and Carskadon (1993) found that bedtime irregularity was related to school functioning as rated by teachers of 5th grade students, with poorer functioning children having more irregularity.

Data from these and other studies provide converging evidence that many adolescents have inadequate sleep patterns both in terms of amount and scheduling of sleep (Wolfson & Carskadon, 1998). Few studies, however, have attempted to assess the unique or relative importance of these two variables for daytime functioning. Manber, Bootzin, Acebo, and Carskadon (1996) reported results from an intervention study in college students that aimed at assessing the effects of increasing sleep time versus increasing schedule regularity. Students in the group given instructions to regularize their sleep patterns showed greater and longer-lasting reductions in self-reported sleepiness and improved self-reported sleep efficiency as compared with students asked only to increase sleep time. The effects were small and based on self-report measures; however, the study provides experimental data supporting an independent contribution of regularity. Furthermore, several laboratory experiments conducted by Taub and colleagues have demonstrated performance and mood deficits in college students when their sleep time was maintained but when the timing was acutely altered (Taub & Berger, 1976).

Data for the present study are taken from a large representative sample of high school students who filled out an anonymous eight-page survey of sleep habits and related behaviors. Previous analyses of this data set have indicated that both low sleep time and irregular bedtimes are related to deficits on measures of daytime functioning (Wolfson & Carskadon, 1998). The purpose of the current analyses was to assess the relative importance of school-night total sleep time, regularity of bedtime schedule, and regularity of sleeping location for predicting a wider range of measures of daytime functioning using multiple regression analysis.

We hypothesized that these three sleep variables would be important and additive predictors of these outcome measures in adolescents even after statistically controlling for demographic and other variables that are expected to have an impact on daytime functioning.

Methods

Subjects

An eight-page sleep habits survey (view the complete survey form at http://www.sleepforscience.org) was administered in the Fall of 1994 to high school students from four public high schools (one urban, two suburban, and one rural) in three Rhode Island school districts. The survey was completed anonymously by 3,119 students during homeroom classes with a response rate of 88%. The sample (13% grade 9, 32% grade 10, 29% grade 11, and 26% grade 12) was 51.6% female and 48.4% male, ranged in age from 13 to 19 years (mean ages = 15.9 ± 1.12 years), and was 86% Caucasian.

Measures

The survey queried students about their usual sleeping and waking behaviors over the past 2 weeks, accidents and injuries over the past 6 months, health, school performance and attendance, frequency of sleep-related behaviors and complaints, and other issues. For this report, we were interested in assessing relationships between 10 outcome measures and 3 measures of sleep and its scheduling. The sleep measures were reported School-Night Total Sleep Time (to assess quantity of sleep), Weekend Bedtime Delay (to assess regularity of timing of sleep), and Number of Nights Sleeping in the Same Bed (to assess regularity of sleeping location).

> *School-Night Total Sleep Time* was obtained from responses to the survey item: "Figure out how long you usually sleep on a night when you do not have school the next day (such as a weekend night) and fill it in here. (Do not include time you spend awake in bed.)"
> *Weekend Bedtime Delay* was derived by subtracting weekend bedtime from school-night bedtime ("What time to you usually go to bed on school days [weekends]?").

Same Bed was a measure obtained from the question "In the last 2 weeks, have you slept in the same bed: (1) every night, (2) almost every night, (3) a few nights, (4) not at all." Scores ranged from 1 (every night) to 4 (not at all).

To control for some of the myriad factors that are assumed to play a role in daytime functioning, eight variables were selected as control variables. These included: Sex; Age; Race (Caucasian, non-Caucasian); highest level of education expected (Expect); self-assessment of Health; self-report of ADHD and/or individualized education program (ADHD/IEP); use of tobacco, alcohol or drugs (Substance); and use of Caffeine. The questions and response sets for these measures are listed in detail on our lab's web site <http://www.sleepforscience.org>. Ten outcome measures of daytime functioning were derived from survey items. These outcome measures are described briefly here. (Cronbach's alpha was calculated from the current data set for scale items.)

Injury: The number of accidents and injuries over the last 6 months (17 types ranging from cuts to gunshots [question 63]; adapted from Starfield et al., 1995).

Alcohol/Drugs: The number of only those accidents and injuries that occurred while using alcohol or drugs.

Homedays: The number of days home from school during the last two weeks because of sickness or any other reason (question 21).

Grades: Self-reported grades in school (question 14, eight-point scale).

Depress: (Coefficient alpha = .79) Depressive mood scale (Kandel & Davies, 1982).

Sleepy 1: (Coefficient alpha = .70) A sleepiness scale consisting of total responses to items in question 43 asking whether the student had fallen asleep or fought sleep in 10 different situations, such as in conversation, while studying, in class at school, driving, etc. (Carskadon, Seifer, & Acebo, 1991).

Sleepy 2: (Coefficient alpha = .68) A sleepiness scale consisting of total responses to four items (c, d, i, and m in question 45) asking about frequency of feeling tired or falling asleep during the day.

Quality: (Coefficient alpha = .80) A scale consisting of total responses to two items (a and o in question 45) querying the frequency of feeling satisfied about sleep.

Delay: (Coefficient alpha = .70) A scale consisting of total responses to six items (b, f, g, h, j, and k of question 45) asking about the frequency of behaviors presumed to be related to a phase delay of sleep.

Owl and Lark: (Coefficient alpha = .78) A 10-item morningness/ eveningness scale (questions 47–56) based on Smith, Reilly, and Midkiff (1989) that assesses time-of-day preferences for activities.

Data Analysis

Hierarchical multiple regression analyses were performed separately for each outcome variable with the set of control variables, as well as School-Night Total Sleep Time, Weekend Bedtime Delay, and Same Bed as the independent variables. The eight control variables (Sex, Age, Race, Expect, Health, ADHD/IEP, Caffeine, and Substances) were entered on the first step, School-Night Total Sleep Time was entered on the second step, Weekend Bedtime Delay on the third, and Same Bed on the fourth. A second analysis entered Weekend Bedtime Delay on the second step, School-Night Total Sleep Time on the third, and Same Bed on the fourth. Results from this second analysis were remarkably similar to the primary analysis and will not be reported.

The increment in R^2 was determined at each step to assess the unique contribution of the variable (or set of variables) upon entry into the equation. This value thus describes the incremental addition of variance accounted for by the variable or set of variables after accounting for those entered on previous steps.

Partial correlation coefficients were also calculated. A partial correlation can be interpreted as the correlation between the independent variable and the dependent variable when the linear effects of the other independent variables have been removed from both the independent and dependent variable; thus, a partial correlation is the correlation between residualized variables.

The very large sample size in this study virtually ensured that all relationships would be statistically significant. Results will be discussed, therefore, from the perspective of effect sizes (Cohen, 1988). A small effect size is equivalent to a multiple R of .14, squared multiple R of .02, and partial correlation of .10; a medium effect size is equivalent to a multiple R of .36, squared multiple R of .13, and partial correlation of .30; a large effect size is a multiple R of .51, squared multiple R of .26, and partial correlation of .50.

Table 13.1. Means, Standard Deviations, Number of Responses (n), and Minimum and Maximum for Interval Measures

Measures	Mean	Standard Deviation	n	Minimum	Maximum
School-Night Total Sleep Time (min)	438.8	66.9	2,887	150	720
Weekend Bedtime Delay (min)	112.0	72.4	2,878	−420	540
Injury	1.4	1.5	2,707	0	8
Alcohol/Drugs	0.2	.6	1,457	0	8
Homedays	0.9	1.5	2,975	0	10
Grades	5.8	1.4	3,060	1	8
Depress	10.2	2.9	2,905	6	18
Sleepy 1	15.0	3.9	2,820	10	40
Sleepy 2	9.4	3.6	2,901	4	20
Quality	6.6	2.3	2,997	5	30
Delay	11.0	4.5	2,994	5	30
Owl and Lark	26.3	5.1	2,885	10	41

Notes: School-Night Sleep Time and Weekend Bedtime Delay are in minutes. Injury, Alcohol/Drugs, and Homedays are the number of incidents. Grades range from 1 to 8 with 1 indicating Ds and Fs and 8 indicating As. Higher scale values for Depress, Sleepy 1, Sleepy 2, and Delay indicate greater numbers of problems. Higher scale values for Quality indicate higher satisfaction with sleep. Higher values on the Owl and Lark scale indicate greater morningness.

Results

Means and standard deviations for each ordinal variable, along with maxima and minima, are presented in Table 13.1. Overall, students reported that they slept slightly more than 7 hours a night on school nights and delayed bedtime nearly 2 hours on weekends (Wolfson & Carskadon, 1998). They reported on average more than 1 injury during the last 6 months and 0.2 injuries while taking alcohol or drugs. Students averaged nearly 1 day home from school for any reason during the past 2 weeks. Average grades for these students were Bs.

Table 13.2 presents the number of students in each category for categorical measures. The majority of students slept in the same bed every night, although over a third of them did not. Most students said that they expected to finish college, that they were in good or excellent health, and that they did not have ADHD, a learning disability, an individualized education program, or special help for difficulties with school work. Less

Table 13.2. Students Responding in Each Category
for Nominal Variables

Variable	Number	Percentage
Same Bed		
Every night	1,963	63.6
Almost every night	947	30.7
A few nights	150	4.9
Not at all	25	0.8
Expect		
May not finish high school	32	1.0
Will finish high school	560	18.2
Will get a college degree	1,156	50.6
Will get a degree beyond college	928	30.2
Health		
Poor	39	1.2
Fair	463	15.1
Good	1,718	55.9
Excellent	856	27.8
ADHD/IEP		
No	2,711	89.0
Yes	336	11.0
Substances		
No use of alcohol, tobacco, or drugs	2,098	69.1
Use 1 of alcohol, tobacco, or drugs	553	18.2
Use 2 of alcohol, tobacco, or drugs	235	7.7
Use 3 of alcohol, tobacco, or drugs	149	4.9
Caffeine		
Never drinks caffeinated beverages	417	13.7
Drinks either caffeinated sodas or coffee/tea	1,612	52.9
Drinks caffeinated sodas and coffee/tea	1,017	33.4

than one-third of students reported using alcohol, tobacco, or drugs, but the majority reported drinking caffeinated beverages.

Table 13.3 presents the multiple R, multiple R^2, and the increment in R^2 upon entry of the variable or set of variables into the equation. The increment in R^2 indicated "small" additive effects for School-Night Total Sleep Time for depressed mood, both sleepiness variables, the quality-of-sleep scale, the delay scale, and the Owl/Lark scale. Thus, *after* the control variables are partialed, School-Night Total Sleep Time accounts for between 2% to 5% of the variance for these measures. Weekend Bedtime Delay and Same Bed showed "small" effect size increments only for the Delay scale. The set of eight control variables accounted for between 4% to 28% of the variance for the dependent variables.

Table 13.3a. Multiple R, R², and the Increment in R² for Variables upon Entry into a Hierarchical Multiple Regression Analysis

Dependent Variable	R	R²	R² Increment
Injury			
Control Variables	.21	.04	.04*
School-Night TST	.21	.04	.00
Weekend Bedtime Delay	.21	.05	.00
Same Bed	.23	.05	.01
Injury with Alcohol/Drugs			
Control Variables	.36	.13	.13**
School-Night TST	.37	.14	.00
Weekend Bedtime Delay	.37	.14	.00
Same Bed	.38	.15	.01
Homeday			
Control Variables	.29	.09	.09*
School-Night TST	.31	.09	.01
Weekend Bedtime Delay	.31	.10	.00
Same Bed	.35	.12	.02*
Grades			
Control Variables	.53	.28	.28***
School-Night TST	.53	.28	.00
Weekend Bedtime Delay	.54	.29	.01
Same Bed	.55	.30	.00
Depressed Mood			
Control Variables	.43	.18	.18**
School-Night TST	.45	.20	.02*
Weekend Bedtime Delay	.45	.20	.00
Same Bed	.45	.21	.00

Notes: * = small effect size; ** = medium effect size; *** = large effect size.

Table 13.4 presents partial correlation coefficients from the analyses. We see from these results that when the linear effects of the independent variables are removed from each other and from the dependent variable, "small" effect size correlations remain between School-Night Total Sleep Time and six of the dependent variables. Thus, after this adjustment for the control variables, lower School-Night Total Sleep Time was related to more symptoms on the depressed-mood scale, more responses on both sleepiness scales, lower satisfaction with sleep, more behaviors indicating delayed sleep phase, and more eveningness on the Owl/Lark scale.

Weekend Bedtime Delay had small effect size partial correlations with grades, the Delay scale, and the Owl/Lark scale. Thus, after adjustment

Table 13.3b. Multiple R, R², and the Increment in R² for Variables upon Entry into a Hierarchical Multiple Regression Analysis

Dependent Variable	R	R^2	R^2 Increment
Sleepy 1			
Control Variables	.37	.13	.13**
School-Night TST	.40	.16	.03*
Weekend Bedtime Delay	.40	.16	.03*
Same Bed	.41	.17	.01
Sleepy 2			
Control Variables	.39	.15	.15**
School-Night TST	.42	.18	.00
Weekend Bedtime Delay	.42	.18	.00
Same Bed	.43	.19	.01
Quality			
Control Variables	.28	.08	.08*
School-Night TST	.36	.13	.05*
Weekend Bedtime Delay	.36	.13	.00
Same Bed	.36	.13	.00
Delay			
Control Variables	.41	.17	.17**
School-Night TST	.44	.20	.03*
Weekend Bedtime Delay	.47	.22	.01
Same Bed	.47	.22	.01
Owl/Lark			
Control Variables	.36	.13	.13**
School-Night TST	.42	.18	.05*
Weekend Bedtime Delay	.43	.19	.01
Same Bed	.44	.19	.00

Notes: * = small effect size; ** = medium effect size; *** = large effect size.

for the control variables, larger bedtime delays on weekends were related to lower grades, more behaviors indicating delayed sleep phase, and more eveningness on the Owl/Lark scale.

Small effect size partial correlations between the dependent variables and Same Bed were evident for Injuries with Alcohol/Drugs, Days Home from School, and the first Sleepiness scale. Thus, students who slept in the same bed every night were less likely to have injuries associated with drugs or alcohol, days home from school, and daytime sleepiness.

As expected, many of the control variables were correlated with the dependent variables. Sex was related to Grades, Depressed Mood, and Quality of sleep, with girls on the average showing higher grades,

Table 13.4a. Partial Correlation Coefficients from Multiple Regression Analysis

Dependent Variable	Injury	Injury with Alcohol/ Drugs	Homeday	Grades	Depressed Mood
Multiple R	.23*	.38**	.35*	.55***	.45**
Multiple R²	.05*	.15**	.12*	.30***	.21**
Partial Correlations					
Sex	−.07	−.05	.06	.13*	.30**
Age	−.09	−.01	.07	.03	.04
Race	.00	.01	.00	.01	.02
Expect	.03	.04	−.13*	.37**	.01
Health	.00	−.01	−.05	.11*	−.18*
ADHD/IEP	.06	.04	.07	−.14*	.09
Substances	.13*	.31**	.10*	−.16*	.11*
Caffeine	.00	−.05	.03	−.03	.03
School-Night TST	−.05	−.06	−.08	−.05	−.16*
Weekend Bedtime Delay	.02	.00	.03	−.11*	.00
Same Bed	.09	.11*	.16*	−.07	.06

Notes: Partial correlation coefficients from multiple regression analysis for each dependent variable, and multiple R and R² for the set of all variables. * = small effect size; ** = medium effect size; *** = large effect size.

more symptoms of depressed mood, and less satisfaction with sleep. Partial correlations with Age and Race did not reach small effect size criteria for any measure. Expected level of education was related negatively to Days Home from School and positively to Grades. Students who reported better Health tended to report higher grades, less depressed mood, more satisfaction with sleep, and tended toward morningness on the Owl/Lark scale. Students reporting ADHD or help with school work reported lower grades in school. Substance use was related to all variables except Sleep Quality in expected directions. Partial correlations with Caffeine use did not reach small effect size criteria for any measure. Figures 13.1, 13.2, and 13.3 illustrate additive effects and partial correlations between variables for Days Home from School, Grades at School, and Depressed Mood.

The multiple R values estimating the correlation between the 11 independent variables and each outcome variable indicated medium effect

Table 13.4b. Partial Correlation Coefficients from Multiple Regression Analysis

Dependent Variable	Sleepy 1	Sleepy 2	Quality	Delay Scale	Owl/Lark Scale
Multiple R	.41**	.43**	.36**	.47**	.44**
Multiple R²	.17**	.19**	.13**	.22**	.19**
Partial Correlations					
Sex	.09	.08	−.14*	−.01	−.01
Age	.01	.04	−.03	−.03	.02
Race	.00	.00	.03	.01	.01
Expect	.01	−.03	−.01	−.05	.15
Health	−.07	−.08	−.13*	−.07	.12*
ADHD/IEP	.07	.02	−.04	.07	−.05
Substances	.23*	.25*	−.04	.26*	−.18*
Caffeine	.07	.08	−.03	.06	−.07
School-Night TST	−.17*	−.17*	.23*	−.20*	.24*
Weekend Bedtime					
Delay	.00	.03	−.01	.15*	−.10*
Same Bed	.11*	.08	−.05	.09	−.08

Notes: Partial correlation coefficients from multiple regression analysis for each dependent variable, and multiple R and R² for the set of all variables. * = small effect size; ** = medium effect size; *** = large effect size.

size multiple correlations for all variables except the Injury and Days Home from School measures, for which small effect size relationships were found. Across the outcome variables, variance accounted for by the 11 independent variables ranged from .05 to .30.

Discussion

Many factors, such as sex, age, race, educational expectations, health, learning disabilities, and substance use contribute to differences in daytime functioning among adolescents. The results of this analysis indicate that even after controlling for several such factors, sleep measures add to prediction. School-Night Total Sleep Time attained small effect size relationships with six of the outcome measures, compared with three each for Weekend Bedtime Regularity and Same Bed. Thus, over this set of outcome measures, School-Night Total Sleep Time might be considered a more important predictor. The regularity variables, however, were related to variables that were not impacted by School-Night Total Sleep Time, that is, Grades, Injuries associated with Alcohol/Drugs, and

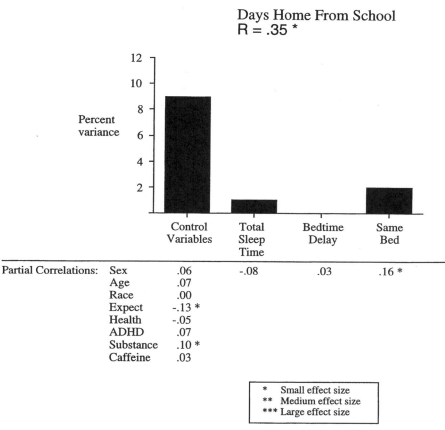

Figure 13.1. Estimated values based on hierarchical multiple regression analysis of Days Home From School with eight control variables entered on step 1, School-Night Total Sleep Time on step 2, Weekend Bedtime Delay on step 3, and Nights in the Same Bed on step 4. The figure illustrates the variance accounted for at each step (the increment in R^2). Partial correlations are tabled for each independent variable.

Days Home from School. All of the relationships were in the expected direction.

The multiple R values for the entire group of independent variables ranged from .23 to .55, indicating at least small effect size relationships for all outcome measures. Thus, the combination of demographic, educational expectation, health, learning disabilities or educational challenge, substance and caffeine use, and sleep measures provide admirable prediction of daytime functioning.

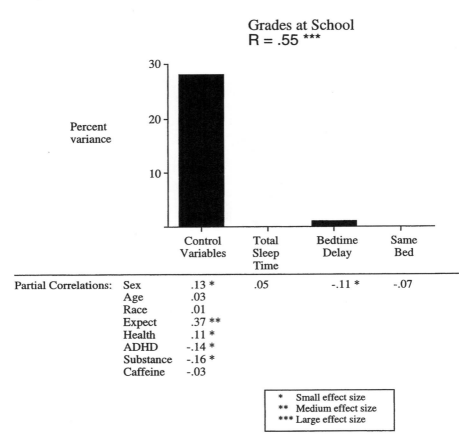

Partial Correlations:		Control Variables	Total Sleep Time	Bedtime Delay	Same Bed
	Sex	.13 *	.05	-.11 *	-.07
	Age	.03			
	Race	.01			
	Expect	.37 **			
	Health	.11 *			
	ADHD	-.14 *			
	Substance	-.16 *			
	Caffeine	-.03			

```
*   Small effect size
**  Medium effect size
*** Large effect size
```

Figure 13.2. Estimated values based on hierarchical multiple regression analysis of Grades at School with eight control variables entered on step 1, School-Night Total Sleep Time on step 2, Weekend Bedtime Delay on step 3, and Nights in the Same Bed on step 4. The figure illustrates the variance accounted for at each step (the increment in R^2). Partial correlations are tabled for each independent variable.

The results of this study are consistent with other reports in the literature linking inadequate sleep with daytime sleepiness, grades, depressed mood, satisfaction with sleep, and morningness-eveningness in adolescents. In addition, this study adds alcohol- and drug-related injuries and school attendance to the list of measures of daytime functioning associated with less adequate sleep. Inadequate sleep measures were also related to behaviors indicating delayed sleep phase and more eveningness on the Owl/Lark scale. Thus, the teenagers who tend to

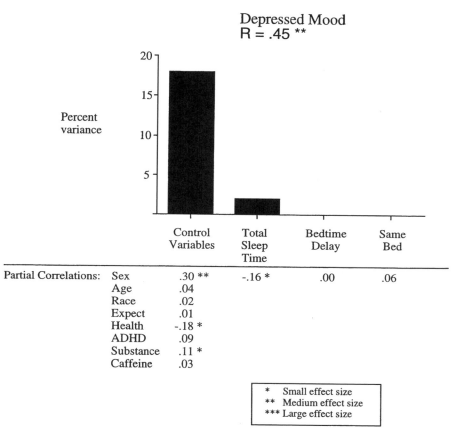

Figure 13.3. Estimated values based on hierarchical multiple regression analysis of Depressed Mood with eight control variables entered on step 1, School-Night Total Sleep Time on step 2, Weekend Bedtime Delay on step 3, and Nights in the Same Bed on step 4. The figure illustrates the variance accounted for at each step (the increment in R^2). Partial correlations are tabled for each independent variable.

have less School-Night Total Sleep Time and who delay bedtime more on weekends on average have a preference for scheduling activities later in the day or night and show more behaviors associated with phase delay, such as difficulty getting up in the morning, oversleeping in the morning, difficulty falling asleep at night, and pulling "all-nighters." Decreased School-Night Total Sleep Time for these teenagers is likely a consequence of nonnegotiable early school start times potentiating sleep loss in a phase delayed subgroup.

Finally, although the amount of sleep appears to be a somewhat stronger predictor of daytime dysfunction, irregularity of sleep scheduling and sleep location was also related to outcome measures. We suggest that disturbances in both the homeostatic and circadian systems regulating sleep-wake behavior are indicators of overall system instability and thus may be useful for predicting adolescent dysfunction. Survey data from a variety of studies paint an increasingly coherent picture of the risks to adolescents of inadequate sleep habits, and, although limited by the self-report nature of measures, they provide a strong rationale for longitudinal and laboratory-based studies aimed at assessing the effects of homeostatic and circadian components of the sleep-wake system on daytime functioning.

REFERENCES

Acebo C, Carskadon MA (1993). An evaluation of children's self-reported sleep measures. *Sleep Research* 22:53.
Allen R (1992). Social factors associated with the amount of school week sleep lag for seniors in an early starting suburban high school. *Sleep Research* 19:114.
Billiard M, Alperovitch A, Perot C, James A (1987). Excessive daytime somnolence in young men, prevalence and contributing factors. *Sleep* 10:297–305.
Carskadon MA (1990). Adolescent sleepiness: Increased risk in a high-risk population. *Alcohol, Drugs and Driving* 5/6:317–328.
Carskadon MA, Seifer R, Acebo C (1991). Reliability of six scales in a sleep questionnaire for adolescents. *Sleep Research* 20:421.
Carskadon MA, Wolfson AR, Acebo C, Tzischinsky O, & Seifer R (1998). Adolescent sleep patterns, circadian timing, and sleepiness at a transition to early school days. *Sleep* 21(8):871–881.
Cohen J (1988). *Statistical Power Analysis for the Behavioral Sciences.* Hillsdale, NJ: Lawrence Erlbaum.
Epstein R, Chillag N, Lavie P (1995). Sleep habits of children and adolescents in Israel: The influence of starting time of school. *Sleep Research* 24A:432.
Kandel DB, Davies M (1982). Epidemiology of depressive mood in adolescents. *Archives of General Psychiatry* 39:1205–1212.
Manber R, Bootzin RR, Acebo C, Carskadon MA (1996). The effects of regularizing sleep-wake schedules on daytime sleepiness. *Sleep* 19(5):432–441.
Smith CS, Reilly C, Midkiff K (1989). Evaluation of three circadian rhythm questionnaires with suggestions for an improved measure of morningness. *Journal of Applied Psychology* 74:728–738.
Starfield B, Riley A, Green B, Ensminger M, Ryan S, Kelleher K, Kim-Harris S, Johnston D, Vogel K (1995). The adolescent child health and illness profile: A population-based measure of health. *Medical Care* 33:553–566.
Strauch I, Meier B (1988). Sleep need in adolescents: A longitudinal approach. *Sleep* 11:378–386.

Szymczak JT, Jasinska M, Pawlak E, Swierzykowska M (1993). Annual and weekly changes in the sleep-wake rhythm of school children. *Sleep* 16(5):433–435.

Taub JM, Berger RJ (1976). The effects of changing the phase and duration of sleep. *Experimental Psychology* 2(1):30–41.

Wolfson AR, Carskadon MA (1998). Sleep schedules and daytime functioning in adolescents. *Child Development* 69(4):875–887.

14. Stress and Sleep in Adolescence: A Clinical-Developmental Perspective

AVI SADEH AND REUT GRUBER

The sleep-wake system during adolescence has been characterized by significant and unique features, including the sleep-phase shift toward delayed bedtime, growing sleep needs, and daytime sleepiness. In addition, many adolescents adopt disorganized sleep-wake patterns including dramatic weekday-weekend variations in their sleep schedule. In light of the debate on the extent of the inherent turmoil and instability of this developmental stage, the striking findings on the adolescent sleep-wake system are particularly interesting, as they demonstrate instability and lack of biobehavioral homeostasis.

The present review addresses two major issues: the relationships between normal adolescent developmental stressors and sleep; and the effects of extraordinary life stressors and traumatic events on sleep in adolescents. These issues are discussed in the context of theoretical models of stress and coping.

Adolescence: A Period of Storm and Stress?

Adolescence is a period of rapid psychosocial and biobehavioral changes and significant emotional turmoil. Adolescents experience many dramatic physical changes associated with the growth spurt and sexual maturation. Pubertal changes are manifested in the appearance of secondary sex signs, in the first episodes of menarche, and in nocturnal emission and ejaculation. In the psychosocial sphere, the adolescent is developing high cognitive skills heavily based on abstract thinking, metacognition, and critical thinking. Psychosocial issues related to identity formation, autonomy, intimacy, sexual behavior and orientation, social status, and academic and professional careers set the stage for intense emotional and cognitive processes. In most youngsters, this results in newly acquired skills and mature adaptation, while in the remainder of youngsters, this results in clinical symptoms or even in the onset of severe psychopathology.

The extent to which adolescence is a period of "storm and stress" is a very controversial issue in the adolescent literature (Hall, 1904; Freud, 1958; Blos, 1962; Erikson, 1968). Early theories, mostly based on psychoanalytic thinking, presented adolescence as a period of turmoil and instability. Perhaps this notion is best illustrated in Anna Freud's writing: "To be normal during the adolescent period is by itself abnormal" (Freud, 1958). In other words, these authors suggested that a serious and prolonged identity crisis during adolescence is essential for healthy and normal development. The view of adolescence as a period of stress and crisis has changed as developmental researchers began to study developmental processes in normal adolescents, as opposed to earlier studies that emphasized clinical populations. Based on recent developmental studies, Offer, Kimberly, and Schonert-Reichl (1992) dismissed some of the basic myths pertaining to the adolescent period. They argued that normal adolescent development is not necessarily tumultuous. On the contrary, these authors claim that teenagers who exhibit little disequilibrium are normal, and that adolescence is a period of development that can be traversed without turmoil. Furthermore, the transition to adulthood is accomplished by most adolescents gradually and without undue upheaval. Another myth that these authors dismiss is that adolescence is a time of increased emotionality. Research revealed no supporting evidence for this myth, although there seems to be a tendency for adolescents to report increased levels of negative feelings. The last important myth dismissed by Offer and his colleagues is that puberty is necessarily a negative event for adolescents. They conclude from recent research findings that pubertal changes have significant psychological impact but that for most adolescents the experience is quite ambivalent, arousing both positive and negative feelings.

Whether adolescence is a period of stress depends to a great extent on the definition of stress. Unfortunately, stress is a very popular but illdefined concept used in a wide range of disciplines and contexts (e.g., the medical and psychosocial literature). Despite the widespread use of the stress concept, its definition has not been crystallized (Engel, 1985). When we discuss stress, we refer to unusual events, change or threat of change, demanding special biobehavioral or psychological adaptive responses by the individual to maintain psychophysiological equilibrium and well-being. The stressor is the event that triggers the change or the threat.

The effects of stress depend on multiple factors: specific characteristics of the event (e.g., intensity, duration, predictability); the adolescent's subjective perception and interpretation of the event; the adolescent's resilience and coping skills; and the adolescent's support systems. In this context, one can view the rapid maturational changes of adolescence as potential stressors. However, these stressors are cognitively mediated and downplayed, as they are mostly perceived as part of the normal maturational processes.

Stress and Sleep: A Conceptual Model

Sleep is very sensitive to transient as well as chronic aspects of emotional status, expectations, anxieties, and psychopatholgy. Sleep disruptions appear in many psychiatric disorders, and sleep-related problems are among the diagnostic criteria of some disorders such as affective disorders, posttraumatic stress disorder (PTSD), and anxiety disorders (American Psychiatric Association, 1994). Despite their relevance, the present review does not address the relationships between sleep and psychopathology in adolescence (for a recent review see Dahl, 1996).

When one examines the sleep-wake phenomena in the wider context of biobehavioral coping and adaptation to stress, one realizes that the sleep-wake system echoes the basic coping mechanisms of fight-or-flight that require hypervigilance and high arousal level along with the withdrawal associated with learned helplessness.

Although there are a variety of definitions of stress, Selye's (1956) unified theory is discussed in relationship to sleep. Selye described the general adaptive syndrome (GAS) as a set of common, nonspecific components of the adaptive response to a wide variety of stressors. This set of responses includes: (1) the alarm phase, in which the activity of the adrenocortical system increases dramatically and facilitates hypervigilance, increased activity, and readiness for action; (2) the stage of resistance, which represents the organism's attempt to regain and maintain homeostasis; and (3) the stage of exhaustion, which results from a depletion of the adaptive energies and may cause irreversible damage to cardiovascular, digestive, immune, and circulatory systems. Within Selye's framework, atypical alternation in rest-activity cycles, hypervigilance, fatigue, and sleep-wake disorders represent nonspecific components of the GAS.

Recently, on the basis of a literature review on sleep, stress, and trauma in children, Sadeh (1996) has identified two underlying antagonistic modes of adaptation of the sleep-wake system in response to stress or traumatic events. The first mode ("turn-on") is compatible with the GAS alarm stage where the organism's adaptational efforts are focused on identifying the stressor and directly coping with it. From the sleep-wake perspective it is not safe to sleep; therefore, hyperarousal is the most protective and evolutionary adaptive response. The second mode ("shut-off"), compatible with the conservation-withdrawal hypothesis (Engel & Schmale, 1967), is the state when the organism realizes that there is no way to influence ongoing stressors and it shuts itself away from further intrusions by withdrawal and energy conservation. In terms of the sleep-wake system this means extending or deepening sleep. This biphasic response to acute and chronic stress is also compatible with Terr's analysis of childhood trauma and its consequences (Terr, 1991; Sadeh, 1996).

Our hypothesis is that the sleep-wake system is an integrated component of a more global biobehavioral stress management system. Sleep could be disrupted by stress when the most adaptive response is hypervigilance, but sleep could also protect the organism from stress when a direct coping response is not optional, thus raising the stimulus barrier and protecting the individual from further bombardment of stimuli and stressors (Emde, Harmon, Metcalf, Koenig, & Wagonfeld, 1971). Sleep and dreaming phenomena also enable cognitive and dynamic processing of the information perceived during wakefulness.

Evidence for the operation of these two modes is mostly derived from infant, child, and adult studies; studies focused specifically on the adolescent period are still lacking. The hypervigilant ("turn-on") mode of response, with the resulting disorders of initiating and maintaining sleep, as well as nightmares, has been well documented in the literature (see Ross, Ball, Sullivan, & Caroff, 1989; Sadeh, 1996). Indeed, the sleep-wake disruptions associated with stress response and PTSD have been recognized as the hallmark of PTSD (Ross, Ball, Sullivan, & Caroff, 1989) and have become an integral part of the psychiatric diagnostic criteria for PTSD (American Psychiatric Association, 1994).

Direct evidence for the second ("shut-off") mode of operation is more sparse. For instance, it has been demonstrated that infants often increase the amount of their quiet or deep sleep in response to stressful events such as circumcision or separation from mother (Emde et al., 1971; Field & Reite, 1984; Field, 1991). From a different perspective it has been demonstrated that, when studied in the sleep laboratory, traumatized adults (such as holocaust survivors and veterans with combat-related PTSD) have unique characteristics that suggest the operation of a protective barrier during sleep. For example, well-adjusted Holocaust survivors had very low dream recall upon awakening from rapid eye movement (REM) sleep (Kaminer & Lavie, 1991), and posttraumatic veterans exhibited higher thresholds for noise-induced awakening in comparison to a control group (Dagan, Lavie, & Bleich, 1991).

Clearly, the relationship between stress and sleep is complex and multidimensional. Sleep and dreaming phenomena are very sensitive to physiological and psychological stress. Sleep and sleep-related issues may arouse significant fears and anxieties in many youngsters and thus represent a significant stressor in their lives.

Stress and Sleep in Adolescence

An integrative model of stress and sleep during adolescence is presented in Figure 14.1. This model represents the bidirectional and circular relationships between sleep and stress. It includes specific factors such as the variations in the sleep-wake system (sleep phase shift, sleep irregularities, and the instability that characterizes the adolescent period) and age-specific psychosocial issues that could be considered as developmental stressors for adolescents.

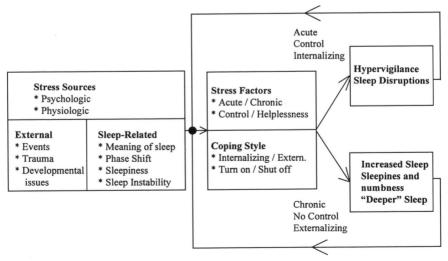

Figure 14.1. An integrative model of stress and sleep: The adolescent period.

The following section is divided into two main topics: specific adolescent issues that may be stressful and negatively impact adolescents' sleep; and the effects of non-age-specific traumatic events during adolescence. Illustrative case reports are appended to this chapter.

Specific Adolescent Issues

Normal adolescent phenomena such as the significant phase shift associated with delayed bedtime, along with the resulting sleep restriction and daytime fatigue, may become a significant source of stress for the adolescent and adversely affect functioning or require intense adaptational efforts. Indeed, as much as 25% of adolescents report a need for more sleep (Morrison, McGee, & Stanton, 1992).

Sleep in itself could be considered a stressor in many situations. For anxious adolescents, going to sleep or falling asleep involves a series of processes that are potentially stressful, such as separation from their parents, discontinuation of daily activity, darkness and its "evil forces," and experiences of loss of control. For other adolescents, different developmental issues predominate the scene. For example, going to sleep is often perceived by adolescents as a counterproductive behavior considering their social and academic pressures. Staying up late at night is also emotionally associated with extended autonomy and independence from the parents. In addition, going to sleep is often linked to other stressful or conflictual issues such as the adolescents' growing awareness of their sexuality and sexual arousal around bedtime.

A number of surveys have reported a high prevalence of sleep and daytime sleepiness problems in adolescents. For instance, Morrison et al. (1992) reported that 33% of their sample of 943 adolescents reported sleep-related problems with a need for more sleep as the most prominent complaint (25%). Other surveys reported prevalence rates ranging between 11% and 38% depending on the exact definition used (Price, Coates, Thoresen, & Grinstead, 1978; Kirmil-Gray, Eagleston, Gibson, & Thoresen, 1984; Bearpark & Michie, 1987; Morrison et al., 1992). These studies also indicated high comorbidity between sleep problems and other behavioral and psychiatric disorders. Considering the fact that a sleep disorder is in itself a severe stressor that can exacerbate further development, Ford and Kamerow (1989) suggested that the treatment of sleep problems may prevent later psychiatric disorders.

The relevant adolescent literature provides very limited direct information on sleep and stress in adolescents. A few adolescent studies

indicated that poor sleep in adolescents is associated with more observable behaviors and feelings of stress (Price et al., 1978; Kirmil-Gray
et al., 1984). For instance, Kirmil-Gray and colleagues (1984) reported
higher frequencies of observable signs and feelings of stress and more
emotional lability, stress-producing ideas, and worries in poor sleepers than in good sleepers. These correlative studies preclude any causal
conclusions, but they are in line with the stress and sleep disruption
link.

Bertelson and Monroe (1979) studied personality characteristics of
good and poor sleepers in a clinical sample of adolescents with emotional disturbances. Their findings indicate that poor sleepers were characterized by neurotic features such as depression, fearfulness, inhibition,
anxiety, and rumination. Good sleepers were characterized by healthy
features. These findings are in line with other findings from the adult literature (e.g., Monroe, 1967) and from the child and adolescent literature
(Dollinger, 1986; Fisher & Rinehart, 1990; Sadeh et al., 1995) indicating
strong ties between sleep disruptions and internalizing characteristics
(Achenbach & Edelbrock, 1978). These findings also imply that adolescents with internalizing presentation are more likely to develop sleep
disruptions in response to significant stressors.

Another interesting finding associating sleep with stress was reported
by Williamson, Dahl, Birmaher, Goetz, Nelson, and Ryan (1995). In a
study comparing depressed and normal adolescents, they found that
in normal adolescents the presence of stressful life events was significantly associated with reduced REM latency and increased total REM
time. Although the authors emphasize the limitation of their subjective stress measure, they do speculate on the basis of related findings
that there might be two types of responses: (1) the response to acute
stress, which may initially lead to prolongation of REM latency and a
decrease in total REM time; and (2) the response to ongoing chronic
stressful life events, which may lead to decreased REM latency and increased total REM time. This biphasic response to stress is consistent and
complementary to the "turn-on" and "shut-off" responses described
earlier.

Sleep extension or restriction also directly influences daytime alertness and responsiveness. It could be speculated, for instance, that the
adolescent tendency to switch from sleep deprivation and increased
daytime sleepiness during the weekdays to extended sleep during the
weekends is, to some extent, a regulatory process that modulates the
adolescent's daily affective and cognitive functioning.

As described earlier, a number of potential stressors occupy the adolescent period. Most of these developmental stressors, such as those related to family, social, and academic issues, are relevant to younger children and adults as well, but they gain special prominence during adolescence. Puberty, by definition, is certainly a unique developmental shift that triggers or intensifies potentially stressful issues, particularly those related to sexual maturation and sexuality.

Sexual Maturation

The maturational changes associated with puberty are well anticipated and accepted by most adolescents. The development of secondary sexual signs, growth of the sexual organs, pubic hair, breasts, and the first experiences of menarche or ejaculation are exciting and potentially stressful self-discoveries during adolescence. Another relevant issue is that of sexual excitement and masturbation. Being in bed isolated from other family members may lead to increased sexual arousal and masturbatory activity. This may in turn lead to increased tension and arousal particularly in adolescents who have strong ambivalent feelings about their developing sexuality.

Beyond the sense of shame and guilt that adolescents may experience with regard to their sexuality, significant stress may result from cultural attitudes toward sexuality in general and masturbation in particular. The Jewish tradition, for instance, prohibits men from wasting semen in nonfertile activities. A number of adolescent boys seen in our clinic came from religious families and reported serious tensions around bedtime due to their forbidden masturbatory activities or fantasies. These tensions and increased sexual arousal may lead to sleep onset difficulties in otherwise normal and healthy adolescents, as illustrated in the case of Dana in the appendix.

Social versus Family Relationships

Adolescence also extenuates the shift from parents to peers. This shift is gradual and is spread throughout childhood, but the pressure to create and maintain close and intimate relationships with peers seems to be of particular importance during adolescence (Savin-Williams & Berndt, 1992). As a result, many adolescents report increasingly later bedtimes and less time for sleep because of new social demands. Specifically, teenagers spend late night time on the Internet, socializing into the early morning hours, or other peer activities that change and interfere with their sleep patterns. Studies have assessed this interaction; however, the case of Ronit in the appendix provides a sense of the ways the interaction can play out.

Relationships with Siblings

Studies focused on adolescents' relationships with their siblings suggest that these relationships are unique in nature and distinguishable from the relationships with parents and peers (Furman & Buhrmester, 1985). Sibling relationships were rated similar to those with parents in terms of companionship and importance. In a recent study, the death of a brother or a sister was considered by adolescents to be the most stressful event, even more than the loss of a parent (Zitzow, 1992). An older and close sibling can function as an intimate friend and as a mature guide who is yet not too old to create a generation gap or to be an authority figure, which may create antagonism in the adolescent. Separation issues may therefore involve a close sibling departing from home. A detailed example of an adolescent girl who developed insomnia in response to the departure of her close sister was described elsewhere (Sadeh, 1996).

Academic Pressures

The growing cognitive skills of adolescents widen their horizons, while at the same time they become more aware of the realities of future career choices and the impact of their current academic achievements on their future choices. Academic pressure becomes more intense, and academic difficulties or failures begin to have a strong impact on self-esteem and peer relations, as well as a risk factor for psychopathology (e.g., Hurrelmann, Engel, & Weidman, 1992; Lewinsohn, Gotlib, & Seeley, 1995). Because these pressures often become very intense, adolescents use different strategies to cope with them. On the one hand, academic anxieties may lead to insomnia, and on the other hand, other adolescents develop sleep-phase delay problems and an inability to wake up in the morning and attend school at all. Often, delayed sleep phase syndrome in adolescents creates tremendous academic and psychological pressures on the youngster who is usually blamed by both parents and the school authorities for lack of motivation and a desire to avoid school.

The Effects of Non-Age-Specific Traumatic Events

The literature on the aftermath of severe stress and trauma is in general not specific to the adolescent period. Trauma is generally defined as a stress that is out of the range of a "normal" human experience. The most traumatic experiences involve assaults on human attachment and bonding (see Bowlby, 1969, 1973, for a comprehensive review of the biological and psychosocial processes involved). Animal and human studies with infants and young children indicate that the initial response to loss or separation is usually manifested in search behavior, increased vigilance, and disrupted sleep. If the contact with the attachment figure is not restored, then a second phase of depression, withdrawal, and increased sleep appears (for a review of these studies, see Sadeh, 1996). Studies indicate that sleep disturbances are among the nonspecific responses in grieving adolescents (e.g., Harris, 1991; Meshot & Leitner, 1993).

Child abuse is a relatively well documented area of traumatic experiences endured by both children and adolescents. Again, sleep disruptions are among the nonspecific symptoms presented by sexually and physically abused children and adolescents (Goodwin, 1988; Rimsza, Berg, & Locke, 1988; Goldston, Turnquist, & Knutson, 1989; Moore, 1989; Hillary & Schare, 1993; Sadeh, Hayden, McGuire, Sachs, & Civita, 1994; Sadeh et al., 1995).

Significant modifications in sleep and dreaming patterns in response to other traumatic events such as violence and natural disasters have been reported (Rofe & Lewin, 1982; Raviv & Klingman, 1983; Dollinger, O'Donnell & Staley, 1984; Dollinger, 1986; Pynoos et al., 1987; Lavie, Carmeli, Merorach, & Liberman, 1991; Shannon, Lonigan, Finch, & Taylor, 1994). Most of these studies included children and young adolescents but were not specific to the adolescent period. Interestingly, in most reports, the specific response was that of fears and anxieties related to the specific nature of the trauma, and the most common nonspecific response was that of disrupted sleep, with a few exceptions. One exception, for example, was reported by Rofe and Lewin (1982), who found that children living under constant threat of terror activities slept longer and had fewer bad dreams compared with children living in more secure areas. They concluded that these findings may represent a repressive coping style in response to ongoing chronic threat. These findings are compatible with those reported earlier for adults and may represent the "shut off" protective mode of the sleep-wake system. Furthermore,

Shannon et al. (1994) reported that the incidence of reported sleep problems and bad dreams in response to a disaster decreased with age, thus
suggesting that adolescents may be less prone to biobehavioral changes
of their sleep-wake system in response to traumatic events.

Another exceptional finding is that when sleep is measured by objective methods (e.g., activity-based monitoring), sleep is not necessarily
altered as much as subjective reports may indicate. Lavie and colleagues
(1991, 1993) reported no significant changes in sleep patterns of children
under the threat of ballistic missiles during the Gulf War. These and
other findings from the adult literature indicate that subjective reports
on changes in sleep patterns in response to stress and trauma should
be considered with great caution because it is commonly known and
thus expected that sleep would be disrupted in stressful situations and
these expectations could sensitize and bias subjective reports under such
circumstances.

Conclusions and Future Directions

The present review raises a number of methodological and theoretical issues concerning stress and sleep in the adolescent period. The
central theoretical issues are those related to adolescence as a unique
developmental period and to the relationships between stress and the
sleep-wake system:

- Adolescence is a period of rapid developmental changes that are
  potentially stressful to many adolescents. These age-specific stressors can adversely affect the sleep-wake system. We speculate that
  some of the changes in sleep patterns and arousal level could be
  considered as adaptive maneuvers and attempts to regulate mood
  and affects.
- Adolescence is a period of physiologically driven changes and an
  instability of the sleep-wake system, which could be considered as
  an age-specific stressor.
- Adolescent psychosocial issues such as those related to bodily
  changes, sexuality, family and peer relationships are interwoven
  and interact with biobehavioral mechanisms, including the sleep-
  wake system. Some of the psychosocial issues have special relevance to sleep itself and related issues. In clinical practice, it is
  very important to identify the adolescent state of mind and the
  psychodynamic issues and motivations in addition to diagnosing

the "objective" sleep problem and prescribing the appropriate solutions.

- The sleep-wake system has two modes of response to stress and trauma: the most prevalent response is the hypervigilant "turn-on" mode, which leads to disorders of initiating and maintaining sleep. A less common, but nonetheless important, response is the "shut-off" protective mode, which is manifested in longer and deeper sleep and appears to be more relevant to chronic and inescapable stressors (see model in Figure 14.1).

The following methodological issues have been identified:

- Research focused on stress and sleep during the adolescent period is very sparse. Most studies include adolescents among child or adult samples and therefore preclude a clearer understanding of adolescence as a unique developmental period.
- Prospective studies on specific adolescent stressors and their effects on sleep are needed to elucidate the links between the debated emotional storm and stress and the documented instability in the sleep-wake system.
- Research on stress and sleep is still too heavily based on subjective reports, which may be biased by lack of awareness of the sleep phenomena, by subjective expectations, and by the adolescent's inclinations to report or deny personal difficulties.

Appendix: Case Vignettes

Case Vignette 1, Dana

The following case illustrates the involvement of sexuality in what initially was seen as a sleep-phase delay problem.

Dana, a 10-year-old girl, was referred to our sleep laboratory because of difficulties in initiating sleep and waking up, as well as daytime fatigue. During the first hours of school she was "floating"; then it took her the rest of the school day to get adjusted. Dana was a thin, attractive girl who appeared self-confident, fluent, and happy. She came with her mother to the sleep lab and was able to introduce the sleep problem herself. A week of actigraphic monitoring revealed what appeared to be a delayed sleep phase. Psychological evaluation led to the conclusion that she was a well-adjusted and a highly functioning youngster. In order to cope with the phase delay problem the therapist initiated an early morning bright-light treatment and made a behavioral contract. After a few weeks of light treatment and weekly meetings with Dana and the mother, her sleep schedule was stabilized, Dana woke up easily, and she was not tired during the day. However, she still insisted on continuing with the meetings. At this point it was rather clear that she wanted something else and that her sleep difficulties had some underlying psychological meaning. The therapist suggested a short-term psychotherapy that would be focused on sleep issues. Dana accepted it immediately, not enabling her mother to refuse. The therapist indicated that Dana would have individual meetings without the involvement of the mother.

At the first meeting Dana disclosed she had a secret "she cannot tell anybody in the world," other than her dog and one of her friends, because she was too embarrassed, ashamed, and afraid. She described to the therapist her pleasure time before falling asleep; she enjoyed being sleepy, letting herself follow her falling-asleep hallucinations, sometimes even setting the snooze-button so it would be possible for her to enjoy it as long as possible. Then she switched to other issues. During the next meetings, Dana and the therapist discussed the split between the Dana who insists on being rational and in control, an aspect of her personality named "Dana of the day," and the Dana who wanted to loosen control and follow her emotions, or the "Dana of the night."

A related issue was her fear of growing up. She felt that although she trusted her mother, she couldn't tell her everything anymore. She felt that she needed to struggle for her independence at home, but yet was not willing to give up her place as the youngest child in her family.

Then she disclosed her secret. She wrote it on a piece of paper because it was too embarrassing for her to speak about it. She had started to masturbate but had stopped already. She was later able to connect the issue of sleep to these first confusing signs and feelings of her sexuality. This topic was linked to her ambivalence toward the emerging feeling of a more mature self.

It is very difficult to conclude from this clinical case the real source of the sleep difficulties. It seems, however, that a tendency to develop a phase shift was interwoven with a struggle to cope with developmental issues, both of which led to sleep onset difficulties.

Case Vignette 2, David

The case of David is an example of the way these processes affect sleep. Although the axis of autonomy versus dependence is ubiquitous, this case exemplifies the need to assess and reassess continuously family relationships and parental involvement while working with adolescents.

David, a 17-year-old youngster, arrived at our clinic because of a very delayed sleep onset (3 A.M.) associated with serious difficulties in waking up in the morning and attending school. David appeared to be intrinsically motivated to receive help and due to his age he was seen individually. Actigraphic evaluation confirmed David's descriptions and provided additional information on the instability of his sleep-wake schedule. David would sometimes nap in the afternoon or fall asleep at an earlier bedtime (e.g., 11 P.M.) after accumulating a significant sleep debt due to his very late sleep onset on previous nights. The therapist worked with David on his sleep hygiene and recommended early morning bright-light therapy to facilitate the desired phase advance. At this point it became apparent that David was not able to conform and follow the therapeutic guidelines. He reported having a serious conflict with his father who was very skeptical about his son's efforts and the therapist's ability to help. The father's skepticism led David to doubt if his parents would finance his clinical sessions and he was on the verge of quitting the treatment program. The therapist then intervened and engaged the father in the therapeutic process. The therapist provided the father with information about the treatment process and asked him to support David emotionally and technically in his efforts to reset his clock. The father agreed to help. This was the turning point of the treatment. Collaborating with his father, David was able to comply fully with the sleep hygiene and light treatment requirements, and he shifted his schedule to a normal one in a fairly short period. It was clear from the joint sessions with David and his father that their renewed male bonding was an important emotional reward for both of them in light of the growing detachment and antagonism that preceded the treatment. This emotional reward motivated and energized David to comply with the treatment guidelines with rapid success.

Case Vignette 3, Ronit

The following example demonstrates how a typical sleep problem involved complex stressors and adaptational efforts related to the need to overcome dependency on the parents and develop social ties with peers.

Ronit, a 13-year-old girl, was referred to our sleep clinic. She was overweight, wearing heavy glasses, sloppily dressed with large clothes blurring her body figure. She reported falling asleep only during early morning hours, sleeping until the afternoon hours, and missing school. Every morning there was a battle to wake her up. The family tried everything it could to solve the problem. In the interview it turned out that Ronit slept with her grandmother ever since she was a young child. Whenever the grandmother was not sleeping at home, Ronit insisted on cosleeping with one of her two siblings. In addition, until half a year before the interview took place she used to sleep with a lot of toy puppets. Then, one day, she decided that she wanted to have a double bed and she got rid of the toys. The family also reported that Ronit had significant social problems. The mother indicated that she did not have friends at all since the beginning of that year when she started junior high school. Ronit protested and said that she did not have friends whom she could meet, but that she had "friends." It turned out that Ronit was an "Internet freak," working all night long, exploiting the cheaper night tariff, and mainly contacting peer networks. The Internet correspondence was her main source of "social" contacts. It helped her to cope with her loneliness and to overcome her lack of confidence and low self-esteem. After the first interview with the family, Ronit was invited for an individual session, and her sleep was assessed with an actigraphic evaluation. A week of actigraphic monitoring revealed what appeared to be a severe delayed sleep phase. In the individual session it was clear that Ronit felt like an outsider at school, and she did not know most of her classmates "because I sleep during the day." It appeared that her sleep difficulty became an efficient way to avoid the pain and anxiety that was involved with being at school. She needed peer company, she was desperate about it, and she created her special way to protect herself by finding a "virtual" substitute. She was not satisfied with her Internet contacts, but at least she felt that she could make it there. So the night became her shelter from the day, and a way to fulfill partially her intense social needs.

Another developmental issue that was expressed in the interview was her fear of being alone at night. It seemed that Ronit had troubles with separating from her parents. She usually spent time at night with her father, and she felt that he was her most intimate friend. Ronit's family was involved and supportive; however, because she did not have friends she could not let herself grow and distance from the family. The sleep problem, on the one hand, reflected this theme, and on the other hand, enabled her to get a "parental supply" at night. She wanted to be able to grow up, so she expressed those feelings in the act of throwing the toy puppets out of the bed and in requesting a double bed. However, she then became frightened because she was insecure about her ability to cope with the separation. The world was too destructive for her, full of frustrations; even though it was very compelling for her, at the same time life felt impossible. Therefore, instead of starting the second separation process, she found the "sleep path" that enabled her to cling to her family and escape from the stressful developmental task.

REFERENCES

Achenbach TM, Edelbrock CS (1978). The classification of child psychopathology: A review and analysis of empirical efforts. *Psychol Bull* 85:1275–1301.

American Psychiatric Association (1994). *Diagnostic and Statistical Manual of Mental Disorders*, 4th ed. Washington, DC: American Psychiatric Association.

Bearpark HM, Michie PT (1987). Prevalence of sleep/wake disturbances in Sydney adolescents. *Sleep Research* 16:304.

Bertelson AD, Monroe LJ (1979). Personality patterns of adolescent poor and good sleepers. *J Abn Child Psychol* 7:191–197.

Blos P (1962). *On Adolescence*. New York: Free Press.

Bowlby J (1969). *Attachment and Loss*. Vol. 1, *Attachment*. London: Hogarth.
    (1973). *Attachment and Loss*. Vol. 2, *Separation Anxiety and Anger*. New York: Basic Books.

Dagan Y, Lavie P, Bleich A (1991). Elevated awakening thresholds in sleep stage 3–4 in war-related post-traumatic stress disorder. *Biol Psychiatry* 30:618–622.

Dahl RE (1996). The regulation of sleep and arousal: Development and psychopathology. *Development and Psychopathology* 8:3–27.

Dollinger SJ (1986). The measurement of children's sleep disturbances and somatic complaints following a disaster. *Child Psychiat Hum Dev* 16:148–153.

Dollinger SJ, O'Donnell, Staley AA (1984). Lightning-strike disaster: Effects on children's fears and worries. *J Consult Clin Psychol* 52:1028–1038.

Emde RH, Harmon R, Metcalf D, Koenig KL, Wagonfeld S (1971). Stress and neonatal sleep. *Psychosomatic Medicine* 33:491–497.

Engel BT (1985). Stress is a noun! No, a verb! No, an adjective! In T. F. Field, P. M. McCabe, & N. Schneiderman, eds., *Stress and Coping*, pp. 3–12. Hillsdale, NJ: Lawrence Erlbaum Associates.

Engel GL & Schmale AH (1967). Psychoanalytic theory of somatic disorder: Conversion, specificity, and the disease onset situation. *Journal of the American Psychoanalytic Association* 15:344–365.

Erickson EH (1968). *Identity, Youth and Crisis*. New York: W. W. Norton.

Field T (1991). Young children's adaptations to repeated separation from their mothers. *Child Develop* 62:539–547.

Field T, Reite M (1984). Children's responses to the separation from mother during the birth of another child. *Child Develop* 55:1308–1316.

Fisher BE, Rinehart S (1990). Stress, arousal, psychopathology and temperament: A multidimensional approach to sleep disturbances in children. *Personality and Individual Differences* 11:431–438.

Ford DE, Kamerow DB (1989). Epidemiologic study of sleep disturbances and psychiatric disorders: An opportunity for prevention? *J Am Med Assoc* 262:1479–1484.

Freud A (1958). Adolescence. *Psychoanalytic Study of the Child* 13:255–278.

Furman W, Buhrmester D (1985). Children's perceptions of the personal relationships in their social networks. *Develop Psychol* 21:1016–1024.

Goldston DB, Turnquist DC, Knutson JF (1989). Presenting problem of sexually abused girls receiving psychiatric services. *J Abn Psychol* 98:314–317.

Goodwin J (1988). Post-traumatic symptoms in abused children. *J Traumatic Stress* 1:465–488.

Hall GS (1904). *Adolescence.* Vols. 1 and 2. Englewood Cliffs, NJ: Prentice-Hall.

Harris ES (1991). Adolescent bereavement following the death of a parent: An exploratory study. *Child Psychiatry Hum Develop* 21:267–281.

Hillary BE, Schare ML (1993). Sexually and physically abused adolescents: An empirical search for PTSD. *J Clinical Psychol* 49:161–165.

Hurrelmann K, Engel U, Weidman JC (1992). Impacts of school pressure, conflict with parents, and career uncertainty on adolescent stress in the Federal Republic of Germany. *Int J Adolesc Youth* 4:33–50.

Kaminer H, Lavie P (1991). Sleep and dreaming in Holocaust survivors: Dramatic decrease in dream recall in well-adjusted survivors. *J Nerv Ment Dis* 179:664–669.

Kirmil-Gray K, Eagleston JR, Gibson E, Thoresen CE (1984). Sleep disturbances in adolescents: Sleep quality, sleep habits, beliefs about sleep, and daytime functioning. *J Youth Adolesc* 13:375–384.

Lavie P, Amit Y, Epstein R, Tzischinsky O (1993). Children's sleep under the threat of attack by ballistic missiles. *Journal Sleep Research* 2:34–37.

Lavie P, Carmeli A, Merorach L, Liberman N (1991). To sleep under the threat of the Scud: Characteristics of war-related insomnia. *Israel Journal Medical Science* 27:681–686.

Lewinsohn PM, Gotlib IH, Seeley JR (1995). Adolescent psychopathology: IV. Specificity of psychosocial risk factors for depression and substance abuse in older adolescents. *J Am Acad Child Adolesc Psychiatry* 34:1221–1229.

Meshot CM, Leitner LM (1993). Adolescent mourning and parental death. *Omega J Death Dying* 26:287–299.

Monroe LJ (1967). Psychological and physiological differences between good and poor sleepers. *J Abn Psychol* 72:255–264.

Moore MS (1989). Disturbed attachment in children: A function in sleep disturbance, altered dream production and immune dysfunction. Not safe to sleep: Chronic sleep disturbances in anxious attachment. *J Child Psychotherapy* 15: 99–111.

Morrison DN, McGee R, Stanton WR (1992). Sleep problems in adolescence. *J Am Acad Child Adolesc Psychiatry* 31:94–99.

Offer D, Kimberly A, Schonert-Reichl (1992). Debunking the myths of adolescence: Findings from recent research. *J Am Acad Child Adolesc Psychiatry* 31:1003–1014.

Price VA, Coates TJ, Thoresen CE, Grinstead OA (1978). Prevalence and correlates of poor sleep among adolescents. *American Journal of Diseases of Children* 132:583–586.

Pynoos RS, Frederick C, Nader K, Arroyo W, Steinberg A, Eth S, Nunez F, Fairbanks L (1987). Life threat and posttraumatic stress in school-age children. *Archives General Psychiatry* 44:1057–1063.

Raviv A, Klingman A (1983). Children under stress. In S. Breznitz, ed., *Stress in Israel*, pp. 138–162. New York: Van Nostrand Reinhold.

Rimsza ME, Berg RA, Locke C (1988). Sexual abuse: Somatic and emotional reactions. *Child Abuse Negl* 12:201–208.

Rofe Y, Lewin I (1982). The effect of war environment on dreams and sleep habits. In C. D. Spielberger, I. G. Sarason, & N. A. Milgram, eds., *Stress and Anxiety* 8:59–75. Washington, DC: Hemisphere.

Ross RJ, Ball WA, Sullivan KA, Caroff SN (1989). Sleep disturbances as the hallmark of Posttraumatic Stress Disorder. *Am J Psychiatry* 146:697–707.

Sadeh A (1996). Stress, trauma and sleep in children. R. E. Dahl, ed. *Child Adolesc Psychiatric Clinics N Am* 5:685–700.

Sadeh A, Hayden RM, McGuire J, Sachs H, Civita R (1994). Somatic, cognitive and emotional characteristics of abused children hospitalized in a psychiatric hospital. *Child Psychiatry Human Development* 24:191–200.

Sadeh A, McGuire JPD, Sachs H, et al. (1995). Sleep and psychological characteristics of children on a psychiatric inpatient unit. *J Am Acad Child Adolesc Psychiatry* 34:813–819.

Savin-Williams RC, Berndt TJ (1992). Friendship and peer relations. In S. S. Feldman & G. R. Elliott, eds., *At the Threshold: The Developing Adolescent*, pp. 277–307. Cambridge, MA: Harvard University Press.

Selye H (1956). *The Stress of Life.* New York: McGraw-Hill.

Shannon MP, Lonigan CJ, Finch AJ, Taylor CM (1994). Children exposed to disaster: I. Epidemiology of post-traumatic symptoms and symptoms profiles. *J Am Acad Child Adolesc Psychiatry* 33:80–93.

Terr LC (1991). Childhood traumas: An outline and overview. *Am J Psychiatry* 148:10–12.

Williamson DE, Dahl RE, Birmaher B, Goetz RR, Nelson B, Ryan ND (1995). Stressful life events and EEG sleep in depressed and normal control adolescents. *Biol Psychiatry* 37:859–865.

Zitzow D (1992). Assessing student stress: School adjustment rating by self-report. *School Counselor* 40:20–23.

15. The Search for Vulnerability Signatures for Depression in High-Risk Adolescents: Mechanisms and Significance

JAMES T. McCRACKEN

The association of a constellation of sleep disturbances in adults with major depressive episodes is perhaps the most robust and widely replicated abnormality in psychobiological studies of psychiatric disorders. Reduced sleep efficiency, deficits of slow wave sleep (SWS), reduced latency to the first rapid eye movement (REM) period, an increase of REM sleep time, and increased density of rapid eye movements (REMD) during REM sleep are strongly associated with depressive illness in most samples (Benca, Obermeyer, Thisted, & Gillin, 1992). Studies of children, adolescents, and young adults with major depressive episodes find similar sleep disruptions, although only partially expressed relative to findings in adults. As Table 15.1 summarizes, certain studies of adolescents with major depression have reported increased REM density, reduced sleep latency, increased time to sleep onset, and increased arousals, whereas others have found mixed results or no differences with nondepressed controls. Even in adults, the specificity of the association of disturbed sleep parameters with the state of depression has been questioned (Benca, Obermeyer, Thisted, & Gillin, 1992). In general, however, the changes in sleep macroarchitecture have been strongly connected to core features of depressive illness and likely parallel aspects of the underlying pathophysiology of severe depression.

More controversial have been claims that certain components of the depression-related sleep disturbances may point toward trait characteristics relating to vulnerability for depression in individuals. The impetus for finding such markers is driven by data indicating that the greatest number of new onsets of major depression occur during the second decade of life (Weissman et al., 1988) and that the experience of depression in adolescence is associated with a variety of adverse outcomes, including depression recurrence, school underachievement, substance

Table 15.1. Sleep Findings from Studies of Depressed Adolescents

	Increased or Reduced	No Difference
Sleep latency[a]	Lahmeyer et al., 1983	Appelboom-Fondu et al., 1988
	Dahl et al., 1990	Kutcher et al., 1992
	Goetz et al., 1987	McCracken et al., 1997
	Emslie et al., 1994	
REM latency[b]	Gillin et al., 1981	Cashman et al., 1986
	Lahmeyer et al., 1983	Goetz et al., 1987
	Kutcher et al., 1992	Dahl et al., 1990
	Emslie et al., 1994	McCracken et al., 1997
	Dahl et al., 1996	
REM density[a]	Lahmeyer et al., 1983	Dahl et al., 1990
	Cashman et al., 1986	Kutcher et al., 1992
	Emslie et al., 1994	
	Goetz et al., 1996	
	McCracken et al., 1997	

[a] Increased in depressives.
[b] Reduced in depressives.

abuse, other psychopathology, and even suicide (Rohde, Lewinsohn, & Seeley, 1994). These issues raise the interest in identifying clinically relevant markers of vulnerability for depression that could be applied to groups of adolescents *prior* to the development of depressive illness. Furthermore, the precise mechanisms leading to the development of major depression are also unknown. Therefore, studies of putative physiologic changes that may themselves create risk for future psychopathology would be of importance for possible approaches for prevention, as well as to expand our understanding of the causes of the illness across the life-span.

The purpose of this chapter is to explore data from adults and adolescents examining whether early vulnerability markers for depressive illness are found in studies of sleep in young people and to articulate the hypothesis that subtle disruptions of sleep may themselves represent a risk for depressive illness if experienced over time and during a critical period of physiologic and emotional development.

Sleep Changes and Depression

Although the majority of sleep studies of depression have emphasized associations during the acute phase of depressive illness (Reynolds & Kupfer, 1987; Benca et al., 1992), other studies of adult depressives studied after remission from depressive illness suggest that at least some aspects of disrupted sleep may not normalize with improvement of depressive symptoms (Hauri, Chernik, Hawkins, & Mendels, 1974; Giles, Jarrett, Roffwarg, & Rush, 1987; Rush, Giles, Jarrett, & Feldman-Koffler, 1989; Thase et al., 1994). Frank, Kupfer, Hamer, Grochocinski, and McEachran (1992) studied 19 patients during an episode of major depression and again following recovery after treatment with interpersonal psychotherapy. Comparison of sleep measures at recovery of depressive symptoms to baseline values found relative stability from the disease state to remission as shown by strong correlations for SWS, REM density, and automated analysis of delta electroencephalographic (EEG) counts and REM activity. The study of Thase and colleagues (1994) of adults with major depression undergoing treatment with cognitive behavioral therapy suggested a disassociation of state-related sleep variables from measures that appear more persistent, possibly representing trait measures of vulnerability to depression (Thase et al., 1994). In particular, these investigators suggested that the stability of reduced SWS and reduced REM latency are candidates for vulnerability markers or possible scars of earlier depressive episodes, as opposed to more reversible disturbances such as increased REM density. Conversely, other reports find near normalization of all sleep parameters with remission of depression (Berger, Reimann, Hochli, & Speigel, 1989).

Another approach to this issue has been to test predictors of depression recurrence from sleep EEG measures. Giles et al. (1987) observed that increased risk for depressive recurrence on follow-up was associated with persistence of reduced REM latency. Similarly, an automated measure of delta sleep power from the first non-REM sleep period showed that lower delta sleep ratios were associated with earlier return of depression (Kupfer, Frank, McEachran, & Grochocinski, 1990).

Few studies have attempted to identify possible sleep trait markers in samples of children or adolescents with depressive illness. An earlier study by Puig-Antich, Goetz, Hanlon, Tabrizi, Davies, & Weitzman (1983) found few differences between a sample of prepubertal children with current major depressive episodes versus controls; however, restudy of sleep profiles following remission in a drug-free sample found for the first time an apparent reduction in REM period latency in the remitted group. A similar pilot study of adolescents with major depression studied during the acute depressive episode and repeated following remission showed greater stability for sleep measures, particularly REM sleep variables. By contrast, measures of the activity of the hypothalamic pituitary adrenal axis (HPA axis) were less stable. For example, reduction in nocturnal urinary-free cortisol secretion was observed in patients during remission versus when actively ill (Rao, McCracken, Lutchmansingh, Edwards, & Poland, 1997).

Although the literature is not always consistent as to which specific sleep variables are most strongly linked with recurrence or which are more stubborn in normalizing with recovery, most important to this chapter is the recognition that not all sleep differences associated with the acute episode of depressive illness resolve completely with the normalization of clinical state. Furthermore, the disassociation of sleep differences from the acute episode of depression has been observed in child, adolescent, and adult samples. Admittedly, these persistent sleep differences observed in remitted patients may be explained as trait markers that possibly existed prior to the episode or as biological "scars" from the acute illness. Regardless, these data suggest that a feature of risk for depression may involve persistent difficulties in the homeostatic regulation of sleep-wake processes.

An additional approach to link sleep parameters to depressive illness is to examine whether baseline sleep measures during acute illness are predictive of response to treatment interventions. Several reports have found that reduced REM latency predicted response to tricyclic antidepressants in adults with major depression (Rush et al., 1989). Similarly, increased sleep latency was also found to be predictive of differential treatment response in another sample (Frank et al., 1990). In a sample of children and adolescents with major depression, 10 of 12 subjects with shortest night REM latency values less than 70 minutes responded to treatment with fluoxetine versus 5 of 17 subjects with similarly short REM latency improving with placebo administration (Emslie & Kowatch, 1996). Taken together, these data finding relationships between baseline sleep differences and treatment outcomes, as with the data revealing associations between sleep parameters after recovery with course of illness, suggest that these observed sleep differences are not simply epiphenomena of mood disorders. More likely, they reflect a biological vulnerability directly associated with etiologic pathways leading to the development and expression of depressive illness.

Familiality of Sleep Measures

Within samples of children, adolescents, and adults with depressive illness, the degree of expression of depression-related sleep abnormalities varies widely, although the source of this variability is unknown. Similarly, the course of depressive illness varies from complete remission to frequent recurrence to chronicity. The variability across individuals in the expression of EEG differences associated with depression has been suggested to relate to a variety of variables, including type of illness, severity, number of episodes, presence or absence of stressors, and possible family-genetic factors. Indeed, a significant literature supports the heritability of subjective reports of sleep, as well as some parameters of EEG recorded sleep (Giles, Roffwarg, Dahl, & Kupfer, 1992). Given the role of genetics in the transmission of depressive illness, the possibility exists that sleep measures could have some utility in identifying individual genetic susceptibility to mood disorders.

Studies examining the heritability of sleep include reports of greater concordance in monozygotic twins over dizygotic twins for measures of sleep architecture, continuity, body movements, and some parameters of REM sleep (Webb & Campbell, 1983; Hori, 1986; Linkowski, Kerkhofs, Hauspie, & Mendlewicz, 1991). A few studies have explored parent-child correlations for EEG verified sleep measures. One small study in depressed children noted significant correlations for a wide variety of EEG sleep measures, including number of arousals ($r = .82$), percentage of stage 1 ($r = .56$), stage 2 ($r = .55$), and slow-wave sleep ($r = .66$); strength of parent-child correlations increased when only parents with reduced REM latency and their offspring were included in the analyses (Giles et al., 1992). Interestingly, this report found nonsignificant correlations for REM measures of latency, density, and REM sleep percentage, even after the effect of age was removed.

Within families identified through probands with a history of adult major depression, important patterns of concordance between sleep measures and the history of depressive illness in relatives have been found. One major study examined family members identified through probands with histories of unipolar depression versus normal controls (Giles, Biggs, Rush, & Roffwarg, 1988). Family members of probands with unipolar depression and shortened REM latency showed striking increases in lifetime risk for depression. In addition, short REM latency appeared to "breed true" and was highly associated with the increased risk of major depression among first-degree relatives of depressed probands with short REM latency. Although these findings have yet to be replicated, alongside other research on the heritability of sleep, these data strongly suggest that certain sleep variables may represent genetically transmitted features that carry with them the heightened risk for depressive illness and that such a marker might be identifiable even prior to the development of a mood disorder. The number of individuals in these family studies tested prior to the development of illness has been small, however, limiting any conclusions on the predictive power of any sleep marker within individuals. These data also raise other interesting questions. For example, do subtle changes in aspects of sleep themselves play a role in heightening risk for mood disorder? Although possibly mediated by genetic influences, could the sleep differences associated within families be influenced by other latent epigenetic variables?

Sleep Disturbance and Subsequent Depression: Epidemiologic Clues

Apart from the smaller, intensively studied samples of mood disorder patients and their relatives and controls suggesting an association between sleep disruption and depression, other data consistently document that reports of poor sleep may precede – in some cases by many months or years – the later development of depression in young adults. Among patients with prior histories of mood disorder, the complaint of sleep disturbance following remission with successful treatment has been shown to be predictive of depression recurrence (Perlis, Giles, Buysse, Tu, & Kupfer, 1997). More important, several large-scale reports of longitudinal community samples of young adults have revealed that the self-report of sleep disturbances was strongly associated with an increased relative risk for subsequent new onset of major depression during the follow-up (Ford & Kamerow, 1989; Breslau, Roth, Rosenthal, & Andreski, 1996; Chang, Ford, Mead, Cooper-Patrick, & Klag, 1997). The nature of sleep complaints included the self-report of difficulty with insomnia during stressful periods, report of chronic poor sleep quality, and sleep duration less than 7 hours per night. All were associated with varying degrees of increased incidence of subsequent depression; however, not all subjects who subsequently developed depression reported insomnia during the initial assessment period (Chang et al., 1997). The relationship between increased risk for new onset of major depression was maintained even after the history of other prior depressive symptoms – including psychomotor change and suicidal ideation – were controlled. Furthermore, the relationship showed a high degree of specificity for affective illness rather than associating with other forms of psychopathology. Such findings from epidemiologic studies do not provide possible explanations of mechanisms for the observed associations. One might speculate that the experience of chronic insomnia and sleep disruption itself represents one pathway or physiologic stressor that cumulatively may increase an individual's vulnerability to develop depressive illness. Such a conclusion would be consistent with the high rates of mood disorders well described among populations of patients with a variety of sleep disorders, including sleep apnea, narcolepsy, and delayed sleep phase syndromes. It is likely that only through investigations of subjects identified at high risk for depression can detailed information about mechanisms of this association be revealed.

Sleep Studies of High-Risk Samples

In spite of early studies suggesting the possibility of familial transmission of sleep markers associated with depression (Giles et al., 1987), surprisingly few studies have examined sleep markers in samples of adolescents or adults deemed to be at high risk for depressive illness. The few existing studies, though with somewhat disparate results, suggest that sleep EEG profiles of a variety of high-risk samples consistently deviate from the sleep of comparison subjects. In the family sleep study of Giles et al. (1988), those adult relatives of probands with unipolar depression who themselves were identified as having short REM latency were compared by virtue of their personal histories of the presence or absence of major depression. Twenty-eight relatives with short REM latency were identified who themselves had no prior history of depression and were compared to 27 relatives with short REM latency and identified histories of depression. The affected and unaffected subgroups were then compared on a variety of sleep measures. Examination of sleep continuity measures, sleep stage percentage, and slow-wave sleep showed no differences across the groups. Only REM minutes and non-REM time distinguished affected from unaffected related relatives, with unaffected short REM latency relatives demonstrating more REM minutes and reduced non-REM sleep. REM latency values were nearly indistinguishable (52 vs. 50 minutes). The investigators argue that these apparent similarities of sleep profiles between those relatives unaffected versus affected suggest that the observed constellation of sleep changes exist prior to the initial unfolding of depressive illness, consistent with these measures reflecting a vulnerability marker for future depression.

Another report focused on a group well known for their risk for depressive disorder by virtue of the presence of borderline personality disorder. Sleep profile variables of 10 subjects with the diagnosis of borderline personality disorder without histories of prior mood disorder were compared with those of a group of matched normal controls. A variety of sleep differences were noted, including increased sleep latency, increased wakefulness, increased awakenings, reduced sleep efficiency, and reduced REM latency (Battaglia, Ferini-Strambi, Smirne, Bernardeschi, & Bellodi, 1993).

The largest study to date of adults at increased risk for mood disorder was published by Lauer, Schreiber, Holsboer, and Krieg (1995). This study included 54 adults with no lifetime or current diagnosis of psychiatric disorder who had at least one first-degree relative with a history of major depression or bipolar disorder and with at least one additional relative with major psychopathology. Individual sleep EEG profiles were compared to 20 unrelated controls without a personal or family history of psychiatric disorder and a small group of 18 inpatients with major depression. Results of sleep data showed prominent differences between controls and high-risk subjects, who differed by virtue of reduced overall SWS percentage, increased first REM period density, and reduced SWS percentage of the second sleep cycle. A discriminate function constructed from selected sleep variables correctly identified 100 percent of control subjects and 94 percent of depressed patients. Nineteen percent of high-risk patients shared the depression-related sleep pattern.

Other studies of adult samples identified at high risk for development of major depression have adopted pharmacologic probe paradigms as a means of better identifying vulnerability. Schreiber, Lauer, Krumrey, Holsboer, and Krieg (1992) explored effects of the cholinergic agonist RS 86 on EEG sleep in 21 high-risk probands and 17 healthy control subjects. In susceptible individuals, sleep variables change in response to such stimulation of the cholinergic system. The study hypothesis was that high-risk individuals would demonstrate increased cholinergic sensitivity as measured by advancement of REM latency, as has been documented in a variety of acutely depressed and remitted adult and child depressives (Sitaram & Gillin, 1980; Gillin et al., 1991). Following RS 86 administration, robust differences were observed between high-risk patients and controls on variables of REM latency, SWS, REM sleep percentage, and SWS latency, consistent with greater cholinergic sensitivity in the high-risk subjects. Sitaram, Dube, Keshavan, Davies, and Reynal (1987) reported a similar association of greater sensitivity to cholinergic agonist administration using arecoline within families identified through probands with depressive illness. In summary, existing studies of baseline sleep of high-risk adults and observations of the effects of cholinergic agonist administration on sleep in high-risk subjects identify a variety of sleep differences between high-risk subjects and controls. These differences do not cluster around a single variable or process; indeed, depending upon the sample and paradigm applied, differences involve measures of sleep continuity and SWS, as well as REM sleep. Some differences in high-risk samples may be due to differences in the sensitivity of cholinergically mediated arousal and REM regulatory systems, as seen in the increased responsiveness to cholinergic muscarinic agonism in these studies.

Few data have been reported on sleep profiles obtained from high-risk samples of children or adolescents. One preliminary note reported no differences in sleep measures between normal controls and prepubertal children at high risk for major depression by virtue of parental histories of depressive illness (Dahl et al., 1994). Coble, Scher, Reynolds, Day, and Kupfer (1988) reported differences in measures of quiet versus active sleep between neonates of mothers with or without histories of depression.

Pharmacologic Probe in High-Risk Adolescents

We have performed a pilot study comparing sleep profiles in high-risk adolescents and normal control adolescents screened for personal and family histories of affective illness. EEG sleep recordings were obtained on baseline (placebo) nights and nights immediately following the administration of scopolamine, a muscarinic cholinergic antagonist. We based the assessment of elevated risk for depression in this sample from studies documenting two- to threefold increased rates of depression in offspring of major depressives (Weissman, Fendrich, Warner, & Wickramrante, 1992; Kovacs, Devlin, Pollock, Richards, & Mukerji, 1997). Based on our findings from studies of acutely depressed adolescents (McCracken, Poland, Lutchmansingh, & Edwards, 1997), we hypothesized that certain high-risk adolescents would share the partially expressed sleep abnormalities seen in some depressed adolescents. We further hypothesized that scopolamine administration would produce a differential pattern of REM sleep effects in high-risk adolescents versus controls. Such a pattern of differential cholinergic sensitivity among high-risk adolescents would be consistent with a vulnerability to depression associated in part with central nervous system cholinergic neurotransmission and shared across child, adolescent, and adult depressed

Table 15.2. Effects of Scopolamine on Selected Sleep Architecture and Continuity Variables in Normal Adolescents versus Adolescents at High Risk for Depression

	Controls (N = 13)		High Risk (N = 11)	
	Placebo Session	SCOP Session	Placebo Session	SCOP Session
Stage 4%	22.0 ± 1.6	22.3 ± 1.5	17.8 ± 2.3	19.1 ± 1.6
Sleep latency, min	19.1 ± 6.2	11.1 ± 1.7	17.4 ± 3.6	8.6 ± 1.5
Number of arousals	6.4 ± 2.4	12.9 ± 4.2	13.6 ± 2.8	10.6 ± 2.9
First REM episode density, units/min	.71 ± .08	.90 ± 1.7	1.45 ± .23	1.14 ± .09

and high-risk subjects (Sitaram et al., 1987; Schreiber et al., 1992; Dahl et al., 1994).

Our high-risk and control subjects were between the ages of 12 and 18 years (mean ages 15.5 vs. 15.6 years; high risk vs. control, respectively). Although non-mood-disorder psychopathology was not an exclusion criteria, few positive histories of psychopathology were noted among high-risk adolescents; one high-risk subject had a history of separation anxiety disorder, and another high-risk subject had a specific developmental disorder. High-risk and control groups were comparable in gender and ethnicity. Data were analyzed by group and by treatment effect for placebo and scopolamine nights. Selected sleep variables are presented in Table 15.2.

Significant group effects were found for first REM period activity and density; both were greater in the high-risk subjects on the placebo night. Total night REM density and activity were also greater in the high-risk sample. In addition, a strong trend for reduced total delta minutes was observed in the high-risk group for pooled means ($p < 0.07$). While scopolamine showed expected robust effects on a variety of REM sleep measures in both groups, several interesting differential effects of scopolamine were observed between the high-risk and control samples. Repeated-measures analyses showed that arousals during sleep were more frequent on the placebo night in the high-risk group ($p < .004$) and that sleep latency on the scopolamine night was shorter in the high-risk group. A further exploratory analysis applied a procedure suggested by the study of Lauer and colleagues (1995) who attempted to identify at-risk subgroups showing greatest separation from control values. Using two standard deviations from the mean of the controls as a threshold, we identified 36% of high-risk subjects showing extreme values for first REM period density and 27% of high-risk subjects showing extreme values for arousals.

Although preliminary, our small but well-characterized sample of high-risk children and adolescents showed robust differences in several sleep variables, as well as in cholinergic sensitivity. In every instance, the significant differences were in agreement with the well-established adult pattern of depression-related sleep changes (Lauer, Schreiber, Holsboer, & Krieg, 1991; Benca et al., 1992), as well as our previous observations of sleep abnormalities in acutely depressed adolescents (McCracken et al., 1997). Specifically, we have observed increased REM density and activity measures in our high-risk adolescent sample, as well as an increased sensitivity to the REM suppressing effects of scopolamine. In addition, an unexpected and interesting finding from this high-risk sample was the prominent increase in arousals. This strong group difference also correlated highly with sleep efficiency for the total sample. This preliminary investigation suggests that within samples of adolescents at high risk for major depressive disorder, prominent sleep differences may indeed exist prior to the development of illness. These findings are novel, at least in this age group, and argue for efforts to replicate and extend these observations.

Are Subtle Sleep Disruptions Pathways to Depression?

Much effort has gone into attempts to explain the mechanisms underlying observed sleep disruptions most notable in studies of adults with major depressive illness. The emphasis on disruption in the regulation of REM latency has led to proposals for two types or two different pathways for the production of reduced REM latency that differ in etiology. As described by Kupfer and Ehlers (1989), a proposed type 1 pathway might involve a stable traitlike deficit of reduced slow-wave sleep releasing REM sleep and allowing shortened REM latency to occur. A type 1 mechanism would be predicted not to vary with recovery from a depressive episode and to be associated with greater family-genetic aggregation of illness. The type 2 reduced REM latency pathway is considered to be more state-dependent. The description of this pathway invokes the possible role of psychosocial stress, activations of the HPA axis, and the production of reduced sleep efficacy and increased phasic REM activity. Although some studies have suggested that depression-related sleep changes can be disassociated with recovery, the construct of two pathways to depression-related sleep disturbances remains largely untested. These models have merit in suggesting that there may be multiple etiologies for the wide variations in sleep profiles observed to accompany depression. Rather than emphasizing the precise mechanism of genesis of change within individual sleep variables, however, we believe that the epidemiologic data and sleep data from high-risk samples suggest an equally important hypothesis of the relation between sleep and depression.

We suggest that for some individuals, one pathway of risk consists of a chronic, possibly inherited, sleep pattern consisting of subtle disruptions of sleep. Such a pattern of subtle but discernible sleep changes in REM regulation and sleep continuity variables may represent a type of loss of homeostatic capacity, itself a physiologic vulnerability to the development of mood disorder. Such a physiologic vulnerability of sleep homeostasis would likely require the interaction with other stressors and risk factors in order to produce the disorder, consistent with contemporary multivariate etiologic models of depression (see Goodman & Gotlib, 1999). Although the exact mechanism underlying such a physiologic risk factor is still obscure, it may relate to alterations in central nervous system cholinergic neurotransmission.

If such a physiologic risk factor involving sleep does indeed exist, it could point directly to possible strategies for prevention of depression that focus on amelioration of sleep changes. Additional studies of sleep variables as well as other physiologic variables are needed in samples of children at high risk for depression in order to clarify these suggested risk factors.

REFERENCES

Appelboom-Fondu J, Kerkhofs M, Mendlewicz J (1988). Depression in adolescents and young adults – polysomnographic and neuroendocrine aspects. *Journal of Affective Disorders* 14:35–40.

Battaglia M, Ferini-Strambi L, Smirne S, Bernardeschi L, Bellodi L (1993). Ambulatory polysomnography of never-depressed borderline subjects: A high-risk approach to rapid eye movement latency. *Biological Psychiatry* 33: 326–334.

Benca RM, Obermeyer WH, Thisted RA, Gillin JC (1992). Sleep and psychiatric disorders: A meta-analysis. *Archives of General Psychiatry* 49:651–668.

Berger M, Reimann D, Hochli D, Speigel R (1989). The cholinergic rapid eye movement sleep induction test with RS-86. State or trait marker of depression? *Archives of General Psychiatry* 46:421–428.

Breslau N, Roth T, Rosenthal L, Andreski P (1996). Sleep disturbance and psychiatric disorders: A longitudinal epidemiological study of young adults. *Biological Psychiatry* 39:411–418.

266   JAMES T. McCRACKEN

Cashman MA, Coble P, McCann BS, Taska L, Reynolds CF, Kupfer DJ (1986). Sleep markers for major depressive disorder in adolescent patients. *Sleep Research* 13:91.

Chang PP, Ford DE, Mead LA, Cooper-Patrick L, Klag MJ (1997). Insomnia in young men and subsequent depression. Johns Hopkins Precursor Study. *American Journal of Epidemiology,* 146:105–114.

Coble PA, Foster FG, Kupfer DJ (1976). Electroencephalographic sleep diagnosis of primary depression. *Archives of General Psychiatry* 33:1124–1127.

Coble PA, Scher MS, Reynolds CF, Day NL, Kupfer DJ (1988). Preliminary findings on the neonatal sleep of offspring of women with and without a prior history of affective disorder. *Sleep Research* 16:120.

Dahl RE, Puig-Antich J, Ryan, ND, Nelson B, Dachille S, Cunningham SL, Trubnik L, Klepper TP (1990). EEG sleep in adolescents with major depression: The role of suicidality and inpatient status. *Journal of Affective Disorders* 19:63–75.

Dahl RE, Ryan ND, Matty MK, Birmaher B, al-Shabbout M, Williamson DE, Kupfer DJ (1996). Sleep onset abnormalities in depressed adolescents. *Biological Psychiatry* 39:400–410.

Dahl RE, Ryan ND, Perel J, Birmaher B, al-Shabbout M, Nelson B, Puig-Antich J (1994). Cholinergic REM induction test with arecoline in depressed children. *Psychiatry Research* 51:269–282.

Emslie GJ, Kowatch R (1996). Predictors of remission and recurrence in depressed children and adolescents. S-3b, *Scientific Proceedings of the 43rd Annual Meeting of the American Academy of Child and Adolescent Psychiatry,* p. 38. Philadelphia, October.

Emslie GJ, Rush AJ, Weinberg WA, Rintelmann J, Roffwarg HP (1994). Sleep EEG features of adolescents with major depression. *Biological Psychiatry* 36:573–581.

Ford DE, Kamerow DB (1989). Epidemiologic study of sleep disturbances and psychiatric disorders. An opportunity for prevention? *Journal of the American Medical Association,* 262:1479–1484.

Frank E, Kupfer DJ, Hamer T, Grochocinski VJ, McEachron AB (1992). Maintenance treatment and psychobiologic correlates of endogenous subtypes. *Journal of Affective Disorders* 25:181–189.

Frank E, Kupfer DJ, Perel JM, Cornes C, Jarrett DB, Mallinger AG, Thase ME, McEachron AB, Grochocinski VJ (1990). Three-year outcomes for maintenance therapies in recurrent depression. *Archives of General Psychiatry* 47:1093–1099.

Giles DE, Biggs MM, Rush AJ, Roffwarg HP (1988). Risk factors in families of unipolar depression, I: Psychiatric illness and reduced REM latency. *Journal of Affective Disorders* 14:51–59.

Giles DE, Jarrett RB, Roffwarg HP, Rush AJ (1987). Reduced REM latency: A predictor of recurrence in depression. *Neuropsychopharmacology* 1:33–39.

Giles DE, Roffwarg HP, Dahl RE, Kupfer DJ (1992). Electroencephalographic sleep abnormalities in depressed children: A hypothesis. *Psychiatry Research* 41:53–63.

Gillin JC, Duncan WC, Murphy DL, Post RM, Wehr TA, Goodwin FK, Wyatt RJ, Bunney WE (1981). Age-related changes in depressed and normal subjects. *Psychiatry Research* 4:73–78.

Gillin JC, Sutton L, Ruiz C, Darko D, Golshan S, Risch SC, Janowsky D (1991). The effects of scopolamine on sleep and mood in depressed patients with a history of alcoholism and a normal comparison group. *Biological Psychiatry* 30:157–169.

Goetz R, Puig-Antich J, Ryan N, Rabinovich H, Ambrosini PJ, Nelson B, Krawiec V (1987). Electroencephalographic sleep of adolescents with major depression and normal controls. *Archives of General Psychiatry* 44:61–68.

Goetz RR, Wolk SI, Coplan JD, Weissman MM, Dahl RE, Ryan ND (1996). Rapid eye movement density among adolescents with major depressive disorder revisited. *Archives of General Psychiatry* 53:1066–1067.

Goodman SH, Gotlib IH (1999). Risk for psychopathology in the children of depressed mothers: A developmental model for understanding mechanisms of transmission. *Psychol Rev* 106(3):458–90.

Hauri P, Chernik D, Hawkins D, Mendels J (1974). Sleep of depressed patients in remission. *Archives of General Psychiatry* 31:386–391.

Hori A (1986). Sleep characteristics in twins. *Japanese Journal of Psychiatry* 40: 35–46.

Kovacs M, Devlin B, Pollock M, Richards C, Mukerji P (1997). A controlled family history study of childhood major depressive disorder. *Archives of General Psychiatry* 54:613–623.

Kupfer DJ, Ehlers CL (1989). Two roads to rapid eye movement latency. *Archives of General Psychiatry* 48:279–280.

Kupfer DJ, Frank E, McEachran C, Grochocinski V (1990). Delta sleep ratio: A biological correlate of early recurrence in unipolar affective disorder. *Archives of General Psychiatry* 47:1100–1105.

Kutcher S, Williamson P, Marton P, Szalai J (1992). REM latency in endogenously depressed adolescents. *British Journal of Psychiatry* 161:399–402.

Lahmeyer HW, Poznanski EO, Bellur SN (1983). EEG sleep in depressed adolescents. *American Journal of Psychiatry* 140:1150–1153.

Lauer CJ, Riemann D, Wiegand M, Berger M (1991). From early to late adulthood: Changes in EEG sleep of depressed patients and healthy volunteers. *Biological Psychiatry* 29:979–993.

Lauer CJ, Schreiber W, Holsboer F, Krieg J-C (1995). In quest of identifying vulnerability markers for psychiatric disorders by all-night polysomnography. *Archives of General Psychiatry* 52:145–153.

Linkowski P, Kerkhofs M, Hauspie R, Mendlewicz J (1991). Genetic determinants of EEG sleep: A study of twins living apart. *Journal of Electroencephalography and Clinical Neurophysiology* 79:114–118.

McCracken JT, Poland RE, Lutchmansingh P, Edwards C (1997). Sleep EEG abnormalities in depressed adolescents: Effects of scopolamine. *Biological Psychiatry* 42:577–584.

Perlis ML, Giles DE, Buysse DJ, Tu X, Kupfer DJ (1997). Self-reported sleep disturbance as a prodromal symptom in recurrent depression. *Journal of Affective Disorders* 42:209–212.

Puig-Antich J, Goetz R, Hanlon C, Davies M, Thompson J, Chambers WJ, Tabrizi MA, Weitzman ED (1982). Sleep architecture and REM sleep measures in prepubertal children with major depression. *Archives of General Psychiatry* 39:932–939.

Puig-Antich J, Goetz R, Hanlon C, Tabrizi MA, Davies M, Weitzman ED (1983). Sleep architecture and REM sleep measures in prepubertal major depressives: Studies during recovery from the depressive episode in a drug-free state. *Archives of General Psychiatry* 40:187–192.

Rao U, McCracken JT, Lutchmansingh P, Edwards C, Poland RE (1997). Electroencephalographic sleep and urinary free cortisol in adolescent depression: A preliminary report of changes from episode to recovery. *Biological Psychiatry* 41:369–373.

Reynolds CF, Kupfer DJ (1987). Sleep research in affective illness: State of the art circa 1987. *Sleep* 10:199–215.

Rohde P, Lewinsohn PM, Seeley JR (1994). Are adolescents changed by an episode of major depression? *Journal of the American Academy of Child and Adolescent Psychiatry* 33:1289–1298.

Rush AJR, Giles DE, Jarrett RB, Feldman-Koffler F, Debus JR, Weissenburger J, Orsulak PJ, Roffwarg HP (1989). Reduced REM latency predicts response to tricyclic medication in depressed outpatients. *Biological Psychiatry* 26:61–72.

Schreiber W, Lauer CJ, Krumrey K, Holsboer F, Krieg J-C (1992). Cholinergic REM sleep induction test in subjects at high risk for psychiatric disorders. *Biological Psychiatry* 32:79–90.

Sitaram N, Dube S, Keshavan M, Davies A, Reynal P (1987). The association of supersensitive cholinergic REM-induction and affective illness within pedigrees. *Journal of Psychiatric Research* 21:487–497.

Sitaram N, Gillin JC (1980). Development and use of pharmacological probes of the CNS in man: Evidence of cholinergic abnormality in primary affective illness. *Biological Psychiatry* 15:925–932.

Thase ME, Reynolds CF, Frank E, Jennings JR, Nofzinger E, Fasiczka AL, Garamoni G, Kupfer DJ (1994). Polysomnographic studies of unmedicated depressed men before and after cognitive behavioral therapy. *American Journal of Psychiatry* 151:1615–1622.

Webb WB, Campbell SS (1983). Relationships in sleep characteristics of identical and fraternal twins. *Archives of General Psychiatry* 40:1093–1095.

Weissman MM, Fendrich M, Warner V, Wickramrante P (1992). Incidence of psychiatric disorder in offspring at high and low risk for depression. *Journal of the American Academy of Child and Adolescent Psychiatry* 31:640–648.

Weissman MM, Leaf PJ, Tischler GL, Blazer DG, Karno M, Bruce ML, Florio LP (1988). Affective disorders in five United States communities. *Psychological Medicine* 18:141–153.

16. The Regulation of Sleep-Arousal, Affect, and Attention in Adolescence: Some Questions and Speculations

RONALD E. DAHL

Pubertal maturation includes an enormous array of changes in social and biological domains. Among these changes are developmental shifts in the control of sleep, arousal, affect, and attention – including both physiologic and behavioral changes. One major theme running through these various developmental changes is the relatively increased influence of executive functions (the use of higher cognitive processes involving regions of prefrontal cortex to guide behaviors according to social rules and long-term goals). The integration of higher cognitive processes with emotional regulation (e.g., learning to inhibit or modulate arousal, attention, and behavior to serve higher cognitive goals) creates the basis for *social competence* – perhaps the most important outcome variable in adolescent development. However, increased cognitive abilities to override lower levels of regulation also confer a greater capacity for cognitive ideas or attitudes to cause *dysregulation* at subcortical levels. In a number of ways, adolescence thus appears to represent a vulnerable period regarding the maturational integration of cognitive and emotional processes. It also appears that this highest level of cognitive-emotional integration is most sensitive to the effects of sleep deprivation or inadequate sleep. Within this general frame a few specific questions are considered, which may be addressed by current or future lines of investigation: (1) What are the neurobiologic underpinnings of these maturational changes (and the likely involvement of alterations in prefrontal cortex [PFC] and limbic circuitry)? (2) Why do some adolescents appear to be particularly vulnerable in these domains (and why may vulnerability in affect regulation confer vulnerability toward sleep deprivation effects)? (3) What is the potential to prevent some types of dysfunction through early cognitive-behavioral or educational interventions in vulnerable adolescents?

Preface (Or, Why This Chapter Digresses So Far from Sleep Patterns)

This chapter focuses on a model of affect regulation emphasizing the developing links between cognitive and emotional processes during adolescence. The relevance of this model to a book on adolescent sleep patterns may not, at first, be readily apparent. However, the model itself grew out of 10 years of investigating the links between sleep-arousal regulation and affective dysregulation (primarily through psychobiologic studies in child and adolescent depression). The bridge from sleep patterns to this cognitive-emotional model is built on two premises. (1) The aspects of affect regulation that require the integration of high cognitive and emotional processing are *particularly sensitive to inadequate or insufficient sleep*, and may represent one of the most significant consequences of poor sleep patterns. (2) These aspects of affect regulation are critically important in the development of social competence and represent a *highly vulnerable period in adolescent development*. Clinical studies designed to test hypotheses directly along these lines are in progress (and some preliminary data are presented here). However, most of this chapter attempts to step back and consider a broader overview of the cognitive-emotional development, and it does not return directly to the link to sleep-arousal regulation until the end. The model is in a preliminary form, makes numerous speculative jumps across domains, and is offered not as a source of explanations, but primarily as a means to generate further questions and discussion.

Defining Adolescence

Adolescence encompasses a complex array of changes that do not fit into any single category or domain of measures. A definition that captures the key aspects of this process relevant to this chapter is: Adolescence is that awkward period between sexual maturation and attaining adult status in society. This conceptualization helps to introduce five points about adolescence that fit a developmental model of cognitive-emotional integration.

1. Adolescence exists within the boundaries of two contrasting domains: it begins with physical changes (sexual maturation) but ends in the realm of social-cultural determinants. Further, there is evidence that the timing of physical maturity and the attainment of adult status in society have moved in opposite directions in recent history. The mean

age of menarche in the United States and Europe has decreased from 15.5 years in the late nineteenth century to 13 years at the current time (Petersen & Crockett, 1985; Rutter & Rutter, 1993). A recent longitudinal study found that 15% of middle-class American girls had reached menarche by 11.7 years of age (Ge, Conger, & Elder, 1996). Yet the average age of leaving school, marrying, beginning a career, and becoming a parent has increased over this same interval (Modell & Goodman, 1990). Historically, puberty coincided with taking on adult roles, whereas in contemporary society many sexually mature 12- to 13-year-olds will not assume adult responsibilities or status for another 10–15 years. Lengthy periods with sexually mature bodies (and sexually active brains) in the context of still-developing frontal lobe (executive) functions, as well as ill-defined social roles, create special challenges and vulnerabilities – particularly with respect to emotion and arousal regulation.

2. The *awkwardness* so strongly associated with adolescence is, in many ways, closely related to the incomplete emergence of *social competence* combined with the new drives, impulses, emotions, and physical changes occurring with puberty (as described in the third point). Social competence, here, is conceptualized as the integration of cognitive and emotional skills involved in the self-regulation of behavior according to learned rules, societal constraints, and the pursuit of long-term goals. There are three primary components to developing these abilities: (a) the cognitive skills needed to process complex abstract information (particularly with respect to learned social rules, holding long-term goals in working memory, imagining future likelihoods-consequences, making complex plans, strategizing, etc.); (b) the cognitive power to use these skills to guide behavior (learning to inhibit, modify, or delay behaviors linked to impulses, drives, or other subcortical influences, as well as initiating and persisting with sequences of behaviors to achieve goals); and (c) a fluency in using these abilities together in a variety of complex social situations. The integration of these higher cognitive skills with lower levels of influence (including drives and emotions) is associated with the maturation of regions of the prefrontal cortex (PFC), executive functions, and affect regulation. This chapter focuses on the close links between these developing regulatory systems and neurobehavioral systems underlying sleep-arousal regulation and attention.

3. Adolescents encounter a new set of challenges at puberty with the activation of subcortical circuits (and their cortical connections) involved in reproductive physiology and behavior. These changes

activate new drives, impulses, emotions, and arousal patterns at a point when most adolescents have a limited cognitive ability to exert control over behavior. These new emotions and drives control and possess a direct influence on cognitive processes (e.g., girls spending increasing amounts of time *thinking about* boys). The establishment of new connections between cognitive processes (executive functions), and these newly activated drives-emotions-arousals represent a potentially important period of neural plasticity relevant to affect regulation and social competence. That is, the particular experiences (and early habits) of the individual as these new patterns of interconnections are being established may have long-term influences across neurobehavioral systems involved in affect-arousal regulation, social competence, and adolescent vulnerabilities to some types of psychopathology.

4. The increase in cognitive abilities (and cognitive power over lower levels of influence) that emerges during adolescence also confers new vulnerabilities regarding the capacity to override lower-level control systems. For example, adolescents develop the ability to hold a goal in working memory with sufficient focus and motivation to go without eating or sleeping for long periods of time in pursuit of the goal. To extend this example, a goal to be extremely thin in pursuit of social status brings with it the vulnerability of severe self-deprecation of food or extreme levels of exercise to the detriment of health. While short-term periods of overriding drives and impulses may lead to some rewarding experiences, this pattern may lead to ignoring physiologic drives over sustained intervals, providing additional routes to developing pathology.

5. Individual differences (either genetic or acquired very early in the developmental process) in affect and arousal regulation may lead to additional vulnerability during adolescent development. Specifically, this chapter focuses on evidence for two factors that may influence the development of affect dysregulation in adolescence: (a) a low threshold to activate threat-related arousal; and (b) a negative affective bias in cognitive and attentional processing.

Cognitive-Emotional Interface from a Literary Perspective (Or, What Happens When Teenage Brains Fall in Love?)

Before proceeding with a more analytic and neurocircuitry-level approach to the early integration of these cognitive-emotional processes during adolescence, it may be helpful to consider a few literary

descriptions of adolescent cognitive-emotional turmoil as these neurobehavioral systems become activated during romantic experiences.

First, consider the most frequently retold description of adolescent
tempest: Shakespeare's *Romeo and Juliet*. From an objective perspective,
it is the story of two adolescents who, having exchanged less than 100
words, decide they are mortally in Love, and would give up not only
sleep and food but also sacrifice their lives, their families, and the world
rather than exist without each other. This play, in its variations over the
centuries, has struck a deep emotional chord for millions of people – to
a large extent because it captures something universal (albeit extreme)
about this set of experiences.

A less dramatic but poignant example is given by Gutterson in
Snow Falling on Cedars, describing an innocent but completely enamored
14-year-old boy: "He noticed her fingernails, the shape of her toes, the
hollow place at her throat. It made him unhappy when he thought about
her lately and he had passed a lot of time, all spring long, mulling how
to tell her about his unhappiness. He'd sat on top of the bluff at South
Beach thinking about it in the afternoons. He'd thought about it during
school. His thoughts yielded no clue how to talk to her . . . words evaded
him completely . . . he couldn't stand another moment without explaining his heart to her . . . he was in pain. . . . He could still feel this pain
20 years later."

A humorous, but equally touching, example is given by Ray Brad-
bury in *One Timeless Spring*, which describes the experience as a 12-
year-old boy struggling with the physical and emotional changes of
early puberty. The boy decides that his parents must be poisoning his
food, and he envisions an elaborate plot against him, which includes his
teachers. He fights the changes in every possible way, avoiding foods
prepared by others, even resorting to induced vomiting. Later, he dis-
covers Clarisse, a girl his age whom he has been (increasingly) notic-
ing – they begin walking together and he experiences the following
scene:

"Clarisse's hand bumped mine as we walked along the trail. I smelled
the moist dank smell of the ravine and the soft new smell of Clarisse
beside me. Very quietly, she put her arm around me. I was so surprised
and bewildered I almost cried out. Then, trembling, her lips kissed me,
and my own hands were moving to hold her and I was shaking and
shouting inside myself. The silence was like a green explosion. The water
bubbled in the creek bed. I couldn't breathe. I knew it was all over. I was
lost . . . forever, now, and I didn't care. But I *did* care, and I was laughing

and crying all in one, and there was nothing to do about it. . . . I could have gone on fighting my war with Mom and Dad, and school and food and things in books, but I couldn't fight this sweetness on my lips."

There are several points about the states described in these passages which are relevant to our later discussion about cognitive-emotional regulation in adolescents. These areas are being increasingly studied by social scientists, and are extremely complex issues in their own right; however, it may be useful to briefly sketch a few of these points here:

1. Early romantic experiences are emotionally powerful and can completely overwhelm most cognitive processes.
2. Many of the experiences are associated with high levels of arousal – even the slightest thought, memory, or association with the "object of desire" can send the heart racing and the brain bathing in new transmitters.
3. Early romantic experiences have profound effects on attentional processes. During these periods, the individual often cannot avoid thoughts directed toward the "coveted other." Even in the middle of competing activities, or any quiet moments, attention quickly returns to thoughts, images, memories, or fantasies, about the desired partner (and, given number 2, this results in frequent and long periods of elevated arousal). James Leckman at Yale University has interviewed students in the early stages of romantic involvement, finding that the obsessional nature of their thought processing was comparable with patients meeting criteria for obsessive-compulsive disorders – many were incapable of going an hour without thinking about their desired partner. Further, the degree of functional impairment (difficulties with concentration, changes in appetite, sleep, school-work difficulties) can frequently reach a clinical threshold in adolescents in the throngs of an initial romance.
4. Any sign of encouragement, reciprocation, or actual contact with the desired person creates an enormous surge of positive affect and *increased sense of self-worth*.
5. Any sign of rejection, lack of reciprocation, or actual separation-loss is strongly associated with enormous levels of negative affect and a *decreased sense of self-worth*.

Neural Plasticity and Sensitive Periods of Development

There has been increasing interest in the field of developmental neuroscience in the principle of critical or sensitive periods of development. There is well-documented evidence of early periods of sensitivity to experimental input in several neurobehavioral systems. The best-investigated example is in the development of binocular vision (Singer, 1986; Greenough, Black, & Wallace, 1987; Miller, Keller, & Styker, 1989). A short interval of time (corresponding to when cortical neurons are crossing over for the two eye fields) is critical for establishing the pattern of interconnection relevant to binocular vision. Well-controlled studies have shown that patching one eye for several days during the sensitive period can result in permanent changes in the visual cortex. Patching one eye for longer intervals prior to or following the sensitive period does not produce these deficits. In brief, what happens is that neurons that "should" become connected to inputs from the patched eye instead develop connections to inputs from the active eye. Later, instead of a *balance of inputs* from each eye, there is always greater influence from the unpatched eye, resulting in suboptimal binocular vision.

The general principle here may be critically important as it applies to other neurobehavioral systems: the particular experiences of the individual during a period when neural systems are first establishing interconnections set the foundation for some aspects of the pattern of later connections. A number of models in developmental neuroscience have focused on this principle. In the model of Greenough (Greenough & Black, 1992), this is called "experience-expectant" learning, meaning that brain processes involved in the overproduction and subsequent pruning of connections *expect* or anticipate certain types of experience during the critical period of development. As a result, the experiences during that period have large and long-standing influences on that particular neurobehavioral system, producing structural changes that may be difficult to alter with later experience.

Analogous findings are seen in some areas of language development. Although the sensitive period occurs over a broader interval of time, the ability to discriminate or produce certain types of sounds relevant to language production becomes fixed by early exposure to a particular language. The most frequently cited example is the finding that Japanese infants easily distinguish *R* versus *L* sounds, but this ability is lost in older children exposed only to the Japanese language (which does not use these distinctions). Similar findings have been shown in other languages. More importantly, the ability to speak fluently in a language has been shown to be extremely difficult in a language learned after puberty – pronunciation patterns and accent are nearly impossible to master after pubertal development.

A full discussion of the complex issues (and controversies) surrounding sensitive periods in development is beyond the scope of this chapter. However, the general principles may be critical to understanding a vulnerable period in cognitive-emotional development – how an individual develops higher cognitive control over affective responses relevant to social competence and social-emotional "fluency." The particular experiences (and affective and arousal state) when the first interconnections are being established between higher cognitive processes and affective regulation may "set" some aspects of the lasting patterns of connection between higher cognition and emotion. These patterns may be much more amenable to change early in development and quite difficult to change later in adulthood (analogous to language fluency). If indeed there is a sensitive period for developing social competence or emotional fluency analogous to visual or language development, this raises a set of important implications regarding early intervention, treatment approaches for some types of psychopathology, and a series of research questions about the specific mechanisms, neurobehavioral systems, and timing involved in the structuring of the systems during the critical period.

Studies from Early Child Development Relevant to the Cognitive-Emotional Interface (Or, How to Get Johnny to Put Away His Toys)

Before moving to more specific speculations about critical periods in the adolescent development of cognitive-emotional integration, it is worth reviewing some studies addressing the earlier developmental roots of cognitive-emotional regulation. Some key investigations in this area have been performed under the rubric of "the development of self-control" in preschool ages. The work of Kochanska and colleagues (Kochanska, DeVet, Goldman, Murray, & Putnam, 1994; Kochanska, Murray, Jacques, & Koening, 1996) shows a fascinating pattern of findings regarding the early development of self-regulatory capacities. This work examines two specific aspects of early self-regulation: (1) the ability to inhibit (by internal volition) a class of prohibited behaviors (e.g., not taking candy from an off-limits location), and (2) the ability to produce a class of requested behavior (e.g., cleaning up the toys after a play session). Investigations into the acquisition of these skills have emphasized the importance of an optimal link between the relevant cognitive processes and the appropriate emotional processes. That is, to reliably produce these behaviors (in the absence of direct supervision), it is necessary to link functionally the cognitive knowledge of the boundary of principle with sufficient affect to motivate remembering and producing the behavior without immediate threat of punishment or imminent reward. Even more important, the process of learning the skill requires experiences of emotional salience to be coupled with the cognitive experience (e.g., a parent's affectively laden response to the child producing the requested or prohibited behavior). The particular way in which parents impart the affective cues (facial expression, tone of voice, verbal threat, or actual punishment) exerts marked influences on the way the child learns the skill. Either too much affect or too little can interfere with skill acquisition. Too much affect apparently interferes with the cognitive aspects of learning while too little affect produces insufficient motivation to internalize the skill. Further, as Kochanska et al. (1996) demonstrated, the optimal level of affective arousal varies considerably across children – with fearful or highly reactive children learning best with relatively low levels of affective input. Clearly, the acquisition of self-regulation and self-control requires an optimal balance of cognitive *and* affective processes. The same issues are relevant to learning to produce prosocial or requested behaviors or a long sequence of steps toward a goal. The cognitive processes include understanding the goal or requested behavior, and linking this to the affective influence to provide sufficient motivation to produce the necessary behaviors (despite distraction or competing shorter-term goals).

The central point here, relevant to adolescent development, is that there is every reason to believe that more complex levels of self-regulation and self-control involve similar processes linking higher cognitive processes with affective states, rewards, and punishments. For example, learning behavioral control with respect to abstract rules or codes of moral behavior requires even higher levels of abstract thought to be linked to affective systems in the guidance of more complex behaviors. Similarly, the goals being held in working memory become more complex and require a greater sequence of behavioral steps, planning, and strategy to achieve the goal (e.g., graduating *cum laude* versus cleaning up the toys). The selection of optimal behaviors in these contexts requires inhibiting many options while augmenting a selected few in the appropriate sequence of what one is "supposed to do" (according to social context or to achieve a long-term goal), *and* this requires *affective regulation*, not simply knowing what to do. These processes almost certainly involve interconnections of higher-order abstract processing (in areas of prefrontal cortex) with neurobehavioral systems involved in affect and motivation. Clearly, these higher-order connections initially develop in adolescence, as these areas of PFC mature and begin to harness the more intense affective states during puberty.

Damasio (1995) and others argue that, even in adulthood, these higher-order cognitive processes cannot be separated from their emotional links. Damasio's research group has studied patients with cortical lesions at the linkage point between higher-order cognitive processes and limbic circuits. These patients show completely normal performance on complex cognitive tasks and can even describe appropriate social responses in objective questions; however, in real-life situations they show marked impairments in social functioning (Damasio, 1995). Damasio and others have convincingly argued that the highest level of cognitive processing *requires* affective input. The connections between these systems are among the last areas of the brain to develop, showing significant changes into late adolescence and early adulthood (Pennington & Welsh, 1995).

Vulnerability to Affect Dysregulation

Our group has been involved in a large program of research examining the developmental psychobiology of child and adolescent depression. We have been investigating a stress-diathesis model of early onset depression, building on evidence for a genetic vulnerability combined with a set of adverse early experiences leading to a syndrome of affective dysregulation (see Dahl & Ryan, 1996; Dahl, 1996). A full discussion of the model will not fit in this chapter; however, there are two major themes related to vulnerability that are relevant to the model. First, there is increasing evidence that one component of the story is related to early anxiety symptoms and a very early pattern of low threshold to activate threat-related arousal (depressed infants and young children show a large threat and arousal response to neutral or novel stimuli) (Kagan, Reznick, Snidman, Gibbons, & Johnson, 1988; Davidson, 1994). These children show early traits of shyness, withdrawal, and fear (Kagan et al., 1988), have higher rates of anxiety disorders at school ages (Biederman et al., 1995), and have elevated rates of anxiety disorders in their families (Hirshfeld, Rosenbaum, & Biederman, 1992).

A second major theme regarding vulnerability is a negative affective bias in cognitive and attentional processing. There are various ways that a negative attentional bias may confer vulnerability toward developing an affective illness. Briefly, there are three sets of data supporting this concept: (1) Rothbart and colleagues showed that infants with difficulty breaking off visual attention toward a novel or threatening visual cue showed increased anxiety and depressive symptoms as children (Rothbart, Posner, & Rosicky, 1994); (2) Nolen-Hoeksema and colleagues demonstrated that children with a tendency to ruminate about negative or stressful events had higher rates of depressive symptoms in early adolescence (Nolen-Hoeksema, Girgus, & Seligman, 1992; Nolen-Hoeksema, Parker, & Larson, 1994); and (3) Seligman and colleagues (1984) have presented data showing that children with negative attributional style in interpreting events (taking undue blame for problems, insufficient credit for successes) predicted depression. Although each of these lines of investigation addresses quite different elements of negative bias, there is a more general theme across these studies regarding a tendency to shift mental processes in a direction toward negative affect. A tendency to link cognitive processes with negative affect may strengthen the connections between these systems through early periods of development.

We have hypothesized (Dahl & Ryan, 1996) that one pathway to early onset depression may evolve from strong connections between goal-directed cognitive processes and negative affect. Specifically, we have been interested in the role of negative affective biases in cross-temporal processing in goal-directed behaviors and social interactions. For example, when a young adolescent considers going to a social event, some of the cross-temporal processing involves the remembering of similar social events in the past and projecting these memories into images of future events; if this cross-temporal processing is biased toward negative affect, the adolescent is more likely to remember bad events (or interpret past events as negative), and to imagine that the upcoming social event will also be a negative experience. In other words, if negative affect creates a shadow or bias of the scanning of past experiences into future likelihoods (high cortical functions), then the behavioral outcome is likely to be failure to initiate behaviors toward similar events. We have termed this process anticipatory anhedonia, whereby adolescents will not initiate goal-directed or social behaviors because they imagine they will go poorly (associated with unpleasant affect). On the other hand (in contrast to depressed adults who show anhedonia or the inability to experience pleasure), many depressed adolescents will enjoy experiences such as social events if they are taken to or encouraged to go to such events (even though they will not initiate behaviors toward attending these events). Over time, however, lack of initiation toward pleasurable or goal-directed behaviors may result in a more traditional form of anhedonia.

Links to Sleep-Arousal Regulation (Or, Back to Sleep)

During adolescence, the pendulum of sleep and arousal regulation tends to get pushed very hard in one direction – toward high arousal and away from sleep – for several reasons. These reasons include adolescents' social schedules, school start times, employment hours, stressors, and sleep and circadian changes at puberty. As presented in this chapter, there are several additional factors leading to frequent and sustained elevations of emotional arousal during adolescence. These factors appear to be particularly marked in some individuals who may have a genetically based decrease in their threshold to activate arousal in response to threat or novelty, resulting in more frequent elevations in arousal with even mild to moderate stressors. Further, negative cognitive biases (a second source of vulnerability to depression) further amplify these problems: diverting internal attention toward threatening, distressing, or painful memories and anticipating negative events in future interactions. One specific example of these tendencies is the pattern of distressing cognitive ruminations at bedtime in depressed adolescents. Although the images and memories are uncomfortable, the adolescent repeatedly revisits them in the interval before falling asleep. It is a bit like pressing one's tongue against a toothache – even though it hurts, they do it again and again, replaying the mental tape of the remembered or imagined stressful experience. These distressing images cause increases in arousal at a time when the sleep and circadian physiology are trying to push arousal to nadir levels to meet other physiologic needs. This creates yet another route of sleep disruption-deprivation and pushes arousal to higher levels. As with the many other sources of decreased sleep and elevated arousal described earlier, there is a capacity for a vicious cycle.

With multiple sources of elevated arousal and decreasing opportunities for sleep, many adolescents end up with profound imbalances in sleep-arousal regulation, which returns the discussion to the consequences of sleep deprivation.

The Consequences of Sleep Deprivation

As has been argued elsewhere (Dahl, Matty, Birmaher, Al-Shabbout, Williamson, & Ryan, 1996; Schlesinger, Redfern, Dahl, & Jennings, 1998), there is increasing evidence that sleep deprivation effects are particularly prevalent in measures of higher cortical functions (Horne, 1993). Further, we have shown in pilot studies that the tasks that simultaneously challenge cognitive and emotional processing appear to be particularly sensitive to sleep deprivation effects. We recently extended this work to a more easily quantifiable domain, looking at higher cognitive processes and another subcortical regulatory system – the maintenance of postural balance – which confirmed our predictions regarding sleep deprivation effects. That study (Schlesinger et al., 1998) showed that, in young healthy university students, one night of sleep deprivation caused no significant effect on performance of either an inhibitory cognitive or postural balance task; however, there was a marked effect on the ability to perform both the cognitive task and the balance task simultaneously after sleep deprivation. In a similar way, sleep deprivation may impair the ability to perform both a cognitive and emotional task at the same time. In summary, there appears to be a vicious negative cycle with sleep deprivation impairing cognitive-emotional regulation, impaired cognitive-emotional regulation leading to increased stress and arousal, and stress and arousal further interfering with sleep, leading to further impairments in affective regulation and emotional well-being.

The Role of Attention (Or, How Can We Teach Highly Aroused-Stressed Kids to Relax?)

In the middle of neurobehavioral systems interconnecting in the regulation of cognition, affect, and behavior, the control of attention sits center stage. In many ways, attention is the selective pattern of linking higher cognitive processes with specific inputs and outputs. In particular, the anterior or executive attentional network (involved in voluntary or effortful control of attention) appears to play a critical role in the patterning of linkage or connections between neurobehavioral systems. These processes are quite amenable to learning or cognitive-behavioral therapy – that is, one can intervene to alter patterns of attention or how attention is used in maladaptive ways. Teaching or training children to avoid the tendency to overattend to threatening stimuli may have positive effects on both mood and sleep-arousal imbalances so commonly slanted toward high arousal and sleep deprivation in adolescents. If children or adolescents learn to expect that bad things will happen, tend to remember the negative things that occurred (out of proportion to the positive ones), and dwell on the negative implications regarding self-worth, these may contribute enormously to poor regulation of emotions and possibly development of psychopathology, such as depression. Early intervention to alter these patterns of cognitive-emotional linkages may prevent some of these vicious cycles. These strategies may also be effective in having a positive effect on sleep-wake patterns among troubled adolescents. Cognitive-behavioral interventions focused on the interval preceding sleep onset may have effects not only on mood but also on the frequently observed difficulties with sleep onset seen in adolescent depression (Dahl et al., 1996).

Clinical programs (early intervention-prevention with high-risk populations) are in early stages of progress and will help to answer at least some of the questions and speculations outlined in this chapter. Similarly, studies involving the use of f-MRI are also being conducted to examine more specific models of the underlying neurocircuitry involved in affect dysregulation in adolescent depression. Other studies using sleep deprivation as a probe to examine affect regulation are also being conducted.

REFERENCES

Biederman J, Rosenbaum JF, Bolduc-Murphy EA, Faraone SV, Chaloff J, Hirshfeld DR, Kagan J (1995). Behavioral inhibition as a temperamental risk factor for anxiety disorders. *Child and Adolescent Psychiatric Clinics of North America* 2:667–683.

Dahl RE (1996). The regulation of sleep and arousal: Development and psychopathology. *Development and Psychopathology* 8(1):3–27.

Dahl RE, Matty MK, Birmaher B, Al-Shabbout M, Williamson DE, Ryan ND (1996). Sleep onset abnormalities in depressed adolescents. *Biological Psychiatry* 39:400–410.

Dahl RE, Ryan ND (1996). The psychobiology of adolescent depression. In D. Cicchetti & S. L. Toth, eds., *Rochester Symposium on Developmental Psychopathology*, vol. 7, *Adolescence: Opportunities and Challenges*, pp. 197–232. Rochester, NY: University of Rochester Press.

Damasio AR (1995). *Descartes' Error: Emotion, Reason and the Human Brain*. New York: G. P. Putnam's Sons.

Davidson RJ (1994). Asymmetric brain function, affective style, and psychopathology: The role of early experience and plasticity. In D. Cicchetti & B. Nurcombe, eds., *Development and Psychopathology*, pp. 741–758. Cambridge: Cambridge University Press.

Ge X, Conger RD, Elder GH (1996). Coming of age too early: Pubertal influences on girls' vulnerability to psychological distress. *Child Development* 67:3386–3400.

Greenough WT, Black JE (1992). *Induction of Brain Structure by Experience: Substrates for Cognitive Development.* Minnesota Symposia on Child Psychology. Hillsdale, NJ: Erlbaum.

Greenough WT, Black JE, Wallace CS (1987). Experience and brain development. *Child Development* 58:539–559.

Hirshfeld DR, Rosenbaum JF, Biederman J (1992). Stable behavioral inhibition and its association with anxiety disorders. *Journal of the American Academy of Child and Adolescent Psychiatry* 31:103–111.

Horne J (1993). Human sleep, sleep loss and behavior implications for the prefrontal cortex and psychiatric disorder. *British Journal of Psychiatry* 162:413–419.

Kagan J, Reznick JS, Snidman N, Gibbons J, Johnson MO (1988). Childhood derivatives of inhibition and lack of inhibition to the unfamiliar. *Child Development* 59:1580–1589.

Kochanska G, DeVet K, Goldman M, Murray K, Putnam SP (1994). Maternal reports of conscience development and temperament in young children. *Child Development* 65(3):852–868.

Kochanska G, Murray K, Jacques TY, Koening AL (1996). Inhibitory control in young children and its role in emerging internalization. *Child Development* 67(2):490–507.

Miller KD, Keller JB, Styker MP (1989). Ocular dominance column development: Analysis and simulation. *Science* 245:605–615.

Modell J, Goodman M (1990). At the threshold: The developing adolescent. In S. S. Feldman & G. R. Elliott, eds., *Historical Perspectives*, pp. 93–122. Cambridge, MA: Harvard University Press.

Nolen-Hoeksema S, Girgus JS, Seligman ME (1992). Predictors and consequences of childhood depressive symptoms: A 5-year longitudinal study. *Journal of Abnormal Psychology* 101(3):405–422.

Nolen-Hoeksema S, Parker LE, Larson J (1994). Ruminative coping with depressed mood following loss. *Journal of Personality and Social Psychology* 67(1):92–104.

Pennington BF, Welsh M (1995). Neuropsychology and developmental psychopathology. In D. Cicchetti & D. Cohen, eds., *Developmental Psychopathology*, vol. 1: *Theory and Methods*, pp. 254–290. Wiley series on personality processes. New York: John Wiley & Sons.

Petersen AC, Crockett L (1985). Pubertal timing and grade effects on adjustment. *Journal of Youth and Adolescence* 14:191–206.

Rothbart MK, Posner MI (1994). Orienting in normal and pathological development. *Development and Psychopathology*, 6(4):635–652.

Rutter M, Rutter M (1993). *Developing Minds: Challenge and Continuity across the Life Span.* New York: Harper Collins.

Schlesinger A, Redfern MS, Dahl RE, Jennings JR (1998). Postural control, attention, and sleep deprivation. *Neuroreport* 9(1):49–52.

Seligman ME, Peterson C, Kaslow NJ, Tanenbaum RL, Alloy LB, Abramson LY (1984). Attributional style and depressive symptoms among children. *Journal of Abnormal Psychology* 93(2):235–238.

Singer W (1986). Neuronal activity as a shaping factor in postnatal development of visual cortex. In W. T. Greenough & J. M. Juraska, eds., *Developing Neuropsychobiology*, pp. 271–293. New York: Academic Press.

Index

absenteeism, 203, 223–34
academic difficulties, 199, 207
academic pressure and sleep patterns, 204, 241, 244
academics, 8–9, 132
accidents: employment and increased risk for, 159; extended work hours and risk for, 169; irregular sleep and, 136; risk associated with sleep deprivation, 173; sleep patterns in Italian students and, 141; survey of, 222
acetylcholine, 32
Ache, 72; bedding, 73; fire, 75; infant breast feeding and lap sitting, 95–6; panther predator tale, 81, 90
actigraph: in delayed sleep phase case vignettes, 247, 248, 250; in rhesus monkeys, 59–61; school transition study, 17; shiftwork study and, 162–3
actimeter, *see* actigraph
active learning, 213
activity offset in rhesus monkeys, 61–3
activity onset, 14; in *Octodon degus*, 43, 46f
activity rhythms: effects of sex steroids on, 36; in *Octodon degus*, 43; in rhesus monkeys, 16
actograms: of *Octodon degus*, 45f; of rhesus monkeys, 60f
adaptation to stress, 238
ADHD/IEP, 223–34
adolescence, definition of, 270
adolescent development, 237; changes in sleep timing and evolutionary ecology of sleep, 103; circadian timing system and, 16; homeostatic process and, 12–13
adult enrichment and school start time, 179
adult status, 270
affect regulation, 270–82
affective arousal, 277

affective disorders, 238, 259, 262, 279
affective dysregulation, 278
afternoon performance, 174
age, 229t; adjustment to early start, 161,164; effects with work delay, 164; hours spent working and, 205f; relaxation to sleep habits, 134–6, 140; shift work, sleep, and tiredness, 163; sleep and dream response to trauma, 246
aggressive behavior: REM sleep loss, 20
agriculturalist, 71–2
air quality, pollution, 74–5, 82
alarm clock, 6
alcohol: academic performance and, 140; avoidance, 215; consumption in adolescents, 122; drugs and, 223; sleep deprivation and, 173; working and, 203, 206
alertness, 8, 41, 148–9, 173; computerized test for, 162, 166; as a continuum in traditional societies, 101–2; effects of naps on, 214; employment and, 159, 165; school and work start time and, 161, 213
allergen producers, 74
American Automobile Association Foundation for Traffic Safety, 157
American students, 126, 128, 142, 144
Anders, Thomas, xiii
animal models of puberty, 27–8, 33, 42–3, 47–8, 51–4
animals' influence on sleep, 80–1
anthropologist, anthropology, xv, 70
anticipatory anhedonia, 279
anxiety: acidents and, 141; scale, 133; school achievement and, 140; sleep and, 118, 140, 144, 173, 209, 238, 241, 242; sleeping pill use and, 145; symptoms and depression vulnerability, 278
anxiolytics, 138–9

ecology of sleep: biotic microecology,
80–3; comparative developmental,
69–112; components of, 71–2;
developmental, 95–102; emotion
regulation and, 109–10; evolutionary,
70–1, 102; influence of physical ecology,
92–3; microecology, 73–80; protection
and safety, 71–2; sleep structure, 76–7
ectoparasites, 74, 82
Edina, Minnesota, 172; case study of
school start time, 187–94; focus groups,
187–92; parent written survey, 192–4
Efe, 72; bedding, 73; dogs (bisinje) and
sleep, 80; grooming for ectoparasites,
82; huts, 76–7; lack of bedtime, 79;
napping when sick, 94; nocturnal social
activity, 85; protection by fire, 75; sex
differences in sleeping, 92; sleeping
arrangements , 77
Egypt, zinc deprivation, 55
elderly and sleep, 41, 103
electroencephalogram (EEG): changes, 54;
sleep episodes at work and, 160
elementary school, 172, 180, 186t, 202,
208
emotion regulation: in adolescent
development, 269, 282; sleep ecology
and, 109; well-being, 207–8
emotions: activated at puberty, 272;
feelings, negative and positive, 237;
turmoil, 236
employment, x, 1, 21, 199; comparison of
adolescents and adults, 169; double
shifts, 165; early start time and, 160;
effects on sleep, 9–10, 210f; effects of
work patterns, 83–5, 104, 107; extended
work hours, 165, 168–9, 203; part-time,
133, 159, 198; positive impact of, 204;
pressure to work, 202; school start time
and, 181–2; sleep regulation and, 280;
work after athletic practice, 177
endocrine changes in puberty, 27–37
environmental exposures, fatigue, sleep
loss, sleepiness and, 169
epinephrine, 32
estradiol, 41; effects on hamster circadian
oscillator, 47; feedback on GnRH pulse
generator, 32; folliculogenesis in the
ovary, 31; receptors in CNS, 33
estrogen: effects on activity onset, 36;
receptors in cortex, 55
ethnographers, ethnography, 71–2, 95
European students, 125, 144
evolution, 69–70; adaptive response to
stress, 239; influence on sleep, 102–4
executive function and adolescent
development, 269, 271–2
exercise and sleep hygiene, 215

expected level of education, 223–34
experience-expectant learning, 275
extracurricular activities, 9, 198, 204;
school start time and, 175–7, 195

falling asleep at night: as a stressor in
anxious adolescents, 241; difficulty,
case vignette 2, 250–1; difficulties in
Italian students, 136–8, 144; relation to
sleep patterns, 124; sleeping pills and,
145; trouble in, 118, 121, 125–6, 128
falling asleep in school, 208; age and sex
effects, 140; driving accident risk and,
155; effects of employment on, 9;
insufficient sleep and, 207; irregular
sleep and, 136; percentage of high
school students, 173; school start time
and, 141
falling asleep while driving, 155t, 156t
familial sleep markers of depression,
257–9
fatigue: as a source of stress, 241; delayed
phase case and, 247; reduced total sleep
time and, 207; reports with delay
start time, 164, 165f; work and, 160,
162, 169
fear, fearfulness: of being alone at night,
250; of growing up, 248; in poor
sleepers, 242; sleep as a source of, 240
fear sleep (*tadoet poeles*), 99–101
fertility, *see* reproductive competence
filarial worms, 82
Finnish Institute of Occupational Health
(FIOH), 160–1
Finnish students, 125, 142, 144
fire, 74–6, 101, 107
fluoxetine, 257
follicle stimulating hormone, GnRH
influence on, 31
follicular phase, *see* menstrual cycle
food intake, 51
food service, 172
forager, 71–2; bedding, 73; dispersed
settlements of, 90; fire as protection
from predators, 74; labor and sleep
patterns in, 83–4; seasonal and diurnal
foraging patterns, 84
"forbidden zones" for sleep, 14
Fore, introduction of blankets, 74
France, 209; students in, 144
frontal cortex, synaptic pruning and
myelination in, 54
fumigant, fire as, 74

Gabra, 72; animal noises in encampment,
80; bedding, beds, 73; bedtimes and rise
times in herders, 83; belief in loss of soul
(*atma*) in dreaming, 91; dogs and sleep,